New Insights into PET and SPECT Imaging

New Insights into PET and SPECT Imaging

Editor: Catheriene Blevins

AMERICAN
MEDICAL PUBLISHERS
www.americanmedicalpublishers.com

AMERICAN
MEDICAL PUBLISHERS
www.americanmedicalpublishers.com

Cataloging-in-Publication Data

New insights into PET and SPECT imaging / edited by Catheriene Blevins.
p. cm.
Includes bibliographical references and index.
ISBN 978-1-63927-751-3
1. Tomography, Emission. 2. Single-photon emission computed tomography. 3. Diagnostic imaging.
4. Imaging systems in medicine. 5. Diagnosis--Data processing. I. Blevins, Catheriene.
RC78.7.T62 N49 2023
616.075 75--dc23

American Medical Publishers,
41 Flatbush Avenue,
1st Floor, New York,
NY 11217, USA

ISBN 978-1-63927-751-3 (Hardback)

Contents

Preface

This book has been an outcome of determined endeavour from a group of educationists in the field. The primary objective was to involve a broad spectrum of professionals from diverse cultural background involved in the field for developing new researches. The book not only targets students but also scholars pursuing higher research for further enhancement of the theoretical and practical applications of the subject.

A positron emission tomography (PET) scan is a type of imaging test that can help reveal the metabolic or biochemical function of the tissues and organs inside the body. A radioactive drug called tracer is used to show both normal and abnormal metabolic activities within the body. There are various diseases including heart disease, brain disorders and cancer that can be diagnosed using a PET scan. A single-photon emission computerized tomography (SPECT) scan is a type of nuclear imaging test that shows the movement of blood towards the tissues and organs. In this medical imaging test, a radioactive substance is used to produce images of the internal structures and organs of the body. It is used to diagnose conditions such as stress fractures, strokes, seizures, infections, and tumors in the spine. This book provides new insights into the field of PET and SPECT imaging. It consists of contributions made by international experts. The book is appropriate for students as well as for experts seeking detailed information in the area of diagnostic imaging.

It was an honour to edit such a profound book and also a challenging task to compile and examine all the relevant data for accuracy and originality. I wish to acknowledge the efforts of the contributors for submitting such brilliant and diverse chapters in the field and for endlessly working for the completion of the book. Last, but not the least; I thank my family for being a constant source of support in all my research endeavours.

Editor

1

Hybrid PET–MRI Imaging in Paediatric and TYA Brain Tumors: Clinical Applications and Challenges

Ananth Shankar [1,*], Jamshed Bomanji [2] and Harpreet Hyare [3,4]

1 Children and Young People's Cancer Services, University College London hospitals NHS Foundation Trust, London NW1 2PG, UK
2 Department of Nuclear Medicine, University College London hospitals NHS Foundation Trust, London NW1 2PG, UK; jamshed.bomanji@nhs.net
3 Department of Radiology, University College London Hospitals NHS Foundation Trust, London NW1 2PG, UK; harpreet.hyare@nhs.net
4 Department of Brain Repair and Rehabilitation, Institute of Neurology, University College London, London WC1N 3BG, UK
* Correspondence: ananth.shankar@nhs.net

Abstract: (1) Background: Standard magnetic resonance imaging (MRI) remains the gold standard for brain tumour imaging in paediatric and teenage and young adult (TYA) patients. Combining positron emission tomography (PET) with MRI offers an opportunity to improve diagnostic accuracy. (2) Method: Our single-centre experience of ^{18}F-fluorocholine (FCho) and ^{18}fluoro-L-phenylalanine (FDOPA) PET–MRI in paediatric/TYA neuro-oncology patients is presented. (3) Results: Hybrid PET–MRI shows promise in the evaluation of gliomas and germ cell tumours in (i) assessing early treatment response and (ii) discriminating tumour from treatment-related changes. (4) Conclusions: Combined PET–MRI shows promise for improved diagnostic and therapeutic assessment in paediatric and TYA brain tumours.

Keywords: PET; MRI; glioma

1. Introduction

Tumours of the Central Nervous System (CNS) are the most common form of solid tumour in children and teenage/young adult (TYA) populations, accounting for more than 25% of all types of cancers and 15% of malignancies in the teenage and young adult population (15–24 years). According to the most recent statistics from Cancer Research UK, tumours of the CNS are the fourth most common cancer type in this age group with astrocytomas forming the largest sub-group followed by embryonal tumours, such as medulloblastoma and ependymoma [1,2]. Treatment is dependent upon histological subtype, tumour molecular genetic profile and staging, with varying combinations of surgery, radiotherapy and chemotherapy. Recent advances in molecular characterization of CNS tumours provide additional information that allow for risk adapted tailored treatment [3–5].

Imaging plays a key role in the management of paediatric/TYA patients with brain tumours at all stages of the diseases: from diagnosis, surgical and radiotherapy planning to the assessment of therapeutic response and detection of recurrent disease. MRI, with its excellent soft tissue contrast, remains the imaging modality of choice in daily practice. However, interpretation of standard anatomical MRI after surgical trauma, disrupting normal CNS anatomy, and treatment with chemoradiation, inducing oedema, necrosis, demyelination and ischaemia, can be challenging. The recently characterised phenomena of *pseudoprogression*, whereby an increase in tumour volume, oedema and enhancement shortly after completion of treatment is often difficult to distinguish from progressive tumour [6,7] and *pseudoresponse*, whereby a dramatic reduction in tumour enhancement following treatment with anti-angiogenic agents is thought to be due to vascular normalisation rather than a true anti-tumour effect [8,9] further compound interpretation. With the recent evidence that non-enhancing WHO grade II and III astrocytomas lacking the IDH1 mutation should be classified as glioblastoma (GBM) [10] and that not all high-grade gliomas enhance [11], there is a need to investigate other imaging technologies to better assess tumour burden.

Various functional imaging techniques depicting specific biological properties of tissues have been introduced to compliment standard MRI, including advanced MRI techniques and positron emission tomography (PET). Each modality is reported as demonstrating increased diagnostic accuracy over standard MRI in neuro-oncology and combining PET with advanced MRI has the potential to further improve diagnostic accuracy and ultimately patient outcomes.

Whilst the role of ^{18}F-fluoro-deoxy-glucose (FDG) PET/CT is well established in oncology, the clinical role of PET–MRI, first introduced in 2008 [12], has yet to be established. Recently, there have been a number of reports exploring the potential of hybrid PET–MRI in neuro-oncology [13–15], but this has been limited to adult patients. Within paediatric and TYA patients, the reported use of hybrid PET–MRI consists of small feasibility studies and case reports [16–18]. Here, we present a critical appraisal of the clinical use of PET–MRI in a group of paediatric/TYA neuro-oncology patients based on over 5 years of experience predominantly using ^{18}F-fluorocholine (FCho) and ^{18}fluoro-L-phenylalanine (FDOPA) on our Siemens mMR system, which performs over 1200 PET–MRI research and clinical studies each year. We present (i) an overview of the current imaging techniques used in clinical practice, (ii) a series of clinical cases at our institution, highlighting the challenges and opportunities of hybrid PET–MRI, and (iii) finally we present recommendations for clinical use on paediatric and TYA neuro-oncology and some limitations.

2. Current Clinical Imaging Methods in Neuro-Oncology

2.1. PET Tracers

Positron emission tomography (PET) is an established imaging modality used commonly in oncology [19]. In the neuro-oncology domain, it is being increasingly used to add incremental value to MRI in the clinical management of glioma [20–22]. The potential to use PET imaging in clinical trials and new strategies for the treatment of glioma, such as immunotherapy, where pseudoprogression is particularly challenging for MRI assessment [23], remains to be explored. An evidence-based recommendation by the PET Response Assessment in Neuro-Oncology (RANO) working group and European Association of Neuro-Oncology (EANO) on the clinical use of PET imaging in gliomas has been published focussing on radiotracers used in clinical practice imaging, i.e., glucose metabolism, 2-deoxy-2-[^{18} F]fluoro-D-glucose (FDG), and system L amino acid transport comprising ^{11}C-methyl-methionine (MET), O-(2-[^{18}F]-fluoroethyl)-L-tyrosine (FET) and 3,4-dihydroxy-6-[^{18}F]-fluoro-L-phenylalanine (FDOPA) [20].

Radiolabelled amino acids have been used in neuro-oncological practice since 1983, and whilst most experience has been gained with MET, radiolabelling with the isotope carbon-11 requires an on-site cyclotron unit. Labelling with the isotope fluorine-18, with a longer half-life, has advantages in clinical practice, and FET is now widely used across Europe with numerous studies reporting increased sensitivity and specificity for differentiating tumour progression from pseudoprogression [24–26]. FDOPA, which was developed to measure dopamine synthesis in the basal ganglia, is increasingly used for brain tumour imaging [21]. Amino acid PET tracers can penetrate the blood–brain or –tumour barrier (BBB/BTB) and thus provide excellent definition of tumours, including those that are non-contrast enhancing [27]. Their uptake is mediated via amino acid transporters LAT1 and LAT 2 [28,29].

Our initial experience has been with FCho, which showed promise as a diagnostic imaging tool in benign and malignant brain tumours [30–32]. Its effectiveness is related to its ability to indirectly evaluate cell proliferation as a measure of the synthesis of lipids required for cell membranes. Additionally, slow-growing tumours such the low-grade gliomas also take up radiolabelled choline. An important feature of radio-labelled choline is its low rate of distribution in normal grey and white matter [33,34]. Our clinical practice is now based on the amino acid tracer FDOPA, which demonstrates superiority over FCho in its ability to provide information on the metabolism of brain tumours, its ability to discriminate low-grade from high-grade gliomas, and the significant impact it has on the management of patients with a suspicion of brain tumour recurrence and the challenging clinical problem of distinguishing pseudoprogression from true progression [35,36].

Other amino acid PET tracers such as α-[^{11}C]-methyl-L-tryptophan (AMT) and [18F]fluciclovie (FACBC) as well as glutamine-based amino acid PET tracers have also been evaluated in gliomas for tumour delineation, prognostication and differentiation of tumour recurrence from radiation injury, but currently, the number of examined subjects is low [37,38].

Promising new PET tracers include ^{18}F-fluoromisonidazole (FMISO) for imaging hypoxia in brain tumours [39,40]; ^{11}C-(R)PK11195, a translocator protein (TSPO) ligand which demonstrates increased binding in high-grade gliomas [41]; and ^{68}Ga-FAPI, which is a labelled fibroblast activating protein inhibitor (FAPI) that binds to cancer associated fibroblasts (FAP) [42]. We plan to evaluate ^{68}Ga-FAPI in our paediatric/TYA glioma population for the monitoring of treatment response.

2.2. MRI

Standard basic minimal anatomical MRI for paediatric brain tumour imaging includes axial fluid-attenuated inversion recovery (FLAIR) and T2-weighted sequences visualizing non-enhancing tumour components, oedema and therapy induced-gliosis, diffusion weighted imaging (DWI) to aid the assessment of therapy response and high-resolution 3D isotropic pre- and post-contrast enhanced T1-weighted sequences to depict contrast leakage from the tumour vessels (Figure 1) [43]. Whilst international standard brain MRI protocols exist for adults [44], no such recommendations exist for paediatric neuro-oncology [45]. At our institution, we follow the adult MRI recommendations but also include a blood sensitive sequence such as T2* or susceptibility weighted imaging (SWI) to depict intra-tumoural haemorrhage and the development of radiation-induced cavernomas, and to depict biopsy tracts [46] and arterial spin labelling (ASL) perfusion to aid in the assessment of gliomas post-treatment [47]. Table 1 demonstrates the parameters for our paediatric/TYA neuro-oncology MRI protocol.

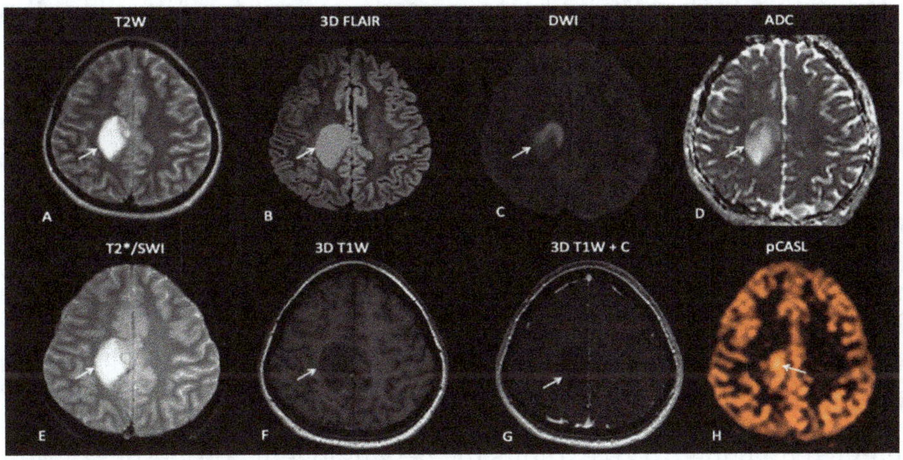

Figure 1. Nineteen-year-old female presenting with epilepsy. MRI demonstrates a well-defined T2W (**A**), FLAIR (**B**), DWI (**C**) and a hyperintense lesion with a medial border of restricted diffusion on an apparent diffusion coefficient (ADC) map (**D**). The lesion demonstrates no areas of susceptibility (**E**) and no pathological enhancement on pre- and post-contrast T1W images (**F**,**G**). The appearances are consistent with low-grade glioma, but pCASL perfusion-weighted imaging (PWI) (**H**) demonstrates medial increased perfusion.

Table 1. Neuro-Oncology MRI protocol sequence parameters.

		TR	TE	FA	FOV	ACQ Matrix	Reconstructed Voxel	Slices
DWI	SE-EPI	2902	95	90	230 × 230	152 × 106	0.9 × 0.9 × 5	22
FLAIR	IR-TSE	11000	125	90/120	230 × 182	352 × 186	0.45 × 0.45 × 5	29
T2WSE	TSE	3000	80	90/120	230 × 184	400 × 255	0.45 × 0.45 × 5	24
T2WFFE	FFE	786	15	18	230 × 183	256 × 164	0.45 × 0.45 × 5	24
pCASL	GEPI	4571	15	90	240 × 240	64 × 64	3 × 3 × 5	20

Note: DWI = diffusion weighted imaging, FLAIR = fluid attenuated inversion recovery, T2WSE = T2-weighted spin echo, T2WFFE = T2-weighted fast field echo, pCASL = pseudo-continuous arterial spin labelling, TR = relaxation time, TE = echo time, FA = flip angle, FOV = field of view, ACQ matrix = acquisition matrix.

Pre- and post-contrast T1-weighted sequences using identical MRI parameters allow voxel-to-voxel image subtraction, which may detect subtle residual enhancement and therefore provide a more accurate and reproducible assessment of the true extent [48]. Whilst this method has been shown to significantly improve visualization and quantification of post-treatment high-grade glioma tumour volume in adults [49], this method needs further validation in paediatric/TYA gliomas.

A variation of this method acquires two high-resolution 3D T1-weighted sequences in the same MRI session, and 3–5 and 60–75 min after the injection of the contrast medium and subsequent subtraction a colour-coded map known as a treatment response assessment map (TRAM) is produced. Areas where contrast accumulates correspond histologically to treatment-induced changes, whilst areas where contrast is cleared rapidly correspond to active tumour [50]. TRAMs are simple to acquire but can be inconvenient to the patient who may have to wait longer to complete the study, a particularly challenging in the paediatric population.

2.2.1. Diffusion-Weighted Imaging (DWI)

Diffusion-weighted imaging (DWI) is sensitive to random microscopic (Brownian) motion of water molecules, which results in signal loss and consequent hyperintensity in areas of restricted diffusion. The apparent diffusion coefficient (ADC) reflects the magnitude of water motion with restricted diffusion having lower ADC values. ADC is inversely correlated with cell density [51] due to reduced water mobility from dense cellular packing and thus is of interest for grading tumours and detection of tumour recurrence. In paediatric neuro-oncology, ADC has been shown to correlate with tumour grade, and in a meta-analysis that included 14 studies of paediatric patients, lower-mean tumour ADC was associated with a higher WHO tumour grade, except for diffuse midline gliomas which demonstrated ADC characteristics similar to low-grade gliomas [52].

One caveat to the application of DWI for identifying non-enhancing tumour is that lower ADC values do not always correlate with increasing tumour infiltration. Low and persistent diffusion restriction can be associated with non-viable tissue necrosis. In adults, these lesions tend to be periventricular, slowly change over several months and are thought to be a type of treatment toxicity, associated with better outcomes. Novel diffusion modelling techniques such as Vascular, Extracellular, and Restricted Diffusion for Cytometry in Tumours (VERDICT) have been developed at our institution that aim to identify diffusion parameters that more accurately reflect tumour microstructure [53] and will be applied to paediatric brain tumours (Figure 2).

2.2.2. Perfusion-Weighted Imaging (PWI)

Perfusion-weighted imaging (PWI) exploits the neoangiogenic properties of proliferating gliomas, and is able to identify areas of high-grade tumour with high accuracy. PWI can be performed in a number of ways; the main techniques in clinical practice are dynamic susceptibility-weighted contrast-enhanced MRI (DSC), dynamic contrast-enhanced MRI (DCE) and arterial spin labelling (ASL).

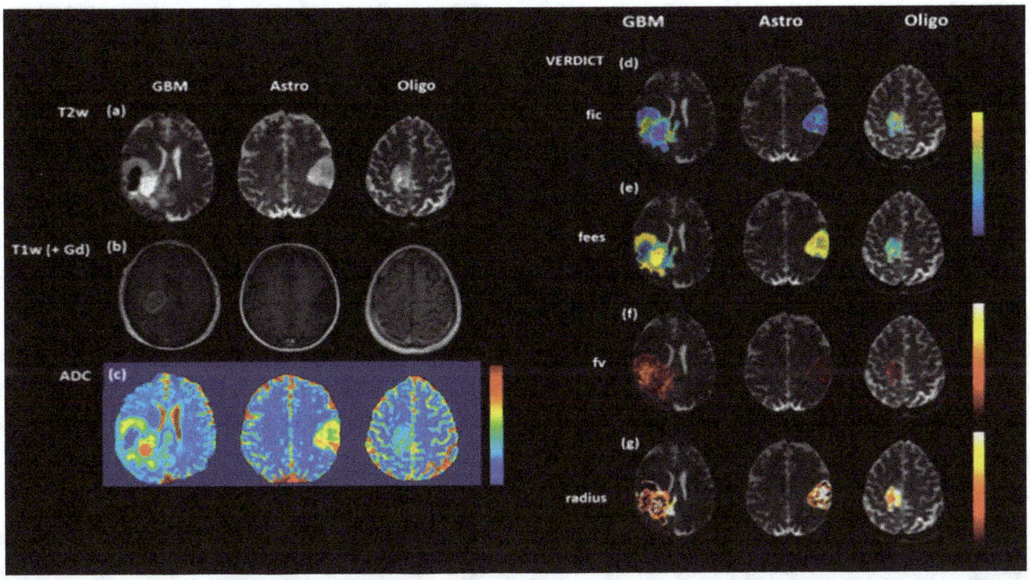

Figure 2. T2-weighted (T2W (**a**), T1-weighted (T1W) post contrast (**b**) and ADC maps (**c**) in a range of brain tumours: glioblastoma multiforme (GBM), diffuse astrocytoma (Astro) and oligodendroglioma (Oligo). Although the ADC map for the oligodendroglioma (**c**) is relatively uniform, the Vascular, Extracellular, and Restricted Diffusion for Cytometry in Tumours (VERDICT) parameter map fic (intracellular fraction) (**d**) demonstrates increased signal at the anterior margin, thought to be a marker of increased cell density. The other VERDICT parameter maps (**e**) fees (extracellular, extravascular fraction), (**f**), fv (vascular fraction) and (**g**) radius (cell radius) also demonstrate tumour heterogeneity which could potentially be used to guide biopsy.

DSC-MRI rapidly acquires gradient echo or spin echo planar images during first-pass transit through the brain of an exogenous paramagnetic gadolinium based-contrast agent that transiently decreases signal intensity. Voxel-wise changes in contrast agent concentration are determined from time–signal curves and processed using kinetic tracer modelling and indicator dilution theory to estimate cerebral blood volume (CBV), cerebral blood flow (CBF) and mean transit time (MTT). Relative CBV (rCBV) is the most common DSC-MRI metric for evaluating brain tumours. To minimize the error caused by contrast extravasation, known to occur in brain tumours, preloading of the contrast agent along with model-based post-processing leakage correction can decrease both T1 and T2* effects [54,55].

DCE-MRI is based on the T1 relaxivity properties of a contrast agent and quantifies various dynamic features of blood–brain barrier contrast agent leakage. After baseline T1 maps are obtained, T1-W DCE-MRI images are acquired before, during and after contrast agent administration. A vascular input function is determined, and pharmacokinetic modelling yields the extravascular extracellular and plasma space volume fractions, transfer constant (K^{trans}) and rate constant. K^{trans} is thought to reflect microvascular permeability but also representative of blood flow and vessel surface area, the most common metric in brain tumour studies [56].

ASL uses endogenous contrast whereby magnetically labelled blood entering the brain can be used to estimate the CBF [57]. The first applications used a long RF pulse simultaneously with a selection gradient, but more recently, a train of short RF pulses combined with a strong gradient has been used (pCASL) [58]. Although, DSC perfusion is most commonly used in clinical practice [59] and numerous studies have demonstrated that rCBV is an early response marker in treated GBMs, pCASL is the favoured PWI technique in paediatric neuro-oncology due to the lack of need for exogenous contrast [60]. pCASL has been shown to correlate with DSC-derived CBF in a study of 15 paediatric gliomas, and numerous studies have demonstrated that increased pCASL-derived CBF is associated with a higher tumour grade [47,52]. pCASL is the preferred PWI technique used at our institution and is part of the neuro-oncology MRI protocol for assessment of treated gliomas (Figure 1).

The role of pCASL in the evaluation of treated paediatric gliomas is yet to be established but is the focus of active research.

2.3. Hybrid PET–MRI

Although combining PET imaging with advanced MRI provides an opportunity to improve overall diagnostic accuracy in neuro-oncology, to date, very few published studies have investigated this potential, mainly focussing on feasibility or agreement of modalities [13,15]. In paediatric neuro-oncology, the literature is even more scarce, limited to case reports and small feasibility studies, but the prevailing literature does support a role for amino acid PET [20]. We have previously shown that 18F-choline PET–MRI improves response assessment in treated gliomas [17,30] and can be used to validate novel MRI techniques such as Amide Proton Transfer-Chemical Exchange Saturation Transfer (APT-CEST) [18] (Figure 3). In addition, we have shown that 18FDOPA PET–MRI improves assessment of post-treatment glioma burden compared to MRI alone [61].

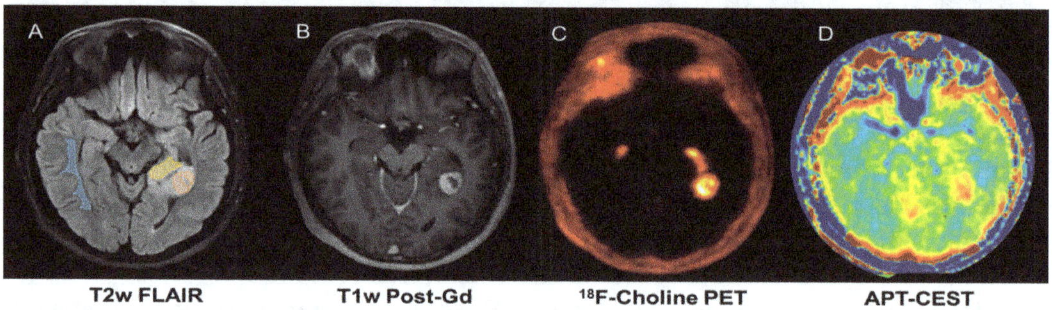

Figure 3. Fifteen-year-old male with pilocytic astrocytoma imaged on hybrid PET/MR which enables exact co-registration of FCho (**C**) with APT-CEST (**D**) showing correlation in enhancing ((**B**), T1 contrast) and non-enhancing tumour components. ((**A**), T2 FLAIR).

3. Clinical Case Studies of Hybrid PET–MRI in Neuro-Oncology

Nevertheless, in paediatric neuro-oncology, hybrid PET–MRI is not routinely used in clinical practice and should be considered as research. At our institution, PET–MRI is a supplementary diagnostic aid performed after an equivocal MRI. In this next section, we present illustrative examples of our experience of PET–MRI in specific tumour types at different timelines during their treatment. For clarity, we have grouped them into 4 groups: high-grade glioma (HGG), low-grade glioma (LGG), intracranial germ cell tumours (ICGCT) and primitive neuroectodermal tumours (PNET):

3.1. High-Grade Gliomas

High-grade gliomas are a challenging group of tumours as they invariably have dismal treatment outcome. While combining the information obtained from conventional MR imaging with the ADC values could increase the accuracy of pre-operative differentiation between low-grade and high-grade paediatric tumours, this is not always possible. Additionally, differentiating pseudoprogression from true progression remains a diagnostic dilemma, as conventional magnetic resonance imaging (MRI) features often cannot discriminate pseudoprogression from early true progression after chemoradiotherapy as contrast-enhancing lesions on MRI that do not reflect true tumour progression.

Patient 1: Diagnostic Biopsy and Radiotherapy Planning

A 16-year-old male presented with a short history of sharp bilateral eye pain that was intermittent in nature. He was seen by an ophthalmologist who detected bilateral swollen optic discs suggestive of papilledema. A diagnostic FCho PET–MRI scan showed an expansile pontine tumour with heterogenous, predominantly high T2-weighted signal abnormality. Choline uptake was seen in the enhancing component (Figure 4). A neuro-navigational stealth-guided biopsy was performed, centred on the choline avid region of the tumour, and the histology confirmed this to be a high-grade astrocytic tumour with a very high proliferative index. A response assessment scan after 6 weeks of chemoradiotherapy showed excellent treatment response with a complete metabolic response.

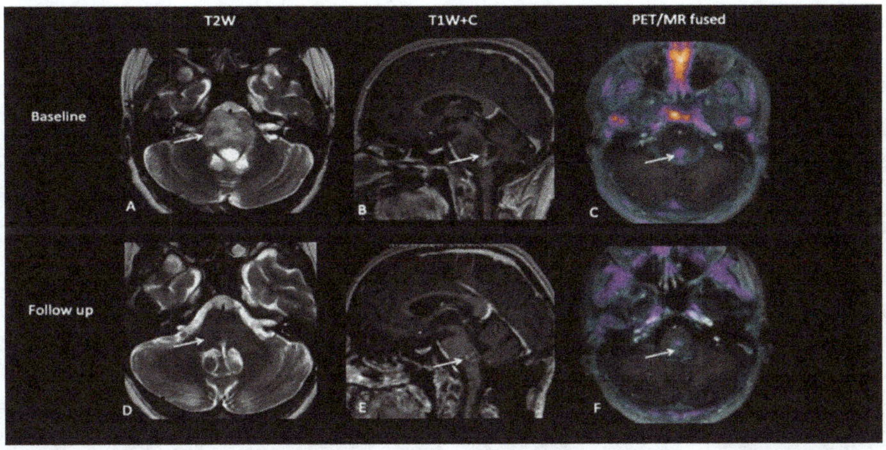

Figure 4. At baseline, there is a large pontine tumour (**A**) with a dorsally exophytic enhancing component (**B**), which shows FCho avidity on the PET/MR fused image (**C**). Follow-up imaging demonstrates residual dorsal enhancement (**D**,**E**), but FCho confirms no avidity (**F**) consistent with complete metabolic response.

Patient 2: Early Response Assessment

A 13-year-old female with a large tumour involving left thalamus and basal ganglia, infiltrating into the adjacent white matter, insular cortex and left aspect of the upper brain stem underwent a biopsy of the thalamic component, which confirmed high-grade astrocytoma with a mutation of the variant H3.3 gene. An early response assessment scan 6 weeks after completion of chemoradiotherapy demonstrated no residual enhancement in the tumour, but FDOPA PET showed residual tracer distribution consistent with residual metabolically active disease (Figure 5).

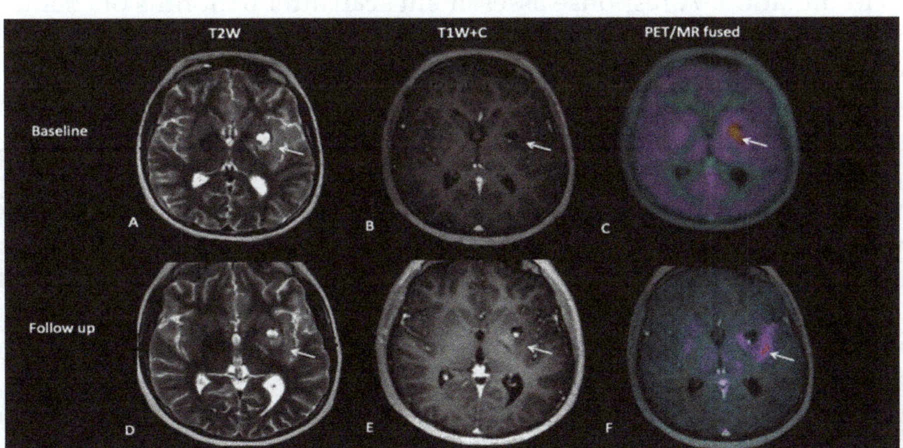

Figure 5. At baseline, there is non-enhancing tumour involving the left basal ganglia (**A**,**B**) with ^{8}F-fluorocholine (FCho) and ^{18}fluoro-L-phenylalanine (FDOPA) avidity (**C**). Follow-up imaging shows residual non-enhancing tumour (**D**,**E**) reported as stable disease, but FDOPA PET demonstrates reduced uptake (**F**) consistent with metabolic partial response.

Patient 3: Tumour Progression Versus Pseudoprogression

A 5-year-old female with diffuse midline glioma (DMG) presented with a short history of headaches, difficulty in walking and double vision. Radiology at diagnosis was consistent with diffuse intrinsic pontine glioma (DIPG). She commenced on 6 week course of focal radiotherapy (RT) to the pontine tumour with good initial response (Figure 6). The patient then went to Mexico for a form of targeted treatment and after four cycles developed clinical signs of disease progression. Whilst follow-up MRI demonstrated increased enhancement and raised the possibility of pseudoprogression, FDOPA PET demonstrated areas of avidity confirming clear progression.

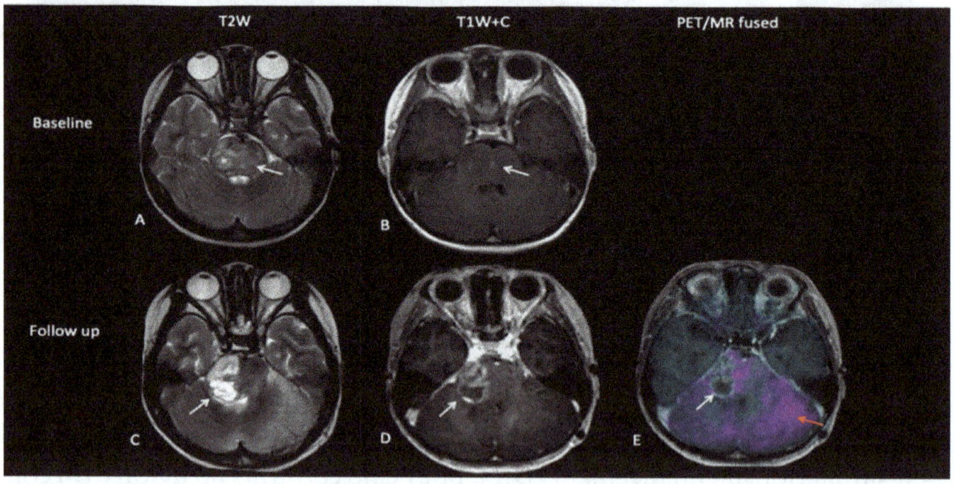

Figure 6. Baseline imaging demonstrates large pontine tumour (**A**) with focus of enhancement (**B**). Follow-up imaging demonstrated a large heterogenous right hemipontine mass (**C**,**D**) suspicious for tumour progression, but FDOPA (**E**) did not show increased uptake (white arrow) and was suggestive of pseudoprogression. However, FDOPA did show increased avidity in the left cerebellar hemisphere (red arrow) confirming non-enhancing tumour progression at that site.

Patient 4: Tumour Progression Versus Pseudoprogression

A 15-year-old male with a large tumour involving the left thalamus underwent gross resection of the thalamic tumour, and the histology confirmed this to be a high-grade astrocytoma with the known histone H3F3A K27M mutation. A response assessment scan after 6 months of chemotherapy (Figure 7) suggested minimal enhancement in the residual tumour that was thought to be pseudoprogression. However, FDOPA showed tracer uptake consistent with tumour progression.

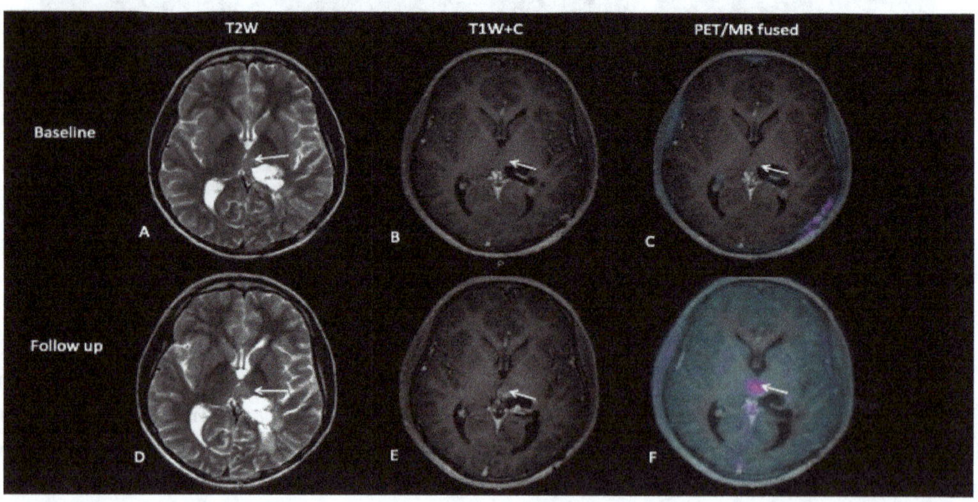

Figure 7. The baseline imaging post-surgery demonstrates residual non-enhancing tumour in the medial right thalamus (**A**–**C**). Follow-up imaging demonstrates the non-enhancing component (**D**) and mild enhancement of this component (**E**), uncertain for tumour progression or pseudoprogression, but the FDOPA (**F**) demonstrates increased uptake consistent with tumour progression.

Patient 5: End of Treatment Assessment

An 18-year-old female presented with a short history of headaches, vomiting and blurred vision. MRI scan at diagnosis (Figure 8) showed a large temporal lobe tumour. She underwent a sub-total resection and then commenced a 6-week course of chemoradiotherapy followed by 14 months of maintenance chemotherapy. Whilst the gadolinium contrast MRI scan at the end of treatment 18 months later demonstrated residual enhancement, FCho demonstrated no uptake, suggesting that the mass was non-viable.

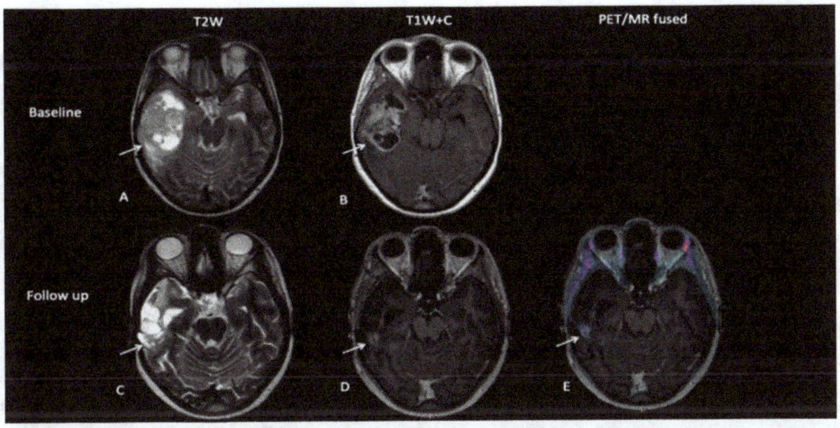

Figure 8. Baseline imaging demonstrates a large heterogenous right temporal lobe tumour (**A**) with avid enhancement (**B**). Follow-up imaging demonstrates the post-surgical resection on the T2W image (**C**) with nodular enhancement at the deep surgical margin (**D**), suspicious for residual tumour, but there is no increased uptake on FCho (**E**).

3.2. Low-Grade Gliomas

Patient 6: Tumour Progression Versus Pseudoprogression

A 10-year-old presented with low-grade glioma with a background of NF1 (neurofibromatosis type 1). A mid treatment MRI scan following disease progression showed enlargement of an enhancing lesion in the right cerebellar hemisphere, but the patient was well and clinically stable, and the radiological changes were thought to reflect pseudoprogression. An FDOPA PET–MRI showed increased tracer activity in the enhancing lesion along with a second FDOPA avid lesion in the right subthalamic region, consistent with metabolically active disease (Figure 9).

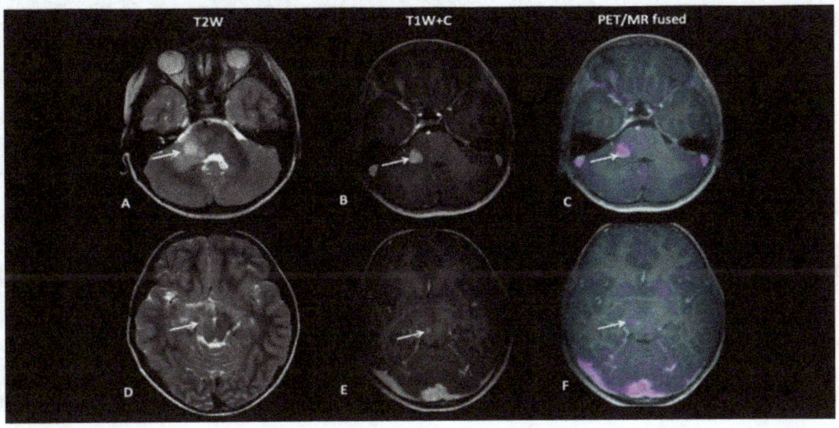

Figure 9. A mid-treatment scan demonstrates an enlarging right cerebellar hemisphere lesion (**A**,**B**) thought to reflect pseudoprogression, but FDOPA demonstrates increased uptake (**C**) and identifies a further lesion in the midbrain (**F**) not obviously apparent on the T2W image (**D**) or T1W post-contrast image (**E**), which is consistent with multifocal tumour progression.

Patient 7: Treatment Response

A 7-year-old female presented with tremors and an upward gaze palsy. A MRI scan showed a large tectal plate tumour involving the right thalamus causing secondary hydrocephalus.

She had a ventriculo-peritoneal (VP) shunt inserted for CSF diversion, but 4 years later following tumour progression, she underwent a biopsy which confirmed low-grade glioma. FDOPA showed intense uptake in both the enhancing and non-enhancing components of the tumour (Figure 10), following which the patient was referred for proton beam treatment PBT]. Post PBT FDOPA at 8 weeks showed complete metabolic response.

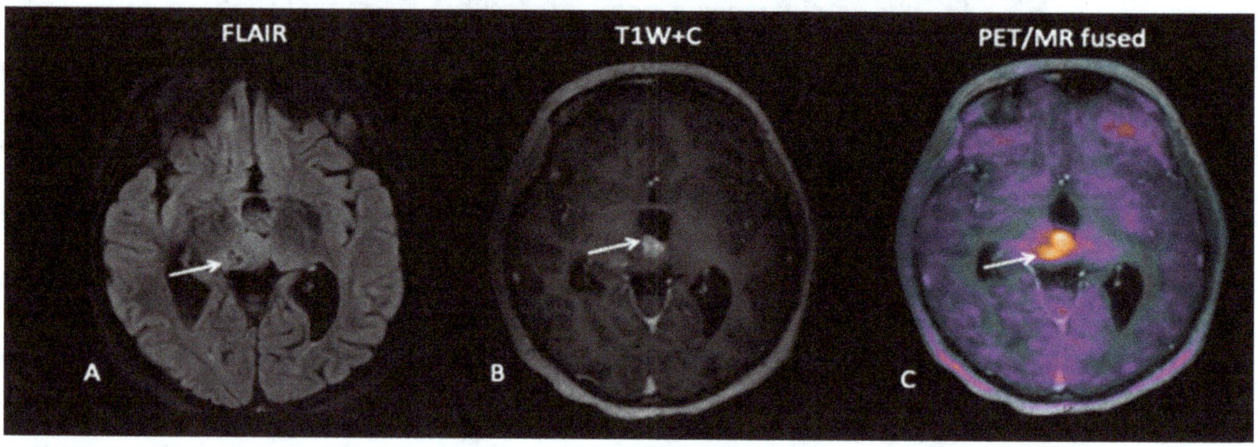

Figure 10. The MRI study demonstrates a large area of signal abnormality in the right thalamus (**A**) associated with a medial enhancing nodule (**B**). However, FDOPA demonstrates increased uptake in the non-enhancing component in addition to the enhancing component (**C**), confirming metabolically active non-enhancing disease in the right thalamus.

Patient 8: Suspicion of Transformation

A 15-year-old female with known low-grade glioma during routine surveillance was noted to have developed a large lesion in the corpus callosum. This occurred 7 years after her initial diagnosis of an optic pathway tumour. The MRI scan raised the possibility of malignant transformation to high-grade glioma. FDOPA (Figure 11) discounted the possibility of transformation as the FDOPA uptake within the corpus callosal lesion was low intensity, unlike that seen in high-grade gliomas.

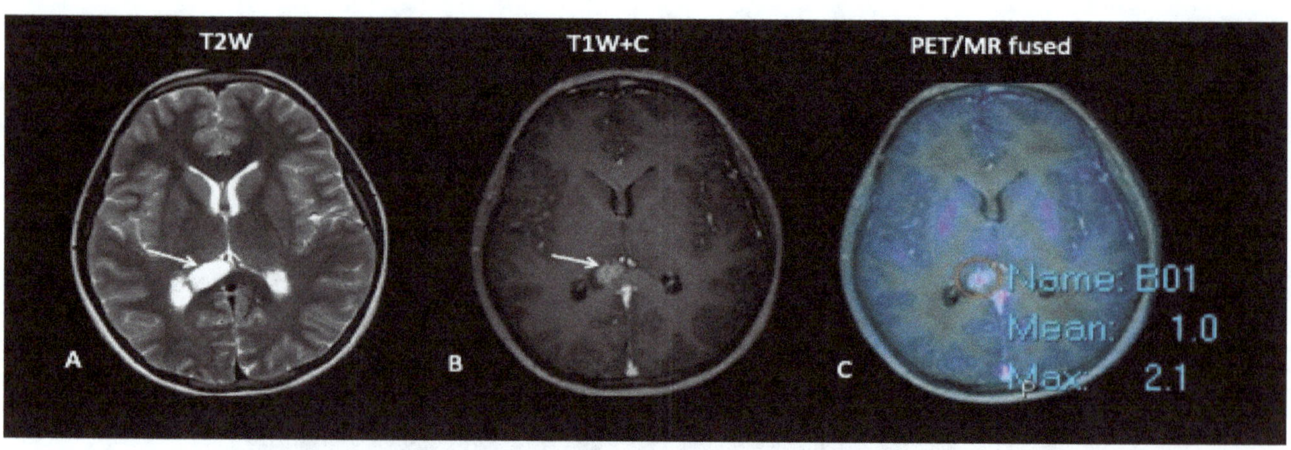

Figure 11. MRI demonstrates an expansile lesion in the right aspect of the splenium (**A**), which demonstrates heterogenous enhancement (**B**), suspicious for malignant transformation. However, FDOPA (**C**) did not demonstrate increased uptake, and the lesion was considered low grade.

3.3. *Intracranial Germ Cell Tumour*

Intracranial germ cell tumours (ICGCTs) are uncommon tumours occurring in children and young adults. They are sub-categorised into germinomas (GGCT) and non-germinomatous tumours (NGGCT). While GGCT are highly curable tumours with multimodality treatment, NGGCTs have a poorer outcome. There are clear differences in the approach to the management of ICGCTs. Current treatment strategies focuses on reducing treatment intensity, particularly the dose and volume of radiotherapy, in order to minimise the risks of late sequelae while maintaining high cure rates. In addition, especially in those with NGGCT, survival outcomes are unsatisfactory, and complete surgical resection combined with more intensive chemotherapy and radiotherapy remains the best available treatment option at this time. Occasionally, second-look surgery is required when the residual tumour increases or remains stable, despite normalized or nearly normalized tumour markers, in order to achieve complete resection and improve outcome.

Patient 9: Response Assessment

A 19-year-old male presented with a short history of headaches and double vision. MRI of the brain and spine showed a multi-cystic tumour pineal region tumour causing obstructive hydrocephalus. As serum AFP and bhCG were elevated, a diagnosis of intracranial NGGCT was made. After four cycles of chemotherapy, 18F-fluoroethylcholine (FEC) PET–MRI showed stable tumour volume with moderate FEC uptake, suggestive of viable tumour (Figure 12). He underwent macroscopic tumour resection that histologically showed the presence of viable tumour and subsequently proceeded to cranio-spinal radiotherapy (CSRT) with a boost to the pineal tumour.

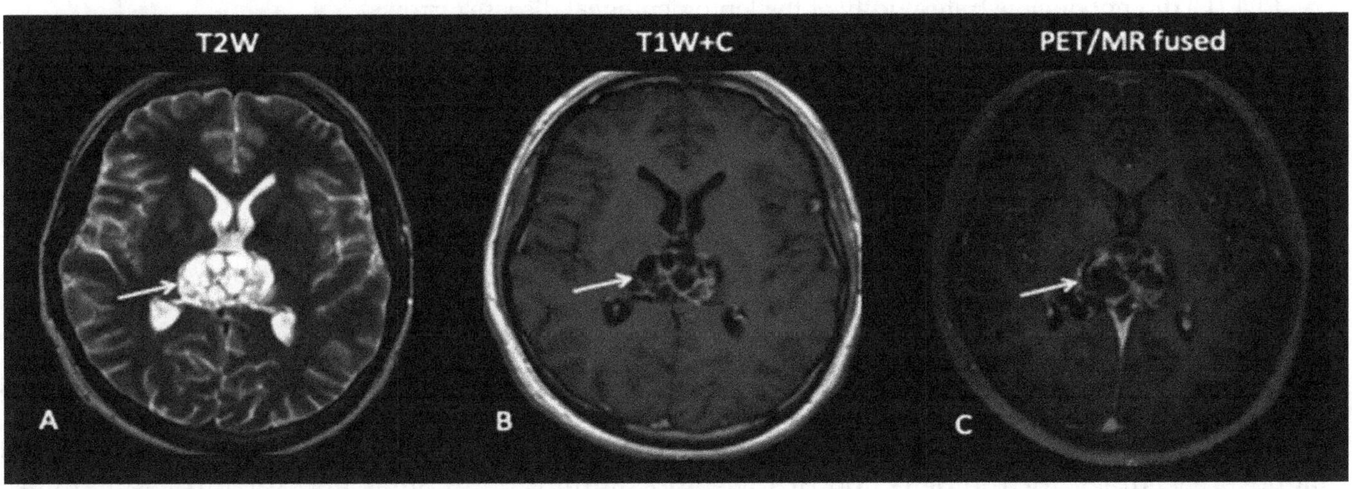

Figure 12. MRI demonstrated a stable residual cystic large pineal region tumour (**A**) with enhancement of the internal septations (**B**) reported as stable disease. However, 18F-fluoroethylcholine (FEC) (**C**) showed increased avidity consistent with metabolically active disease.

3.4. *Primitive Neuro-Ectodermal Tumours (PNET)*

Combining anatomical and functional imaging can improve sensitivity and accuracy of tumour diagnosis in high-grade paediatric embryonal tumours. Although PET using radiolabelled amino acids provides important metabolic information for astrocytic tumours, much less is known of the value of PET in medulloblastomas.

Patient 10: Diagnosis

This 15-year-old female had a short-presenting history of recurrent headaches, vertigo, back ache and a band like numbness around the right breast and chest. She also complained of her legs "giving away". MRI of the brain and spine revealed multiple lesions involving the brain with multiple drop spinal lesions occupying the spinal canal, compressing the spinal cord and nerve roots at all the levels (Figure 13), suggestive of a high-grade tumour. Surprisingly, the FCho PET–MRI showed that all the lesions in the brain and spine were choline non-avid, suggestive of a low-grade tumour, i.e., a low proliferative index, but a subsequent biopsy of the spinal lesion confirmed medulloblastoma.

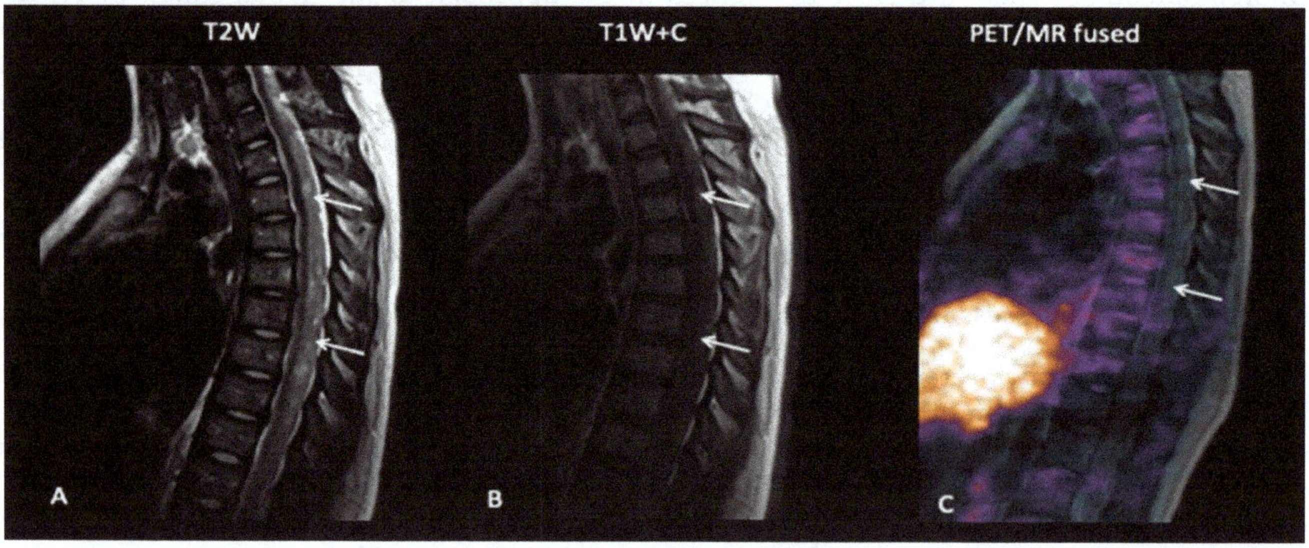

Figure 13. Spinal MRI (**A**,**B**) demonstrates extensive intraspinal-enhancing soft tissue in keeping with leptomeningeal metastatic disease (arrows point out the leptomeningeal disease). However, the FCho PET (**C**) did not demonstrate avidity of the leptomeningeal disease (arrows).

4. Discussion

Imaging is a critical component in the management of brain tumours, with MRI being the modality of choice. While conventional cross-sectional contrast-enhanced MRI provides structural information with regard to tumour size and location, it does not provide complimentary information on tumour metabolism, biological aggressiveness and prognosis. Various functional imaging have been developed that provide information on tissue properties and tumour metabolism, including advanced MR and PET. Combining the techniques in hybrid PET–MRI provides the opportunity to demonstrate structural and metabolic information, improving diagnosis. We have shown that the use of the hybrid PET–MRI imaging platform in our paediatric/TYA neuro-oncology practice has had a decisive bearing on treatment decisions, prognosis and overall outcome.

We have previously shown unequivocal evidence that FDOPA PET and FCho PET have high diagnostic accuracy for the detection of low- and high-grade gliomas and for intracranial germ cell tumours [17,30,31]. In gliomas, while the discrimination between tumour recurrence and radiation-induced changes has been well described [17], the parameters for treatment response assessment need further investigation with standardized imaging protocols in prospective studies.

4.1. FCho

We have previously shown that FCho PET–MRI is a promising and reliable imaging tool for children with astrocytic tumours, as it permits monitoring of morphological and metabolic response and changes during therapy [17,30]. FCho has been shown to be highly effective in confirming the absence of viable residual tumour, as illustrated in patient 5, or the presence of viable residual tumour (patient 9), confirming the predictive value of discrimination of viable from non-viable tumour. In addition, the use of PET is particularly useful to target the malignant foci for biopsy sites in gliomas, which is well illustrated by the case of patient 1 and in the management of patients with recurrent disease when combined with MRI [32]. There are also reports in the literature where PET has been used to improve the diagnostic accuracy [61] and radiation therapy planning in patients with gliomas [20,33].

FCho has been used as an imaging tool for diagnosis, assessment of treatment response and remission status for children and adolescents with intracranial germ cell tumours [31]. Management of intracranial germ cell tumours in TYA patients is complex, as many patients have an incomplete radiological response to standard treatment. These residual radiological lesions could harbour viable tumour, and, hence, surgical resection is recommended to improve survival outcome. In this series report, patient 9 demonstrated moderate FEC uptake, suggestive of residual viable tumour, enabling a decision to proceed with surgical resection that confirmed the presence of residual viable tumour. There were two further patients who had residual pineal lesions on MRI but were FCho PET negative. Both patients underwent surgical resection, and there was complete concordance with choline uptake and histology at resection: both had necrotic non-viable tumour at resection. We have not included these cases here as the scans were not performed on the hybrid PET–MRI scanner, but further details can be found in a previous publication [31].

4.2. FDOPA

Reports in published literature have highlighted the value of FDOPA PET as an imaging tool for early response assessment for high-grade gliomas [62,63]. The ability of FDOPA to better delineate treatment response was illustrated in patients 2 and 5 and differentiation of progression from pseudoprogression are well illustrated in patients 4 and 6. In patients 4 and 6, while treatment-related changes/pseudoprogression could not be excluded on the contrasted MRI, FDOPA was highly discriminatory, and the changes were consistent for true disease progression. While many paediatric low-grade gliomas unlike in adults are contrast-enhancing tumours, they are often heterogenous and do not enhance uniformly. Additionally, contrast enhancement resulting from increased permeability of the blood–brain barrier is nonspecific and does not demarcate tumour extent or treatment effect. Planning treatment, especially radiotherapy, can be difficult in such a situation. The use of a PET tracer such as 18F DOPA can better identify the non-enhancing tumour, as the increased uptake of FDOPA in gliomas appears to be related to increased transport via the amino acid transport system [28,29].

4.3. False Negative Studies

It must be emphasised that not all gliomas or embryonal tumours of the brain are FCho or FDOPA avid. It has been previously shown that while a significant correlation between FDOPA uptake and tumour proliferation in newly diagnosed tumours is usually observed, this correlation is not seen in recurrent tumours [64,65]. The reason attributed for this discordance is because recurrent tumours could have differential blood–brain barrier breakdown due to previous treatments. Therefore, it is not surprising that the correlation between ^{18}FDOPA PET uptake and tumour grade is better seen in treatment-naïve newly diagnosed tumours. However, our patient had no previous treatment other than resection of her spinal astrocytoma at first diagnosis, thus, the latter explanation cannot be applied here. It is therefore important that a negative scan during any phase of treatment cannot be equated to complete metabolic response if there was no previous positive PET scans for comparison.

In our series, FCho demonstrated no uptake in patient 10 with disseminated medulloblastoma at diagnosis. Typically, medulloblastomas are hypermetabolic with a high proliferative index and have been shown to be choline avid [66]. Hence, the lack of choline avidity was surprising, and we can only speculate that this was due to technical failure.

4.4. Recommendations

Based on our experience illustrated here, we consider that combined amino acid PET–MRI is likely to improve the diagnostic accuracy of standard MRI in paediatric and TYA tumours in the following clinical situations:

1. Surveillance imaging in low-grade gliomas.
2. Discriminating tumour progression from treatment effects in high-grade gliomas.

3. Assessment of early and end of treatment response in gliomas and intra-cranial germ cell tumours.
4. Surgical and radiotherapy planning in diffuse gliomas.

Although the clinical situations presented do not necessarily require simultaneous acquisition in a PET–MRI scanner, the advantages, particularly in the paediatric population, are the requirement for only one examination, particularly if sedation or general anaesthetic is planned. Another advantage is the exact co-registration of PET and MRI, which is desirable post-surgery where anatomical distortion is likely to occur. However, there are several disadvantages in that PET–MRI is a lengthier examination process, at approximately 90 min acquisition, compared to MRI or PET alone. There is also likely to be decreased patient comfort due to smaller bore size causing claustrophobia and ear phones not being standard. Finally, the necessity of rigid head fixation for smaller head size can be a cause of increased imaging artefacts. However, next-generation PET–MRI patient scanners will hopefully improve patient comfort and realize the potential of a one-stop non-invasive imaging technique in neuro-oncology. It is important to stress that a one-off negative scan with PET–MRI during any phase of treatment does not equate to a complete metabolic response, and, hence, a baseline scan is mandatory. The ease of availability is a common limitation for both tracers— ^{18}fluorocholine [FCho] and ^{18}fluoro-L-phenylalanine ad will have to be factored in for clinical use.

4.4.1. Premise of This Report

Is PET–MRI an effective tool for oncological imaging of primary brain tumours in children and TYA patients, especially in the delineation tumour extent, monitoring treatment response and post-treatment differentiation between tumour progression or recurrence versus treatment-related changes? The second question is, what is the optimal indication of PET–MRI imaging in brain tumours?

4.4.2. What this Report Adds to Published Literature

Although conventional gadolinium-enhanced magnetic resonance imaging (MRI) is considered the primary imaging modality for patients with brain tumours, it has some limitations, primarily in differentiating tumour grade, its inability to provide metabolic or functional information of the biology of the tumour, and in distinguishing disease recurrence from post-therapy changes. This report corroborates the effectiveness as well as the limitations of PET–MRI in paediatric and TYA neuro-oncology in the following:

1. Facilitating diagnostic neuro-surgical intervention, i.e., the site for pre-operative biopsy planning and navigation in children and TYA patients;
2. The reassurance that metabolically inert post-therapy residual lesions in patients with intracranial germ cell tumours represent non-viable tissue;
3. Defining the tumour and target volumes for radiotherapy by combining metabolic and radiological information of tumour extent and infiltrative margins;
4. The detection of tumour recurrence during clinical and radiological surveillance;
5. In distinguishing tumour recurrence from treatment necrosis/therapy-related changes;
6. That PET–MRI alone is insufficient in providing accurate delineation and diagnostic sensitivity of observed lesions, as not all histological subtypes of brain tumours take up the radiotracers.

4.4.3. Published Evidence

There is limited published evidence of the use of PET–MRI as an imaging modality for diagnostic purposes, early treatment response assessment, end of treatment disease status or as an imaging tool for post-treatment radiological surveillance in a paediatric and TYA patients with brain tumours.

4.4.4. Added Value of This Report

This review highlights the importance of a multi-parametric imaging and that PET–MRI unequivocally is a promising imaging tool for children and TYA patients with a variety of brain tumours. It allows for the diagnosis and monitoring of morphological and metabolic response and changes during therapy and is an effective imaging tool in detecting viable residual tumour at the end of treatment.

4.4.5. Implication of All of the Available Evidence

Overall, the conventional cross-sectional MRI combined with PET is a complementary modality for assessment of tumour burden. Combining and matching both imaging modalities is significantly superior to either imaging modality alone in assessing the presence of viable residual tumour and indicating the radiotherapy target volume. Additionally, PET–MRI generates quantitative measures that may add significant value to conventional SUV image-derived measures.

5. Conclusions

While for primary tumour staging, MRI on its own is sufficient, the use of combined PET and MRI provides additional molecular and functional information for critical treatment decisions. This is highly relevant in clinical neuro-oncology, and the use of PET–MRI will increase in the years to come. Whilst mostly a research tool in paediatric/TYA neuro-oncology, there is enough evidence from the adult neuro-oncology literature to justify its clinical use. We have demonstrated a number of clinical situations where hybrid PET–MRI can improve diagnostic accuracy, and as improvements in PET–MRI scanners are made, the use in paediatric/TYA neuro-oncology is likely to increase.

Author Contributions: H.H.: contributed by evaluating the MRI component of the PET-MRI and writing the manuscript. A.S.: contributed to the concept of the paper, clinical omponent and to the writing of the manuscript. J.B.: contributed by evaluating the PET component of the paper and contributed to the discussion and writing of the manuscript. All authors have read and agreed to the published version of the manuscript.

References

1. Pollack, I.F.; Jakacki, R.I. Childhood brain tumors: Epidemiology, current management and future directions. *Nat. Rev. Neurol.* **2011**, *7*, 495–506. [CrossRef]
2. Udaka, Y.T.; Packer, R.J. Pediatric Brain Tumours. *Neurol. Clin.* **2018**, *36*, 533–556. [CrossRef]
3. Sturm, D.; Pfister, S.M.; Jones, D.T.W. Pediatric gliomas: Current concepts on diagnosis, biology, and clinical management. *J. Clin. Oncol.* **2017**, *35*, 2370–2377. [CrossRef]
4. Pajtler, K.W.; Mack, S.C.; Ramaswamy, V.; Smith, C.A.; Witt, H.; Smith, A.; Hansford, J.R.; von Hoff, K.; Wright, K.D.; Hwang, E.; et al. The current consensus on the clinical management of intracranial ependymoma and its distinct molecular variants. *Acta Neuropathol.* **2017**, *133*, 5–12. [CrossRef]
5. Zapotocky, M.; Ramaswamy, V.; Lassaletta, A.; Bouffet, E. Adolescents and young adults with brain tumors in the context of molecular advances in neuro-oncology. *Pediatr. Blood Cancer* **2018**, *64*, e26861. [CrossRef]
6. Young, R.J.; Gupta, A.; Shah, A.D.; Graber, J.J.; Zhang, Z.; Shi, W.; Holodny, A.I.; Omuro, A.M.P. Potential utility of conventional MRI signs in diagnosing pseudoprogression in glioblastoma. *Neurology* **2011**, *76*, 1918–1924. [CrossRef]
7. Verma, N.; Cowperthwaite, M.C.; Burnett, M.G.; Markey, M.K. Differentiating tumor recurrence from treatment necrosis: A review of neuro-oncologic imaging strategies. *Neuro Oncol.* **2013**, *15*, 515–534. [CrossRef]
8. Norden, A.D.; Drappatz, J.; Wen, P.Y. Antiangiogenic therapies for high-grade glioma. *Nat. Rev. Neurol.* **2009**, *15*, 610–620. [CrossRef] [PubMed]
9. Narayana, A.; Kelly, P.; Golfinos, J.; Parker, E.; Johnson, G.; Knopp, E.; Zagzag, D.; Fischer, I.; Raza, S.; Medabalmi, P.; et al. Antiangiogenic therapy using bevacizumab in recurrent high-grade glioma: Impact on local control and patient survival: Clinical article. *J. Neurosurg.* **2009**, *110*, 173–180. [CrossRef]

10. Hartmann, C.; Hentschel, B.; Wick, W.; Capper, D.; Felsberg, J.; Simon, M.; Westphal, M.; Schackert, G.; Meyermann, R.; Pietsch, T.; et al. Patients with IDH1 wild type anaplastic astrocytomas exhibit worse prognosis than IDH1-mutated glioblastomas, and IDH1 mutation status accounts for the unfavorable prognostic effect of higher age: Implications for classification of gliomas. *Acta Neuropathol.* **2010**, *120*, 707–718. [CrossRef]
11. Metellus, P.; Coulibaly, B.; Colin, C.; De Paula, A.M.; Vasiljevic, A.; Taieb, D.; Barlier, A.; Boisselier, B.; Mokhtari, K.; Wang, X.W.; et al. Absence of IDH mutation identifies a novel radiologic and molecular subtype of WHO grade II gliomas with dismal prognosis. *Acta Neuropathol.* **2010**, *120*, 719–729. [CrossRef]
12. Schlemmer, H.P.W.; Pichler, B.J.; Schmand, M.; Burbar, Z.; Michel, C.; Ladebeck, R.; Jattke, K.; Townsend, D.; Nahmias, C.; Jacob, P.K.; et al. Simultaneous MR/PET imaging of the human brain: Feasibility study. *Radiology* **2008**, *248*, 1028–1035. [CrossRef]
13. Filss, C.P.; Galldiks, N.; Stoffels, G.; Sabel, M.; Wittsack, H.J.; Turowski, B.; Antoch, G.; Zhang, K.; Fink, G.R.; Coenen, H.H.; et al. Comparison of18f-fet pet and perfusion-weighted mr imaging: A pet/mr imaging hybrid study in patients with brain tumors. *J. Nucl. Med.* **2014**, *55*, 540–545. [CrossRef]
14. Jena, A.; Taneja, S.; Gambhir, A.; Mishra, A.K.; D'Souza, M.M.; Verma, S.M.; Hazari, P.P.; Negi, P.; Jhadav, G.K.R.; Sogani, S.K. Glioma recurrence versus radiation necrosis single-session multiparametric approach using simultaneous O-(2-18F-fluoroethyl)-L-tyrosine PET/MRI. *Clin. Nucl. Med.* **2016**, *41*, E228–E236. [CrossRef]
15. Henriksen, O.M.; Larsen, V.A.; Muhic, A.; Hansen, A.E.; Larsson, H.B.W.; Poulsen, H.S.; Law, I. Simultaneous evaluation of brain tumour metabolism, structure and blood volume using [18F]-fluoroethyltyrosine (FET) PET/MRI: Feasibility, agreement and initial experience. *Eur. J. Nucl. Med. Mol. Imaging* **2016**, *43*, 103–112. [CrossRef]
16. Morana, G.; Piccardo, A.; Puntoni, M.; Nozza, P.; Cama, A.; Raso, A.; Mascelli, S.; Massollo, M.; Milanaccio, C.; Garre, M.L.; et al. Diagnostic and prognostic value of 18F-DOPA PET and 1H-MR spectroscopy in pediatric supratentorial infiltrative gliomas: A comparative study. *Neuro Oncol.* **2015**, *17*, 1637–1647. [CrossRef] [PubMed]
17. Fraioli, F.; Shankar, A.; Hyare, H.; Ferrazzoli, V.; Militano, V.; Samandouras, G.; Mankad, K.; Solda, F.; Zaccaagna, F.; Mehdi, E.; et al. The use of Multiparametric 18F-Choline PET/MR in post therapy assessment of patients gliomas. *Nucl. Med. Commun.* **2020**, *41*, 517–525.
18. Rega, M.; Torrealdea, F.; Hearle, J.; Zaiss, M.; Cavalho, A.; Afaq, A.; Punwani, S.; Golay, X.; Dickson, J.; Shankar, A.; et al. Correlation between APT-CEST and 18F-Choline PET in glioma at 3T. *Neuro Oncol.* **2018**, *20*, 170–171. [CrossRef]
19. Boellaard, R.; Delgado-Bolton, R.; Oyen, W.J.; Giammarile, F.; Tatsch, K.; Eschner, W.; Verzijlbergen, F.J.; Barrington, S.F.; Pike, L.C.; Weber, W.A.; et al. FDG PET/CT: EANM procedure guidelines for tumour imaging: Version 2.0. *Eur. J. Nucl. Med. Mol. Imaging* **2015**, *42*, 328–354. [CrossRef]
20. Albert, N.L.; Waller, M.; Suchorska, B.; Galldiks, N.; Soffietti, R.; Kim, M.M.; La Fougere, C.; Pope, W.; Law, I.; Arbizu, J.; et al. Response Assessment in Neuro-Oncology working group and European Association for Neuro-Oncology recommendations for the clinical use of PET imaging in gliomas. *Neuro Oncol.* **2016**, *18*, 1199–1208. [CrossRef]
21. Langen, K.J.; Galldiks, N.; Hattingen, E.; Shah, N.J. Advances in neuro-oncology imaging. *Nat. Rev. Neurol.* **2017**, *13*, 279–289. [CrossRef] [PubMed]
22. Langen, K.J.; Watts, C. Neuro-oncology: Amino acid PET for brain tumours-ready for the clinic? *Nat. Rev. Neurol.* **2016**, *12*, 375–376. [CrossRef]
23. Okada, H.; Weller, M.; Huang, R.; Finocchiaro, G.; Gilbert, M.R.; Wick, W.; Ellingson, B.M.; Hashimoto, N.; Pollack, I.F.; Brandes, A.A.; et al. Immunotherapy response assessment in neuro-oncology: A report of the RANO working group. *Lancet Oncol.* **2015**, *16*, e534–e542. [CrossRef]
24. Cicone, F.; Filss, C.P.; Minniti, G.; Rossi-Espagnet, C.; Papa, A.; Scaringi, C.; Galldiks, N.; Bozzao, A.; Shah, N.J.; Scopinaro, F.; et al. Volumetric assessment of recurrent or progressive gliomas: Comparison between F-DOPA PET and perfusion-weighted MRI. *Eur. J. Nucl. Med. Mol. Imaging* **2015**, *42*, 905–915. [CrossRef]
25. Galldiks, N.; Law, I.; Pope, W.B.; Arbizu, J.; Langen, K.J. The use of amino acid PET and conventional MRI for monitoring of brain tumor therapy. *NeuroImage Clin.* **2017**, *13*, 386–394. [CrossRef]

26. Galldiks, N.; Dunkl, V.; Ceccon, G.; Tscherpel, C.; Stoffels, G.; Law, I.; Henriksen, O.M.; Muhic, A.; Poulsen, H.S.; Steger, J.; et al. Early treatment response evaluation using FET PET compared to MRI in glioblastoma patients at first progression treated with bevacizumab plus lomustine. *Eur. J. Nucl. Med. Mol. Imaging* **2018**, *45*, 2377–2386. [CrossRef]
27. Nowosielski, M.; DiFranco, M.D.; Putzer, D.; Seiz, M.; Recheis, W.; Jacobs, A.H.; Stockhammer, G.; Hutterer, M. An intra-individual comparison of MRI, [18F]-FET and [18F]-FLT PET in patients with high-grade gliomas. *PLoS ONE* **2014**, *9*, e95830. [CrossRef]
28. Wiriyasermkul, P.; Nagamori, S.; Tominaga, H.; Oriuchi, N.; Kaira, K.; Nakao, H.; Kitashoji, T.; Ohgaki, R.; Tanaka, H.; Endou, H.; et al. Transport of 3-fluoro-L-α-methyl-tyrosine by tumor-upregulated L-type amino acid transporter 1: A cause of the tumor uptake in PET. *J. Nucl. Med.* **2012**, *53*, 1253–1261. [CrossRef]
29. Papin-Michault, C.; Bonnetaud, C.; Dufour, M.; Almairac, F.; Coutts, M.; Patouraux, S.; Virolle, T.; Darcourt, J.; Burel-Vandenbos, F. Study of LAT1 expression in brain metastases: Towards a better understanding of the results of positron emission tomography using amino acid tracers. *PLoS ONE* **2016**, *11*, e0157139. [CrossRef]
30. Fraioli, F.; Shankar, A.; Hargrave, D.; Hyare, H.; Gaze, M.N.; Groves, A.M.; Alongi, P.; Stoneham, S.; Michopoulou, S.; Syed, R.; et al. ^{18}F-fluoroethylcholine (^{18}F-cho) PET/MRI functional parameters in pediatric astrocytic brain tumors. *Clin. Nucl. Med.* **2015**, *40*, e40–e45. [CrossRef]
31. Tsouana, E.; Stoneham, S.; Fersht, N.; Kitchen, N.; Gaze, M.; Bomanji, J.; Fraioli, F.; Hargrave, D.; Shankar, A. Evaluation of treatment response using integrated 18F-labeled choline positron emission tomography/magnetic resonance imaging in adolescents with intracranial non-germinomatous germ cell tumours. *Pediatr. Blood Cancer* **2015**, *62*, 1661–1663. [CrossRef] [PubMed]
32. Calabria, F.F.; Barbarisi, M.; Gangemi, V.; Grillea, G.L. Cascini. Molecular imaging of brain tumors with radiolabeled choline PET. *Neurosurg. Rev.* **2018**, *41*, 67–76. [CrossRef] [PubMed]
33. Alongi, P.; Vetrano, I.G.; Fiasconaro, E.; Alaimo, V.; Laudicella, R.; Bellavia, M.; Rubino, F.; Bagnato, S.; Galardi, G. Choline-PET/CT in the Differential Diagnosis Between Cystic Glioblastoma and Intraparenchymal Hemorrhage. *Curr. Radiopharm.* **2019**, *12*, 88–92. [CrossRef] [PubMed]
34. Giovannini, E.; Lazzeri, P.; Milano, A.; Gaeta, M.; Ciarmiello, A. Clinical Applications of Choline PET/CT in Brain Tumors. *Curr. Pharm. Des.* **2015**, *21*, 121–127. [CrossRef] [PubMed]
35. Kim, S.J.; Ryul Shim, S. Diagnostic value of radiolabeled amino acid PET for detection of pseudoprogression of brain tumor after treatment: A meta-analysis. *Nucl. Med. Commun.* **2019**, *40*, 965–972. [CrossRef]
36. Cicone, F.; Minniti, G.; Romano, A.; Papa, A.; Scaringi, C.; Tavanti, F.; Bozzao, A.; Maurizi Enrici, R.; Scopinaro, F. Accuracy of F-DOPA PET and perfusion-MRI for differentiating radionecrotic from progressive brain metastases after radiosurgery. *Eur. J. Nucl. Med. Mol. Imaging* **2015**, *42*, 103–111. [CrossRef]
37. Kondo, A.; Ishii, H.; Aoki, S.; Suzuki, M.; Nagasawa, H.; Kubota, K.; Minamimoto, R.; Arakawa, A.; Tominaga, M.; Arai, H. Phase IIa clinical study of [18F]fluciclovine: Efficacy and safety of a new PET tracer for brain tumors. *Ann. Nucl. Med.* **2016**, *30*, 608–618. [CrossRef]
38. Alkonyi, B.; Barger, G.R.; Mittal, S.; Muzik, O.; Chugani, D.C.; Bahl, G.; Robinette, N.L.; Kupsky, W.J.; Chakraborty, P.K.; Juhasz, C. Accurate differentiation of recurrent gliomas from radiation injury by kinetic analysis of α-11C-methyl-L-tryptophan PET. *J. Nucl. Med.* **2012**, *53*, 1058–1064. [CrossRef]
39. Kawai, N.; Lin, W.; Cao, W.D.; Ogawa, D.; Miyake, K.; Haba, R.; Maeda, Y.; Yamamoto, Y.; Nishiyama, Y.; Tamiya, T. Correlation between 18F-fluoromisonidazole PET and expression of HIF-1α and VEGF in newly diagnosed and recurrent malignant gliomas. *Eur. J. Nucl. Med. Mol. Imaging* **2014**, *41*, 1870–1878. [CrossRef]
40. Bekaert, L.; Valable, S.; Lechapt-Zalcman, E.; Ponte, K.; Collet, S.; Constans, J.M.; Levallet, G.; Bordji, K.; Petit, E.; Branger, P.; et al. [18F]-FMISO PET study of hypoxia in gliomas before surgery: Correlation with molecular markers of hypoxia and angiogenesis. *Eur. J. Nucl. Med. Mol. Imaging* **2017**, *44*, 1383–1392. [CrossRef]
41. Winkeler, A.; Boisgard, R.; Awde, A.; Dubois, A.; Theze, B.; Zheng, J.; Ciobanu, L.; Dolle, F.; Viel, T.; Jacobs, A.H.; et al. The translocator protein ligand [18F]DPA-714 images glioma and activated microglia in vivo. *Eur. J. Nucl. Med. Mol. Imaging* **2012**, *39*, 811–823. [CrossRef]
42. Mentlein, R.; Hattermann, K.; Hemion, C.; Jungbluth, A.A.; Held-Feindt, J. Expression and role of the cell surface protease seprase/fibroblast activation protein-α (FAP-α) in astroglial tumors. *Biol. Chem.* **2011**, *392*, 199–207. [CrossRef]

43. Wen, P.Y.; Macdonald, D.R.; Reardon, D.A.; Cloughesy, T.F.; Sorensen, A.G.; Galanis, E.; DeGroot, J.; Wick, W.; Gilbert, M.R.; Lassman, A.B.; et al. Updated response assessment criteria for high-grade gliomas: Response assessment in neuro-oncology working group. *J. Clin. Oncol.* **2010**, *28*, 1963–1972. [CrossRef]
44. Ellingson, B.M.; Benszus, M.; Boxerman, J.; Barboriak, D.; Erickson, B.J.; Smits, M.; Nelson, S.J.; Gerstner, E.; Alexander, B.; Goldmacher, G.; et al. Consensus recommendations for a standardized Brain Tumor Imaging Protocol in clinical trials. *Neuro Oncol.* **2015**, *17*, 1188–1198. [CrossRef]
45. Craig, E.; Connolly, D.J.; Griffiths, P.D.; Raghavan, A.; Lee, V.; Batty, R. MRI protocols for imaging paediatric brain tumours. *Clin. Radiol.* **2012**, *67*, 829–832. [CrossRef]
46. Wang, X.C.; Zhang, H.; Tan, Y.; Qin, J.B.; Wu, X.F.; Wang, L.; Zhang, L. Combined value of susceptibility-weighted and perfusion-weighted imaging in assessing WHO grade for brain astrocytomas. *J. Magn. Reson. Imaging* **2014**, *39*, 1569–1574. [CrossRef]
47. Keil, V.C.; Hartkamp, N.S.; Connolly, D.J.A.; Morana, G.; Dremmen, M.H.G.; Mutsaerts, H.J.M.M.; Lequin, M.H. Added value of arterial spin labeling magnetic resonance imaging in pediatric neuroradiology: Pitfalls and applications. *Pediatr. Radiol.* **2019**, *49*, 245–253. [CrossRef]
48. Melhem, E.R.; Mehta, N.R. Dynamic T1-weighted spin-echo mr imaging: The role of digital subtraction in the demonstration of enhancing brain lesions. *J. Magn. Reson. Imaging* **1999**, *9*, 503–508. [CrossRef]
49. Ellingson, B.M.; Aftab, D.T.; Schwab, G.M.; Hessel, C.; Harris, R.J.; Woodworth, D.C.; Leu, K.; Chakhoyan, A.; Raymond, C.; Drappatz, J.; et al. Volumetric response quantified using T1 subtraction predicts long-term survival benefit from cabozantinib monotherapy in recurrent glioblastoma. *Neuro Oncol.* **2018**, *20*, 1411–1418. [CrossRef]
50. Daniels, D.; Guez, D.; Last, D.; Hoffmann, C.; Nass, D.; Talianski, A.; Tsarfaty, G.; Saloman, S.; Kanner, A.A.; Blumenthal, D.T.; et al. Early biomarkers from conventional and delayed-contrast MRI to predict the response to bevacizumab in recurrent high-grade gliomas. *Am. J. Neuroradiol.* **2016**, *37*, 2003–2009. [CrossRef]
51. LaViolette, P.S.; Mickevicius, N.J.; Cochran, E.J.; Rand, S.D.; Connelly, J.; Bovi, J.A.; Malkin, M.G.; Mueller, W.M.; Schmainda, K.M. Precise ex vivo histological validation of heightened cellularity and diffusion restricted necrosis in regions of dark apparent diffusion coefficient in 7 cases of high-grade glioma. *Neuro Oncol.* **2014**, *16*, 1599–1606. [CrossRef]
52. Simon, D.; Fritzsche, K.H.; Thieke, C.; Klein, J.; Parzer, P.; Weber, M.A.; Stieltjes, B. Diffusion-weighted imaging-based probabilistic segmentation of high- and low-proliferative areas in high-grade gliomas. *Cancer Imaging* **2012**, *12*, 89–99. [CrossRef]
53. Hales, P.W.; d'Arco, F.; Copper, J.; Pfeuffer, J.; Hargrave, D.; Mankad, K.; Clark, C. Arterial spin labelling and diffusion-weighted imaging in paediatric brain tumours. *Neuroimage Clin.* **2019**, *22*, 101696. [CrossRef] [PubMed]
54. Roberts, T.A.; Hyare, H.; Agliardi, G.; Hipwell, B.; d'Esposito, A.; Ianus, A.; Breen-Norris, J.O.; Ramasawmy, R.; Taylor, V.; Atkinson, D.; et al. Noninvasive diffusion magnetic resonance imaging of brain tumour cell size for the early detection of therapeutic response. *Sci. Rep.* **2020**, *10*, 9223. [CrossRef] [PubMed]
55. Boxerman, J.L.; Shiroishi, M.S.; Ellingson, B.M.; Pope, W.B. Dynamic Susceptibility Contrast MR Imaging in Glioma: Review of Current Clinical Practice. *Magn. Reson. Imaging Clin. N. Am.* **2016**, *24*, 649–670. [CrossRef]
56. Welker, K.; Boxerman, J.; Kalnin, A.; Kaufmann, T.; Shiroishi, M.; Wintermark, M. ASFNR recommendations for clinical performance of MR dynamic susceptibility contrast perfusion imaging of the brain. *Am. J. Neuroradiol.* **2015**, *36*, E41–E51. [CrossRef]
57. Yan, L.F.; Sun, Y.Z.; Zhao, S.S.; Hu, Y.C.; Han, Y.; Li, G.; Zhang, X.; Tian, Q.; Liu, Z.C.; Yang, Y.; et al. Perfusion, Diffusion, Or Brain Tumor Barrier Integrity: Which Represents The Glioma Features Best? *Cancer Manag. Res.* **2019**, *11*, 9989–10000. [CrossRef]
58. Buxton, R.B. Quantifying CBF with arterial spin labeling. *J. Magn. Reson. Imaging* **2005**, *22*, 723–726. [CrossRef]
59. Dai, W.; Garcia, D.; De Bazelaire, C.; Alsop, D.C. Continuous flow-driven inversion for arterial spin labeling using pulsed radio frequency and gradient fields. *Magn. Reson. Med.* **2008**, *60*, 1488–1497. [CrossRef] [PubMed]
60. Thust, S.C.; Heiland, S.; Falini, A.; Jager, H.R.; Waldman, A.D.; Sundgren, P.C.; Godi, C.; Katsaros, V.K.; Ramos, A.; Bargallo, N.; et al. Glioma imaging in Europe: A survey of 220 centres and recommendations for best clinical practice. *Eur. Radiol.* **2018**, *28*, 3306–3317. [CrossRef]

61. Sollini, M.; Sghedoni, R.; Erba, P.A.; Cavuto, S.; Froio, A.; De Berti, G.; Pisanello, A.; Fraternali, A.; Iori, M.; Iaccarino, C.; et al. Diagnostic performances of [18F]fluorocholine positron emission tomography in brain tumors. *Q. J. Nucl. Med. Mol. Imaging* **2018**, *62*, 209–219. [CrossRef]
62. Delgado, A.F.; De Luca, F.; Hanagandi, P.; Van Westen, D. Arterial spin-labeling in children with brain tumor: A meta-analysis. *Am. J. Neuroradiol.* **2018**, *39*, 1536–1542. [CrossRef]
63. Treglia, G.; Muoio, B.; Trevisi, G.; Mattoli, M.V.; Albano, D.; Bertagna, F.; Giovanella, L. Diagnostic performance and prognostic value of PET/CT with different tracers for brain tumors: A systematic review of published meta-analyses. *Int. J. Mol. Sci.* **2019**, *20*, 4669. [CrossRef]
64. Schwarzenberg, J.; Czernin, J.; Cloughesy, T.F.; Ellingson, B.M.; Pope, W.B.; Grogan, T.; Elashoff, D.; Geist, C.; Silverman, D.H.S.; Phelps, M.E.; et al. Treatment response evaluation using 18F-FDOPA PET in patients with recurrent malignant glioma on bevacizumab therapy. *Clin. Cancer Res.* **2014**, *20*, 3550–3559. [CrossRef] [PubMed]
65. Fueger, B.J.; Czernin, J.; Cloughesy, T.; Silverman, D.H.; Geist, C.L.; Walter, M.A.; Schiepers, C.; Nghiemphu, P.; Lai, A.; Phelps, M.E.; et al. Correlation of 6-18F-fluoro-L-dopa PET uptake with proliferation and tumor grade in newly diagnosed and recurrent gliomas. *J. Nucl. Med.* **2010**, *51*, 1532–1538. [CrossRef]
66. Padma, M.V.; Jacobs, M.; Kraus, G.; McDowell, P.; Satter, M.; Adineh, M.; Mantil, J. Radiation-induced medulloblastoma in an adult: A functional imaging study. *Neurol. India* **2004**, *52*, 91–93. [PubMed]

2

Role of 2-[^{18}F]FDG as a Radiopharmaceutical for PET/CT in Patients with COVID-19

Salvatore Annunziata [1], Roberto C. Delgado Bolton [2], Christel-Hermann Kamani [3], John O. Prior [3], Domenico Albano [4], Francesco Bertagna [4] and Giorgio Treglia [3,5,6,*]

1. Nuclear Medicine Unit, IRCSS Regina Elena National Cancer Institute, 00144 Rome, Italy; salvatoreannunziata@live.it
2. Department of Diagnostic Imaging (Radiology) and Nuclear Medicine, University Hospital San Pedro and Centre for Biomedical Research of La Rioja (CIBIR), 26006 Logroño, La Rioja, Spain; rbiolton@gmail.com
3. Department of Nuclear Medicine and Molecular Imaging, Lausanne University Hospital and University of Lausanne, CH-1011 Lausanne, Switzerland; Christel-Hermann.Kamani@chuv.ch (C.-H.K.); John.Prior@chuv.ch (J.O.P.)
4. Nuclear Medicine, University of Brescia and Spedali Civili Brescia, 25123 Brescia, Italy; domenico.albano@unibs.it (D.A.); francesco.bertagna@unibs.it (F.B.)
5. Clinic of Nuclear Medicine and PET/CT Center, Imaging Institute of Southern Switzerland, Ente Ospedaliero Cantonale, 6500 Bellinzona, Switzerland
6. Health Technology Assessment Unit, Academic Education, Research and Innovation Area, Ente Ospedaliero Cantonale, 6500 Bellinzona, Switzerland

* Correspondence: giorgio.treglia@eoc.ch

Abstract: Some recent studies evaluated the role of fluorine-18 fluorodeoxyglucose (2-[^{18}F]FDG) as a radiopharmaceutical for positron emission tomography/computed tomography (PET/CT) imaging in patients with Coronavirus Disease (COVID-19). This article aims to perform a systematic review in this setting. A comprehensive computer literature search in PubMed/MEDLINE and Cochrane library databases regarding the role of 2-[^{18}F]FDG PET/CT in patients with COVID-19 was carried out. This combination of key words was used: (A) "PET" OR "positron emission tomography" AND (B) "COVID" OR "SARS". Only pertinent original articles were selected; case reports and very small case series were excluded. We have selected 11 original studies of 2-[^{18}F]FDG PET/CT in patients with COVID-19. Evidence-based data showed first preliminary applications of this diagnostic tool in this clinical setting, with particular regard to the incidental detection of interstitial pneumonia suspected for COVID-19. To date, according to evidence-based data, 2-[^{18}F]FDG PET/CT cannot substitute or integrate high-resolution CT to diagnose suspicious COVID-19 or for disease monitoring, but it can only be useful to incidentally detect suspicious COVID-19 lesions in patients performing this imaging method for standard oncological and non-oncological indications. Published data about the possible role of 2-[^{18}F]FDG PET/CT in patients with COVID-19 are increasing, but larger studies are warranted.

Keywords: fluorodeoxyglucose; FDG; PET; COVID-19; SARS-CoV-2; infection; systematic review

---

1. Introduction

Coronavirus Disease (COVID-19) is an infectious acute respiratory syndrome caused by the virus SARS-CoV-2 (Severe Acute Respiratory Syndrome Coronavirus 2) able to enter the human cells through the angiotensin-converting enzyme 2 (ACE2) receptor, like the SARS virus [1]. COVID-19 mainly affects the lower respiratory tract and causes several flu-like symptoms. In severe cases, COVID-19 may cause interstitial pneumonia, which can evolve in acute respiratory distress syndrome and subsequently death. Real-time reverse polymerase chain reaction (RT-PCR) is a useful test for the diagnosis of SARS-CoV-2 infection, with several limitations due to possible false-negative results [1].

COVID-19 suspicious patients are usually assessed with radiological investigations, and high-resolution chest computer tomography (CT) is the preferred tool [2]. Usually, in the early phases, single or multiple ground glass opacities, nodules, or plaques may appear. With the disease progression, the lesions may increase, occupying most of the lungs [2]. Furthermore, several authors showed an ever-growing incidental pulmonary findings suggestive of COVID-19 highlighted in the CT component of the predominantly oncological positron emission tomography (PET)/CT studies of patients without a known SARS-CoV-2 infection, COVID-19 diagnosis, or symptoms [3].

Fluorine-18 fluorodeoxyglucose (2-[^{18}F]FDG) is a radiopharmaceutical representing a radiolabelled glucose analogue that can be used to evaluate the glucose metabolism (Figure 1). Its cellular uptake by cells is proportional to their glucose consumption. After the uptake of this radiopharmacetical through the glucose transporters located in the cell membrane, it is phosphorylated by hexokinase [4]. As the cells involved in inflammatory response have high glycolytic activity (with high expression of glucose transporters and increased hexokinase activity) then they are able to take up 2-[^{18}F]FDG and therefore 2-[^{18}F]FDG PET/CT may be able to identify sites of inflammation and infection [4].

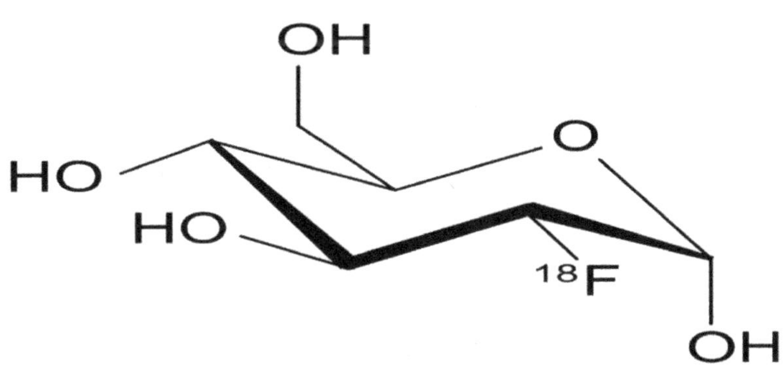

Figure 1. Chemical structure of 2-[^{18}F]FDG.

Several recently published studies have evaluated the role of 2-[^{18}F]FDG PET/CT in patients with COVID-19. This article aims to perform a systematic review according to related guidelines [5,6] to investigate the possible role of 2-[^{18}F]FDG PET/CT in this setting.

2. Results

From the comprehensive computer literature search of PubMed/MEDLINE and Cochrane databases, 169 records were screened. In total, 11 studies were selected and retrieved in full-text version according to the predefined inclusion criteria [7–17]. Conversely, 158 records were excluded because case reports or small case series (n = 51), reviews, editorials, letters (n = 39) or because they were outside the field of interest of this review (n = 68). No additional articles were found checking the references of the selected articles. Figure 2 shows the flowchart of study selection and search results. The characteristics of the selected studies are presented in Table 1 and Figure 3 and summarized here below.

All the studies were published in 2020 during the COVID-19 outbreak from European authors (from Italy, Spain, United Kingdom, France, and Monaco) and all except one of them are retrospective observational studies.

In most of the studies, 2-[^{18}F]FDG PET/CT was performed in patients evaluated for standard indications (mostly oncological indications) and incidental findings suspicious of SARS-CoV-2 infection or COVID-19 at whole-body 2-[^{18}F]FDG PET/CT were described [7–10,12–17]. Only in one study

2-[^{18}F]FDG PET/CT was performed in COVID-19 patients to assess the inflammatory status at the presumed peak of the inflammatory phase [11].

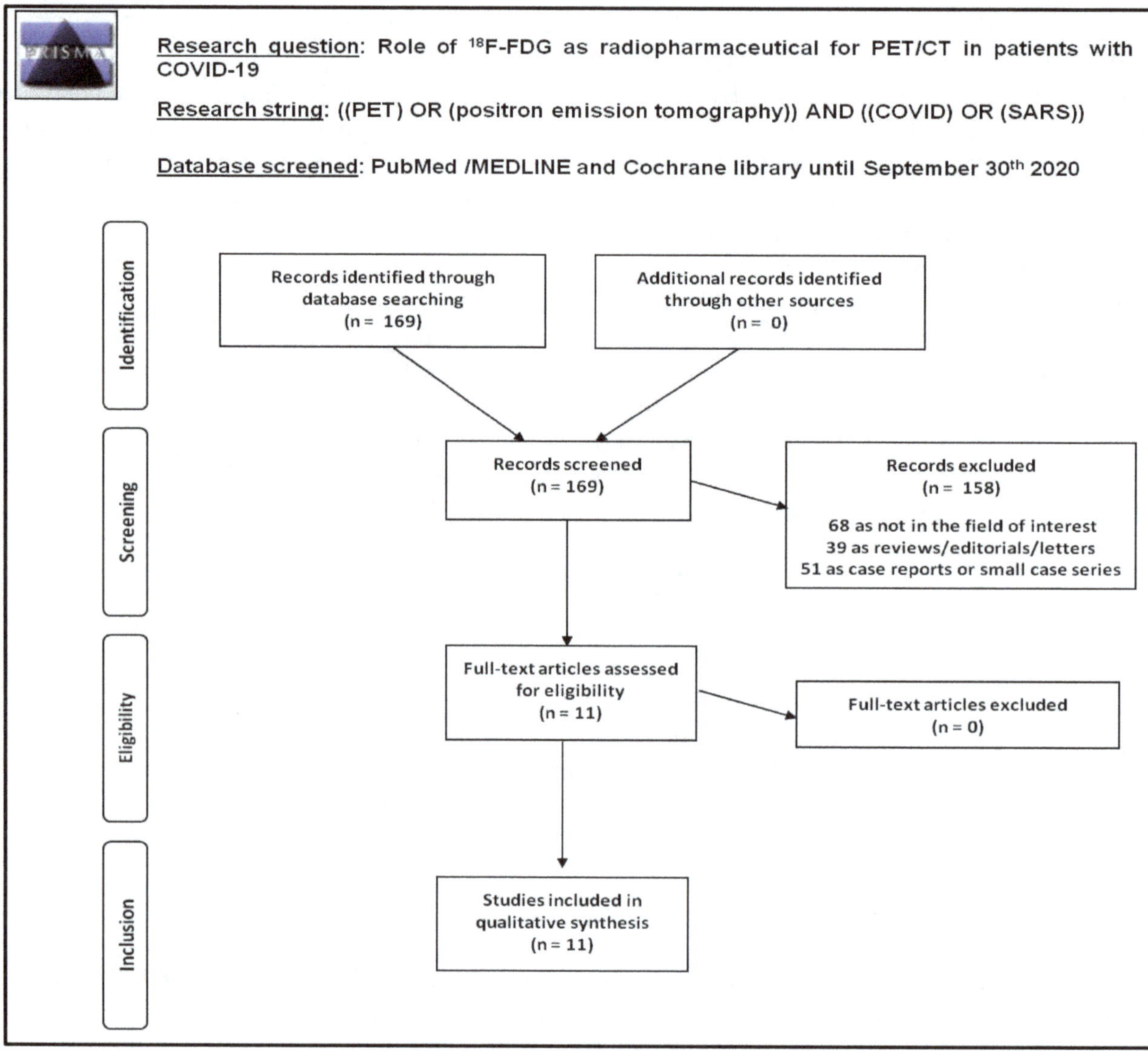

Figure 2. Flowchart of study selection and search results.

Most of the included studies reported the rate of incidental findings suspicious of SARS-CoV-2 infection or COVID-19 at 2-[^{18}F]FDG PET/CT performed for standard indications. This rate largely varied among the included studies from 2.1% to 16.2% of all whole body 2-[^{18}F]FDG PET/CT scans [7–9,12–17], based on the prevalence of SARS-CoV-2 infection or COVID-19 during the examination period in a specific country or region [11,12,16]. A significant association of the appearance of imaging findings suspicious for COVID-19 on 2-[^{18}F]FDG PET/CT with gender, sex, age, or ethnicity was not demonstrated [12]. Only a percentage of suspicious COVID-19 at 2-[^{18}F]FDG PET/CT was finally confirmed by further examinations (e.g., RT-PCR or serological testing) [7–10,12–17].

As reported by all the included studies, the 2-[^{18}F]FDG PET/CT findings suspicious for SARS-CoV-2 infection or COVID-19 are mainly CT signs of interstitial pneumonia (e.g., ground-glass opacities, crazy paving patterns, and/or consolidations) with involvement of both lungs in most of the cases [7–17].

In cases of pulmonary CT findings suspicious for SARS-CoV-2 infection or COVID-19 at 2-[^{18}F]FDG PET/CT, areas of pneumonia were 2-[^{18}F]FDG avid in most of the cases but with heterogeneous 2-[^{18}F]FDG uptake [7–17].

In patients with pulmonary CT findings suspicious for SARS-CoV-2 infection or COVID-19 at 2-[^{18}F]FDG PET/CT, the radiopharmaceutical uptake (measured as maximal standardized uptake value—SUVmax) from pulmonary consolidations was usually higher than radiopharmaceutical uptake from ground-glass opacities and crazy paving patterns [8]. One study found that 2-[^{18}F]FDG uptake of pulmonary CT abnormalities, in particular in cases of consolidation areas, were significantly lower in patients with a final diagnosis of COVID-19 compared to those who were negative for COVID-19 [8]. Conversely, another study did not find a significant difference of 2-[^{18}F]FDG uptake in ground glass pulmonary infiltrates between COVID-19 patients and controls [17].

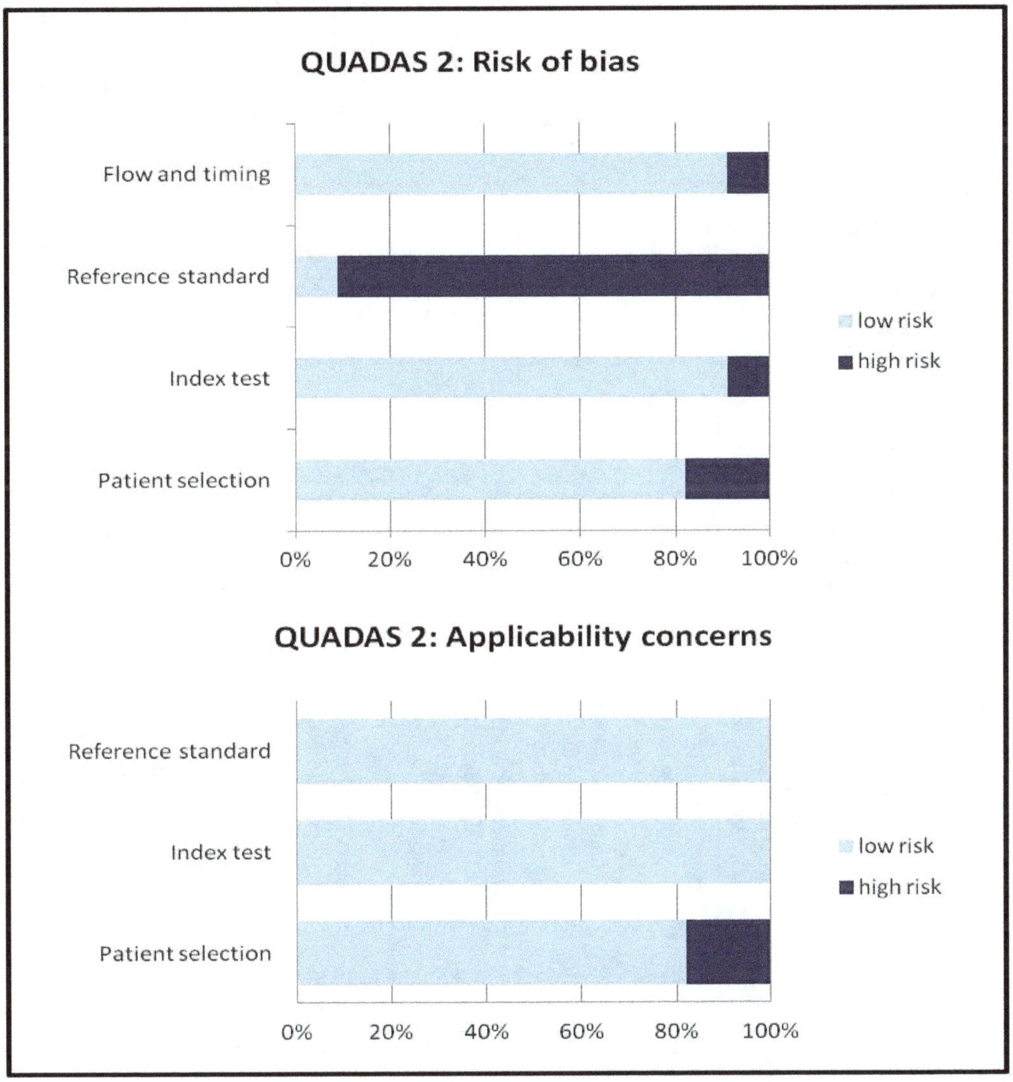

Figure 3. Quality assessment of the included studies according to QUADAS-2 tool.

Some studies reported that the prevalence of incidental pulmonary findings suspicious for interstitial pneumonia by COVID-19 at 2-[^{18}F]FDG PET/CT was higher when compared to 2-[^{18}F]FDG PET/CT scans of the same period one year earlier, without significant differences in 2-[^{18}F]FDG uptake [7,12,13,16].

Beyond the lungs, increased 2-[^{18}F]FDG uptake in patients with suspicious COVID-19 may be frequently detected in lymph nodes (in particular mediastinal lymph nodes) and less frequently in extra-thoracic sites [7,10–13,16,17].

Interestingly, cases with known COVID-19 and negative 2-[^{18}F]FDG PET/CT findings are described, even if less frequently [10].

The only prospective study aimed to assess the inflammatory status by 2-[^{18}F]FDG PET/CT in patients with known COVID-19 demonstrated that there was no correlation between pulmonary inflammatory status at 2-[^{18}F]FDG PET and chest CT evolution or short-term clinical outcome [11].

Table 1. Characteristics of included studies on the role of 2-[^{18}F]FDG PET/CT in patients with COVID-19.

First Author	Country	Type of Study	Period of the Study	Type of Patients Evaluated by 2-[^{18}F]FDG PET/CT	Patients with Suspicious (Confirmed) SARS-CoV-2 Infection or COVID-19 Evaluated by 2-[^{18}F]FDG PET/CT	Rate of Incidental Findings Suspicious of COVID-19 at 2-[^{18}F]FDG PET/CT	Other Endpoints
Albano [7]	Italy	R	March 2020	Asymptomatic patients evaluated for standard indications	6 (4)	9.2% (6/65)	Radiological and metabolic findings in patients with suspicious COVID-19
Bahloul [8]	France	R	March–May 2020	Asymptomatic patients evaluated for standard indications	22 (11)	2.5% (22/884)	Radiological and metabolic findings in patients with suspicious COVID-19
Cabrera Villegas [9]	Spain	R	March–April 2020	Asymptomatic patients evaluated for standard indications	7 (5)	5.3% (7/132)	Radiological and metabolic findings in patients with suspicious COVID-19
Charters [10]	United Kingdom	R	2020 (months N.A.)	Asymptomatic or known COVID-19 patients evaluated for standard indications	6 (4)	N.A.	Radiological and metabolic findings in patients with suspicious or known COVID-19
Dietz [11]	Monaco	P	March–May 2020	Known COVID-19 patients to evaluate the inflammatory status	(13)	N.A.	Radiological and metabolic findings in patients with known COVID-19 and correlation between inflammatory status and CT evolution or short-term outcome
Halsey [12]	United Kingdom	R	March–April 2020	Asymptomatic or symptomatic patients evaluated for standard indications	26 (1)	16.2% (26/160)	Radiological and metabolic findings in patients with suspicious COVID-19
Maurea [13]	Italy	R	February–April 2020	Asymptomatic patients evaluated for standard indications	26 (0)	8.7% (26/299)	Radiological and metabolic findings in patients with suspicious COVID-19

Table 1. *Cont.*

First Author	Country	Type of Study	Period of the Study	Type of Patients Evaluated by 2-[^{18}F]FDG PET/CT	Patients with Suspicious (Confirmed) SARS-CoV-2 Infection or COVID-19 Evaluated by 2-[^{18}F]FDG PET/CT	Rate of Incidental Findings Suspicious of COVID-19 at 2-[^{18}F]FDG PET/CT	Other Endpoints
Mucientes Rasilla [14]	Spain	R	March–April 2020	Asymptomatic patients evaluated for standard indications	11 (5)	8.5% (11/129)	Radiological and metabolic findings in patients with suspicious COVID-19
Olivari [15]	Italy	R	April 2020	Asymptomatic patients evaluated for standard indications	7 (6)	4.1% (7/172)	Radiological and metabolic findings in patients with suspicious COVID-19
Setti [16]	Italy	R	December 2019–May 2020	Asymptomatic patients evaluated for standard indications	24 (4)	4.2% (24/575)	Radiological and metabolic findings in patients with suspicious COVID-19
Wakfie-Corieh [17]	Spain	R	February–May 2020	Asymptomatic patients evaluated for standard indications	23 (14)	2.1% (23/1079)	Radiological and metabolic findings in patients with suspicious COVID-19

Legend: N.A. = not available; P = prospective; R = retrospective.

3. Discussion

2-[^{18}F]FDG is a radiolabelled glucose analogue and the most common PET radiopharmaceutical used in oncology or for detecting inflammatory diseases. An increased uptake of this radiopharmaceutical is expected in inflammatory/infectious sites and tumor lesions due to the usually high glycolytic metabolism of activated inflammatory cells as well as tumor cells [4]. An advantage of 2-[^{18}F]FDG PET as a functional imaging is the possible identification of metabolically active diseases in the early stages, which usually precedes morphological changes appreciated in conventional imaging techniques such as CT. Therefore, by detecting the active phase of an infectious or inflammatory condition, it may be theoretically possible to diagnose and monitor the inflammatory/infectious disease progression [4].

We have performed a systematic review of the literature to evaluate whether a possible role of 2-[^{18}F]FDG as a radiopharmaceutical for PET/CT in patients with suspicious, known, or unknown COVID-19 may be hypothesized. Searching the literature, we found a plethora of case reports and very small case series describing incidental findings of COVID-19 in patients performing 2-[^{18}F]FDG PET/CT for common indications (mainly for oncological purposes). We have excluded these case reports and small case series from our analysis due to their low value on the quality of evidence point of view. Conversely, we have restricted the inclusion criteria only to original articles including more than five patients with suspicious or known COVID-19 evaluated by 2-[^{18}F]FDG PET/CT because these articles provide more reliable information compared to case reports.

However, most of the studies selected about our topic of interest were observational and retrospective studies mainly focused on incidental detection of COVID-19 by 2-[^{18}F]FDG PET/CT (n = 10) [7–10,12–17] and only one study was a prospective analysis of patients with known COVID-19 aimed to assess the inflammatory status by 2-[^{18}F]FDG PET/CT and the possible correlation with CT evolution and short-term clinical outcome [11].

First of all, our review clearly demonstrates that the rate of incidental findings suspicious for COVID-19 in asymptomatic patients undergoing 2-[^{18}F]FDG PET/CT is significant, ranging from 2 to 16 % of 2-[^{18}F]FDG PET/CT examinations performed during the COVID-19 outbreak as reported in the included studies. This rate of incidental findings is also related to the prevalence of COVID-19 in different countries and regions [7–9,12–17]. Due to the relevant heterogeneity among the included studies and some biases in particular about the reference standard (Figure 3), we have not performed a meta-analysis to calculate the pooled prevalence of incidental findings suspicious for COVID-19 at 2-[^{18}F]FDG PET/CT, because this pooled analysis would be not appropriate [5,6,18].

The lungs are the most frequent sites of incidental findings suspicious for COVID-19 at 2-[^{18}F]FDG PET/CT [7–17] and this observation is quite obvious considering the pulmonary tropism of SARS-CoV-2 [1,2]. Most of the pulmonary incidental findings suspicious for COVID-19 at 2-[^{18}F]FDG PET/CT are detected by using the CT component, which may allow to recognize ground-glass opacities, crazy paving patterns, and/or consolidations [7–17]. Nevertheless, it should be underlined that the co-registered CT component of PET/CT is often a low-dose CT (useful for attenuation correction and for anatomical localization of PET findings) not performed on a breath-hold. The diagnostic quality of this low-dose CT is not entirely equivalent to dedicated chest CT having a lower detection rate for smaller pulmonary lesions; furthermore, motion artefacts generated on a free-breathing CT thorax can artificially create ground glass opacities particularly in the lower pulmonary lobes [7–17]. Improving the diagnostic quality of the co-registered CT component of the PET/CT is possible following EANM guidelines [19], by trimming certain aspects of the PET/CT procedure. Including in the protocol a deep-inspiration thoracic CT scan, which is not used for attenuation correction or for PET/CT fusion, but instead to assess the lung parenchyma with thinner slices (2.5 mm), is very useful for studying the lung parenchyma, especially for comparing with previous and/or future studies [19]. In summary, the need for incorporating this CT protocol to the PET/CT should be considered given the relevance of precisely evaluating lung parenchyma, especially in patients who have not had a thoracic CT scan recently.

A recent published meta-analysis focused on the diagnostic performance of CT in the diagnosis of COVID-19 demonstrated that observation of ground glass opacities and other radiological features of viral pneumonia at CT scan had optimum performance in detection of COVID-19 [20]. However, it is suggested to make the final diagnosis based on both CT scan and RT-PCR, as none of these diagnostic tests are reliable alone [20].

In this scenario, the increased 2-[^{18}F]FDG uptake related to the increased metabolic activity of active inflammatory lesions may help to identify COVID-19 lesions at 2-[^{18}F]FDG PET/CT [7–17]. The relatively lower 2-[^{18}F]FDG uptake observed in pulmonary lesions of COVID-19 patients compared to those of COVID-19 negative patients could be explained a trend toward lower rates of CT consolidation patterns in COVID-19 positive than in COVID-19 negative patients. Indeed, consolidation patterns were associated with much higher SUVmax values when compared with ground-glass opacities or crazy paving patterns, which include a non-cellular component and therefore are less likely to take up 2-[^{18}F]FDG [8]. However, as a significant overlap of SUVmax values was demonstrated in pulmonary lesions from COVID-19 positive and COVID-19 negative patients, 2-[^{18}F]FDG PET/CT alone cannot be used to discriminate between COVID-19 and other pulmonary infections [7–17]. Moreover, 2-[^{18}F]FDG PET/CT cannot be used to exclude COVID-19 due to the possibility of a negative 2-[^{18}F]FDG PET/CT in COVID-19 patients. Furthermore, the sensitivity of 2-[^{18}F]FDG PET/CT in detecting post-infective pulmonary lesions that are no longer hypermetabolic is potentially limited [10].

Beyond the lungs, increased 2-[^{18}F]FDG uptake in patients with suspicious COVID-19 may be frequently detected in lymph nodes (in particular mediastinal lymph nodes) and less frequently in extra-thoracic sites [7,10–13,16,17]. Notably, lymph nodal 2-[^{18}F]FDG uptake is probably linked to cytokine-mediated inflammation rather than to direct viral infection, considering the absence of ACE2 (a functional receptor for SARS-CoV-2) on lymphoid cells [11,17].

Overall, literature data have demonstrated an increased prevalence of 2-[^{18}F]FDG PET/CT abnormalities evocative of a pulmonary infection in asymptomatic patients during the COVID-19 outbreak. Therefore, as for other organs [21], PET/CT reading physicians should consider and recognize pulmonary incidental findings, and in particular potential COVID-19 related features, at 2-[^{18}F]FDG PET/CT. These findings should be reported to the referring physicians immediately for appropriate action, as the incidental detection of COVID-19 pneumonia in early stages may help to prevent further spread of the virus [7–10,12–17,22–25].

Even if one article included in our systematic review has reported the possible utility of 2-[^{18}F]FDG PET/CT to monitor the inflammatory status in patients with known COVID-19, and even if 2-[^{18}F]FDG PET/CT may be feasible in patients with confirmed SARS-CoV-2 infection when taking adequate protective measures [10,25], the current available evidence are scarce and not sufficient to justify the use of 2-[^{18}F]FDG PET/CT in patients with suspicious or known COVID-19 in the clinical practice and further research is needed before this can be eventually considered [3]. It should be noted that, in comparison to CT, 2-[^{18}F]FDG PET/CT is a complex procedure requiring more human resources and a long stay in the investigation unit, bearing a certain risk of infectious disease spreading for the health personnel. Moreover, we should be aware about the radiation issue since CT and 2-[^{18}F]FDG PET/CT are both radiating procedure [3].

Regarding future studies, other radiopharmaceuticals beyond 2-[^{18}F]FDG exploring different metabolic pathways or receptor status have been evaluated in patients with COVID-19 but, to date, only preclinical studies or case reports (with low quality of evidence) are currently available [26–32] and more studies are needed in this regard.

The main limitation of our systematic review is that a limited number of articles were included; therefore, more studies with an adequate number of patients are needed to better understand the possible role of 2-[^{18}F]FDG PET/CT in COVID-19 patients or with SARS-CoV-2 infection.

4. Materials and Methods

PubMed/MEDLINE and Cochrane library databases were screened on 30th September 2020 to perform a comprehensive computer literature search according to international guidelines (including PRISMA) [5,6] to find published original studies on the role of 2-[^{18}F]FDG PET/CT in patients with COVID-19. A search algorithm based on the combination of these terms was used: (A) "PET" OR "positron emission tomography" AND (B) "COVID" OR "SARS". The literature search was performed by two authors independently (S.A. and G.T.).

Original studies including more than five patients with suspicious or known COVID-19 evaluated by 2-[^{18}F]FDG PET/CT during the SARS-CoV-2 outbreak were eligible for inclusion. Case reports and small case series ($n \leq 5$ cases with suspicious or known COVID-19), reviews, editorials, letters, and articles outside the field of interest of this review (including preclinical studies) were excluded. No language or time restrictions were used.

Titles and abstracts of the retrieved articles were reviewed by two authors (S.A. and G.T.) applying the inclusion criteria mentioned above. References of the eligible articles were also checked to find potential additional articles. For each selected article information was collected about authors, country, type of study, period of study, type of patients evaluated by 2-[^{18}F]FDG PET/CT, number of patients with known or suspicious SARS-CoV-2 infection or COVID-19 at 2-[^{18}F]FDG PET/CT. The main findings of the selected studies were briefly described and risk of bias assessment of the studies was performed through the QUADAS-2 tool [5,6].

5. Conclusions

To date, according to evidence-based data, 2-[^{18}F]FDG PET/CT cannot substitute or integrate high-resolution CT to diagnose suspicious SARS-CoV-2 infection or COVID-19 or for disease monitoring, but it can only be useful to incidentally detect suspicious COVID-19 lesions in patients performing this imaging method for standard oncological and non-oncological indications. Published data about the possible role of 2-[^{18}F]FDG PET/CT in patients with COVID-19 are increasing, but larger studies are warranted.

Author Contributions: Conceptualization, S.A. and R.C.D.B.; methodology, G.T.; writing—original draft preparation, G.T. and S.A.; writing—review and editing, R.C.D.B., C.-H.K., D.A. and F.B.; supervision, G.T. and J.O.P. All authors have read and agreed to the published version of the manuscript.

References

1. Jarrom, D.; Elston, L.; Washington, J.; Prettyjohns, M.; Cann, K.; Myles, S.; Groves, P. Effectiveness of tests to detect the presence of SARS-CoV-2 virus, and antibodies to SARS-CoV-2, to inform COVID-19 diagnosis: A rapid systematic review. *BMJ Evid. Based Med.* **2020**. [CrossRef]
2. Şendur, H.N. Debate of Chest CT and RT-PCR Test for the Diagnosis of COVID-19. *Radiology* **2020**. [CrossRef] [PubMed]
3. Treglia, G. The role of 18F-FDG PET for COVID-19 infection: Myth versus reality. *Clin. Transl. Imaging* **2020**. [CrossRef] [PubMed]
4. Treglia, G. Diagnostic Performance of 18F-FDG PET/CT in Infectious and Inflammatory Diseases according to Published Meta-Analyses. *Contrast Media Mol. Imaging* **2019**, *2019*, 3018349. [CrossRef] [PubMed]
5. McInnes, M.D.F.; Moher, D.; Thombs, B.D.; McGrath, T.A.; Bossuyt, P.M.; Clifford, T.; Cohen, J.F.; Deeks, J.J.; Gatsonis, C.; Hooft, L.; et al. Preferred Reporting Items for a Systematic Review and Meta-analysis of Diagnostic Test Accuracy Studies: The PRISMA-DTA Statement. *JAMA* **2018**, *319*, 388–396. [CrossRef]
6. Sadeghi, R.; Treglia, G. Systematic reviews and meta-analyses of diagnostic studies: A practical guideline. *Clin. Transl. Imaging* **2017**, *5*, 83–87. [CrossRef]

7. Albano, D.; Bertagna, F.; Bertoli, M.; Bosio, G.; Lucchini, S.; Motta, F.; Panarotto, M.B.; Peli, A.; Camoni, L.; Bengel, F.M.; et al. Incidental Findings Suggestive of COVID-19 in Asymptomatic Patients Undergoing Nuclear Medicine Procedures in a High-Prevalence Region. *J. Nucl. Med.* **2020**, *61*, 632–636. [CrossRef]
8. Bahloul, A.; Boursier, C.; Jeulin, H.; Imbert, L.; Mandry, D.; Karcher, G.; Marie, P.Y.; Verger, A. CT abnormalities evocative of lung infection are associated with lower 18F-FDG uptake in confirmed COVID-19 patients. *Eur. J. Nucl. Med. Mol. Imaging* **2020**. [CrossRef]
9. Cabrera Villegas, A.; Romero Robles, L.G.; Boulvard Chollet, X.L.E.; Albornoz Almada, M.C.; Mangas Losada, M.; Garrastachu, P.; Cañete Sánchez, F.M.; Ramírez Lasanta, R.; Delgado Bolton, R.C. [18F]-FDG PET/CT in oncologic patients with unsuspected asymptomatic infection with SARS-CoV-2. *Eur. J. Nucl. Med. Mol. Imaging* 2020. [CrossRef]
10. Charters, P.F.P.; Little, D.; Rodrigues, J.C.L.; Graham, R.N.; Redman, S.L. 18FDG-PET/CT findings in COVID-19: A single centre retrospective radiological review. *BJR Case Rep.* **2020**, *6*, 20200091. [CrossRef]
11. Dietz, M.; Chironi, G.; Claessens, Y.E.; Farhad, R.L.; Rouquette, I.; Serrano, B.; Nataf, V.; Hugonnet, F.; Paulmier, B.; Berthier, F.; et al. COVID-19 pneumonia: Relationship between inflammation assessed by whole-body FDG PET/CT and short-term clinical outcome. *Eur. J. Nucl. Med. Mol. Imaging* **2020**. [CrossRef] [PubMed]
12. Halsey, R.; Priftakis, D.; Mackenzie, S.; Wan, S.; Davis, L.M.; Lilburn, D.; Thornton, A.; Papathanasiou, N.; Gnanasegaran, G.; Bomanji, J. COVID-19 in the act: Incidental 18F-FDG PET/CT findings in asymptomatic patients and those with symptoms not primarily correlated with COVID-19 during the United Kingdom coronavirus lockdown. *Eur. J. Nucl. Med. Mol. Imaging* **2020**. [CrossRef] [PubMed]
13. Maurea, S.; Mainolfi, C.G.; Bombace, C.; Annunziata, A.; Attanasio, L.; Petretta, M.; Del Vecchio, S.; Cuocolo, A. FDG-PET/CT imaging during the Covid-19 emergency: A southern Italian perspective. *Eur. J. Nucl. Med. Mol. Imaging* **2020**, *47*, 2691–2697. [CrossRef] [PubMed]
14. Mucientes Rasilla, J.; Jimeno Pernett, R.; Cardona Arboniés, J. Diagnóstico de neumonía COVID-19 en pacientes asintomáticos tras la realización de un PET/TC oncológico [Diagnosis of COVID-19 pneumonia in asymptomatic patients after an oncological PET/CT]. *Rev. Esp. Med. Nucl. Imagen. Mol.* **2020**, *39*, 299–302. [CrossRef] [PubMed]
15. Olivari, L.; Riccardi, N.; Rodari, P.; Buonfrate, D.; Diodato, S.; Formenti, F.; Angheben, A.; Salgarello, M. Accidental diagnosis of COVID-19 pneumonia after 18F FDG PET/CT: A case series. *Clin. Transl. Imaging* **2020**. [CrossRef] [PubMed]
16. Setti, L.; Bonacina, M.; Meroni, R.; Kirienko, M.; Galli, F.; Dalto, S.C.; Erba, P.A.; Bombardieri, E. Increased incidence of interstitial pneumonia detected on [18F]-FDG-PET/CT in asymptomatic cancer patients during COVID-19 pandemic in Lombardy: A casualty or COVID-19 infection? *Eur. J. Nucl. Med. Mol. Imaging* **2020**. [CrossRef]
17. Wakfie-Corieh, C.G.; Blanes García, A.M.; Ferrando-Castagnetto, F.; Valhondo-Rama, R.; Ortega Candil, A.; Rodríguez Rey, C.; Cabrera Martín, M.N.; García-Esquinas, M.G.; Couto Caro, R.M.; Pedrera Canal, M.; et al. Assessment of extra-parenchymal lung involvement in asymptomatic cancer patients with COVID-19 pneumonia detected on 18F-FDG PET-CT studies. *Eur. J. Nucl. Med. Mol. Imaging* **2020**. [CrossRef]
18. Treglia, G.; Sadeghi, R. Meta-analyses and systematic reviews on PET and PET/CT in oncology: The state of the art. *Clin. Transl. Imaging* **2013**, *1*, 73–75. [CrossRef]
19. Boellaard, R.; Delgado-Bolton, R.; Oyen, W.J.; Giammarile, F.; Tatsch, K.; Eschner, W.; Verzijlbergen, F.J.; Barrington, S.F.; Pike, L.C.; Weber, W.A.; et al. FDG PET/CT: EANM procedure guidelines for tumour imaging: Version 2.0. *Eur. J. Nucl. Med. Mol. Imaging* **2015**, *42*, 328–354. [CrossRef]
20. Hossein, H.; Ali, K.M.; Hosseini, M.; Sarveazad, A.; Safari, S.; Yousefifard, M. Value of chest computed tomography scan in diagnosis of COVID-19; A systematic review and meta-analysis. *Clin. Transl. Imaging* **2020**. [CrossRef]
21. Tamburello, A.; Treglia, G.; Albano, D.; Bertagna, F.; Giovanella, L. Prevalence and clinical significance of focal incidental ^{18}F-FDG uptake in different organs: An evidence-based summary. *Clin. Transl. Imaging* **2017**, *5*, 525–532. [CrossRef]
22. Annunziata, S.; Albano, D.; Laudicella, R.; Bauckneht, M.; Young Committee of the Italian Association of Nuclear Medicine (AIMN). Surveys on COVID-19 in nuclear medicine: What happened and what we learned. *Clin. Transl. Imaging* **2020**. [CrossRef] [PubMed]

23. Annunziata, S.; Bauckneht, M.; Albano, D.; Argiroffi, G.; Calabrò, D.; Abenavoli, E.; Linguanti, F.; Laudicella, R. Young Committee of the Italian Association of Nuclear Medicine (AIMN). Impact of the COVID-19 pandemic in nuclear medicine departments: Preliminary report of the first international survey. *Eur. J. Nucl. Med. Mol. Imaging* **2020**, *47*, 2090–2099. [CrossRef] [PubMed]
24. Boulvard Chollet, X.L.E.; Romero Robles, L.G.; Garrastachu, P.; Cabrera Villegas, A.; Albornoz Almada, M.C.; Colletti, P.M.; Rubello, D.; Ramírez Lasanta, R.; Delgado Bolton, R.C. 18F-FDG PET/CT in Hodgkin Lymphoma With Unsuspected COVID-19. *Clin. Nucl. Med.* **2020**, *45*, 652–653. [CrossRef] [PubMed]
25. Kamani, C.H.; Jreige, M.; Pappon, M.; Fischbacher, A.; Borens, O.; Monney, P.; Nicod Lalonde, M.; Schaefer, N.; Prior, J.O. Added value of 18F-FDG PET/CT in a SARS-CoV-2-infected complex case with persistent fever. *Eur. J. Nucl. Med. Mol. Imaging* **2020**, *47*, 2036–2037. [CrossRef] [PubMed]
26. Foster, C.C.; Davis, R.A.; Hausner, S.H.; Sutcliffe, J.L. αlphavbeta6 targeted molecular PET/CT imaging of lung post SARS-CoV-2 infection. *J. Nucl. Med.* **2020**. [CrossRef]
27. Müller, C.; Schibli, R.; Maurer, B. Can Nuclear Imaging of Activated Macrophages with Folic Acid-Based Radiotracers Serve as a Prognostic Means to Identify COVID-19 Patients at Risk? *Pharmaceuticals* **2020**, *13*, 238. [CrossRef]
28. Stasiak, C.E.S.; Cardoso, F.R.; de Almeida, S.A.; Rosado-de-Castro, P.H. Incidental finding of COVID-19 infection after [(68)Ga]Ga-PSMA-11 PET/CT imaging in a patient with prostate cancer. *Eur. J. Nucl. Med. Mol. Imaging* **2020**. [CrossRef]
29. Scarlattei, M.; Baldari, G.; Silva, M.; Bola, S.; Sammartano, A.; Migliari, S.; Graziani, T.; Cidda, C.; Sverzellati, N.; Ruffini, L. Unknown SARS-CoV-2 pneumonia detected by PET/CT in patients with cancer. *Tumori* **2020**, *106*, 325–332. [CrossRef] [PubMed]
30. Turpin, L.; Pouliot, Q.; Zhang, J.; Glikman, M.; Gomez, F.; Talbot, J.N.; Montravers, F. (18)F-Fluorocholine uptake matching CT lesions in the lungs of a patient clinically cured from COVID-19 syndrome. *Eur. J. Nucl. Med. Mol. Imaging* **2020**, *47*, 2706–2708. [CrossRef] [PubMed]
31. García Vicente, A.M.; Soriano Castrejón, Á. Incidental COVID-19 Pneumonia on 18F-Fluorocholine PET/CT. *Clin. Nucl. Med.* **2020**, *45*, e376–e377. [CrossRef] [PubMed]
32. Olivari, L.; Riccardi, N.; Rodari, P.; Angheben, A.; Artioli, P.; Salgarello, M. COVID-19 pneumonia: Increased choline uptake with 18F-choline PET/CT. *Eur. J. Nucl. Med. Mol. Imaging* **2020**, *47*, 2476–2477. [CrossRef] [PubMed]

3

Kinetic Modelling of [^{68}Ga]Ga-DOTA-Siglec-9 in Porcine Osteomyelitis and Soft Tissue Infections

Lars Jødal [1,*], Anne Roivainen [2,3], Vesa Oikonen [2,3], Sirpa Jalkanen [4], Søren B. Hansen [5], Pia Afzelius [6], Aage K. O. Alstrup [5], Ole L. Nielsen [7] and Svend B. Jensen [1,8]

1 Department of Nuclear Medicine, Aalborg University Hospital, DK-9000 Aalborg, Denmark; svbj@rn.dk
2 Turku PET Centre, Turku University Hospital, FI-20520 Turku, Finland; aroivan@utu.fi (A.R.); vesa.oikonen@utu.fi (V.O.)
3 Turku PET Centre, University of Turku, FI-20520 Turku, Finland
4 MediCity Research Laboratory and Institute of Biomedicine, University of Turku, FI-20520 Turku, Finland; sirjal@utu.fi
5 Department of Nuclear Medicine and PET, Aarhus University Hospital, DK-8200 Aarhus, Denmark; soerehse@rm.dk (S.B.H.); aagealst@rm.dk (A.K.O.A.)
6 North Zealand Hospital, Hillerød, Copenhagen University Hospital, DK-3400 Hillerød, Denmark; pia.maria.tullia.afzelius@regionh.dk
7 Department of Veterinary and Animal Sciences, University of Copenhagen, DK-1870 Copenhagen, Denmark; ole.lerberg.nielsen@gmail.com
8 Department of Chemistry and Biosciences, Aalborg University, DK-9100 Aalborg, Denmark
* Correspondence: lajo@rn.dk

Academic Editor: Derek J. McPhee

Abstract: Background: [^{68}Ga]Ga-DOTA-Siglec-9 is a positron emission tomography (PET) radioligand for vascular adhesion protein 1 (VAP-1), a protein involved in leukocyte trafficking. The tracer facilitates the imaging of inflammation and infection. Here, we studied the pharmacokinetic modelling of [^{68}Ga]Ga-DOTA-Siglec-9 in osteomyelitis and soft tissue infections in pigs. Methods: Eight pigs with osteomyelitis and soft tissue infections in the right hind limb were dynamically PET scanned for 60 min along with arterial blood sampling. The fraction of radioactivity in the blood accounted for by the parent tracer was evaluated with radio-high-performance liquid chromatography. One- and two-tissue compartment models were used for pharmacokinetic evaluation. Post-mortem soft tissue samples from one pig were analysed with anti-VAP-1 immunofluorescence. In each analysis, the animal's non-infected left hind limb was used as a control. Results: Tracer uptake was elevated in soft tissue infections but remained low in osteomyelitis. The kinetics of [^{68}Ga]Ga-DOTA-Siglec-9 followed a reversible 2-tissue compartment model. The tracer metabolized quickly; however, taking this into account, produced more ambiguous results. Infected soft tissue samples showed endothelial cell surface expression of the Siglec-9 receptor VAP-1. Conclusion: The kinetics of [^{68}Ga]Ga-DOTA-Siglec-9 uptake in porcine soft tissue infections are best described by the 2-tissue compartment model.

Keywords: kinetic analysis; Siglec-9; gallium-68; vascular adhesion protein; VAP-1; infection; inflammation; osteomyelitis; animal model; *Staphylococcus aureus*

---

1. Introduction

Infections causing localized lesions in the body, e.g., osteomyelitis, cannot always be successfully treated by the systemic administration of antibiotics; instead, surgical intervention may be necessary, which requires knowledge of the site(s) of infection. Assuming the availability of a suitable tracer, positron emission tomography (PET) is well suited for the task. However, it has proven difficult to find a tracer with both high and specific uptake in infected tissue.

The current standard tracer used for PET imaging of infectious and inflammatory diseases is the fluorine-18 labelled glucose analogue 2-deoxy-2-[^{18}F]-fluoro-D-glucose ([^{18}F]FDG) [1]. Generally, [^{18}F]FDG shows high uptake in sites of infection and inflammation, but the uptake is not specific: [^{18}F]FDG accumulates in all cells that use glucose as an energy source, including not only activated immune cells but also rapidly proliferating cancer cells, brain tissue and working muscle tissue.

Leukocytes (white blood cells, WBC) are natural seekers of infection. Leukocytes labelled with ^{111}In or ^{99m}Tc have been widely used for scintigraphy imaging of infection, but the labelling procedure is time consuming and requires withdrawing 30–40 mL of blood from the patient [2]. A simpler alternative is anti-granulocyte monoclonal antibodies (anti-G-mAbs) labelled with ^{99m}Tc. However, while the isotopes ^{111}In and ^{99m}Tc are suitable for gamma camera imaging, they cannot be used for PET imaging. This is a technical disadvantage, as the counting efficiency is typically an order of magnitude higher for the PET scanner than for the gamma camera, and the spatial resolution is superior. Labelling of leukocytes with [^{18}F]FDG for PET imaging has been investigated, but the labelling efficiency is lower, and [^{18}F]FDG elutes from the leukocytes over time [3]. Furthermore, the molar activity of labelled leukocytes will be many orders of magnitude higher than in the patient as a whole, for which reason the short-range β^+ radiation (positrons before annihilation) can result in damaging self-irradiation to [^{18}F]FDG-labelled leukocytes [4].

The relationship between time and physical decay must also be noted. Injected leukocytes take hours or more to accumulate at the infection site, and imaging can be performed 3–4 h after injection at the earliest [2]. These delays are acceptable with ^{111}In ($T_{\frac{1}{2}}$ = 2.8 days) and ^{99m}Tc ($T_{\frac{1}{2}}$ = 6 h), but in relation to PET imaging, the shorter physical half-lives of the two most widely used isotopes, ^{18}F ($T_{\frac{1}{2}}$ = 110 min) and ^{68}Ga ($T_{\frac{1}{2}}$ = 68 min), make long uptake times problematic.

Instead of labelled leukocytes, a tracer directly related to the processes causing leukocyte accumulation in infected tissues is being sought. Such a tracer would potentially enable faster imaging, and at the same time, the handling of blood products from the patient would be avoided. A relevant target molecule is vascular adhesion protein 1 (VAP-1), currently known as a primary amine oxidase (AOC3, EC 1.4.3.21), which is acting both as an adhesion molecule and as a regulatory enzyme in the process of leukocyte binding to the endothelium of blood vessels in infected and inflamed tissue [5,6]. Under normal conditions, VAP-1 is stored in intracellular granules. Upon an inflammatory stimulus, VAP-1 is rapidly translocated to the endothelial cell surface, where it is readily accessible to intravenously administered PET ligands.

As reviewed in [7], ^{68}Ga-labelled synthetic peptides that bind to VAP-1 have been investigated in different experimental infection and inflammation models, and some have shown a better distinction than [^{18}F]FDG between cancer and inflammation. Overall, the review considers VAP-1 to be an optimal target for imaging of inflammation. One of the reviewed tracers, [^{68}Ga]Ga-DOTA-Siglec-9, is currently in a phase I clinical trial (trial no. NCT03755245).

It may be noted that VAP-1 imaging will not distinguish between infection and inflammation, but because VAP-1 is involved in leukocyte extravasation, it is directly linked to the body's natural response to infection. Imaging of VAP-1 expression may even be used to study this process, especially if the kinetics of the VAP-1 imaging tracer are known.

Sialic acid-binding immunoglobulin-like lectin 9 (Siglec-9) is a natural ligand for VAP-1 and is expressed on monocytes and neutrophils [8,9]. The PET tracer [^{68}Ga]Ga-DOTA-Siglec-9 contains a modified fraction of the full Siglec-9 protein and has been found to accumulate in infected tissues [10,11] as well as inflammation sites [8,11–13] and certain tumours [8]. However, the kinetics of [^{68}Ga]Ga-DOTA-Siglec-9 have been investigated only in a single study that addressed inflammation [12]; thus studies on the kinetics of this tracer in infections are lacking.

In earlier studies, we investigated the PET imaging of infection in a porcine osteomyelitis model. In this model, *Staphylococcus aureus* (*S. aureus*) bacteria were injected into the right femoral artery of juvenile pigs to haematogenously induce osteomyelitis in the right hind limb without trauma to the bone [14–16]. In a number of animals, both osteomyelitis and soft tissue infections were induced in the limb, allowing us to compare the uptake in these two types of tissues. Each animal was scanned with a series of radioactive tracers within the same day, with planned delays to allow one tracer to physically decay before the next was injected [17].

The present study investigates the kinetics of [^{68}Ga]Ga-DOTA-Siglec-9 in this porcine osteomyelitis model, including a comparison of the uptake in osteomyelitis and in soft tissue infections.

2. Results

The characteristics of the eight pigs in the study are summarized in Table 1.

Table 1. Characteristics of the pigs in the study.

Pig No.*	Body Weight (kg)	Days from Inoculation to Scan	Injected Radioactivity (MBq)
6	22.0	7	178
9	23.0	8	175
10	22.5	7	191
22	19.0	9	208
23	19.0	9	150
24	20.0	8	126
25	20.5	8	253
26 †	24.5	8	227 360

* The numbering follows the order in the overall osteomyelitis project described in the main text. Pigs no. 6, 9, and 10 have been described regarding other tracers in previous publications: [18,19] (same numbers) and [20] (where A–E corresponds to numbers 6–10). All pigs in the table except no. 24 were also included in [21] (with different numbering). Blood sample data on [^{68}Ga]Ga-DOTA-Siglec-9 in pig no. 10 have been described in [22]. † Pig no. 26 was scanned twice with [^{68}Ga]Ga-DOTA-Siglec-9. The second scan was performed 4.6 h (approximately 4 physical half-lives of ^{68}Ga) after the first scan and with a higher level of injected radioactivity. Prior to the second scan, 5 mg of unlabelled ("cold") DOTA-Siglec-9 peptide in 10 mL had been slowly injected intravenously (i.v.) into the pig to block receptors—see main text.

2.1. Visual Uptake

Visually, [^{68}Ga]Ga-DOTA-Siglec-9 showed elevated uptake in inflamed and infected soft tissues, while not being prominent in infected bone (osteomyelitis). As an example, a coronal view of the uptake around the femur in pig no. 25 is shown in Figure 1.

At late time points, the decay-corrected PET signal was markedly reduced in all tissues outside the bladder, indicating that uptake of the tracer is reversible rather than irreversible (see Figure 2).

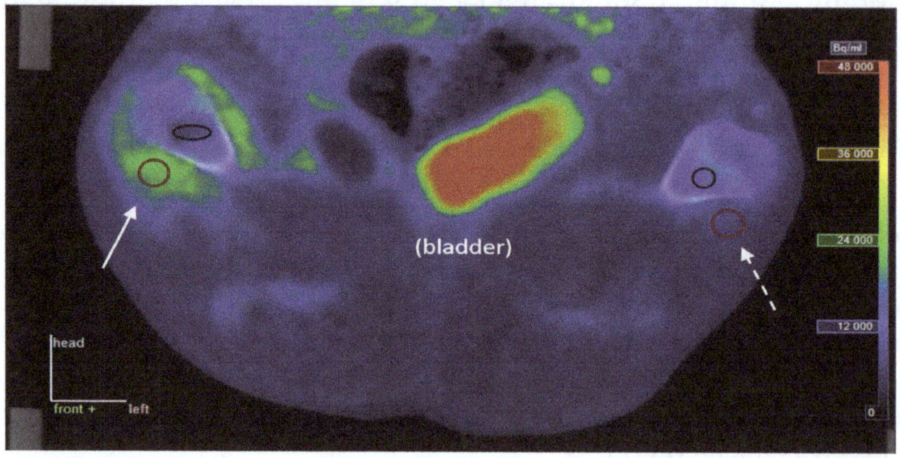

Figure 1. Representative PET/CT image from pig no. 25. The pig was lying supine with roughly upward-pointing limbs, and the view is coronal, seen from the ventral side of the animal ("front" = opposite of back is in the direction of the reader); the top of the image is in the direction of the animal's head. Full arrow: Uptake in phlegmon/early abscess at the right distal femur. Dotted arrow: Similar non-infected tissue for comparison. Red circles show sections of volumes of interest (VOIs) in soft tissue, black ellipse/circle show VOIs in bone tissue. The PET image represents the summed data from 15 to 30 min post-injection (p.i.). The tissue samples presented in Figure 3 were taken from positions approximately corresponding to the soft tissue VOIs.

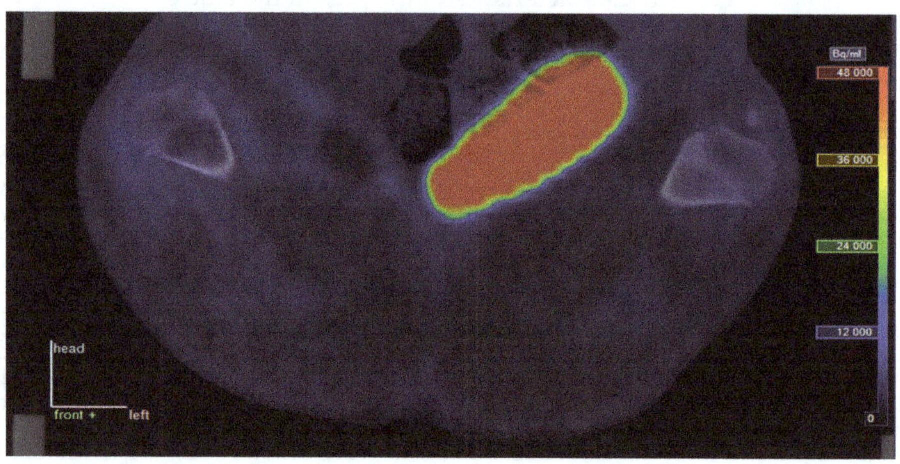

Figure 2. Late PET/CT image from pig no. 25. Static scan with [^{68}Ga]Ga-DOTA-Siglec-9 at approximately 70 min p.i.; position and colour scale correspond to those in Figure 1 (radioactivity is corrected for physical decay).

2.2. *VAP-1 Expression Studied by Immunofluorescence (IF)*

To analyse the expression of VAP-1 in infectious/inflammatory foci and to determine whether VAP-1 is translocated from intracellular granules to the endothelial cell surface, pig no. 25 was administered anti-VAP-1 antibody shortly before euthanasia, as described in the Methods section. The tissue samples were stained either with anti-VAP-1 + secondary antibody or with secondary antibody alone. Together, this pair of stainings allowed us to detect both the total VAP-1 pool and the part of the pool reached by the intravenously injected antibody; presumably only the latter pool is accessible to the imaging peptide. It can be noted that even though Siglec-9 and anti-VAP-1 both bind to VAP-1, their binding sites are different [9]; thus, they do not compete for binding.

VAP-1 was highly expressed in abscess-associated vasculature and a portion of this pool was detected with the intravenously injected antibody (Figure 3A,B). While VAP-1 is intracellularly expressed in certain vessels of normal soft tissue, no signal was detected with the intravenously administered antibody (Figure 3C,D). It thus appears that VAP-1 is accessible to blood-circulating antibodies only in the infected/inflammatory tissue, which can be seen as an indication that the translocation of VAP-1 to the cell surface is inflammation-induced.

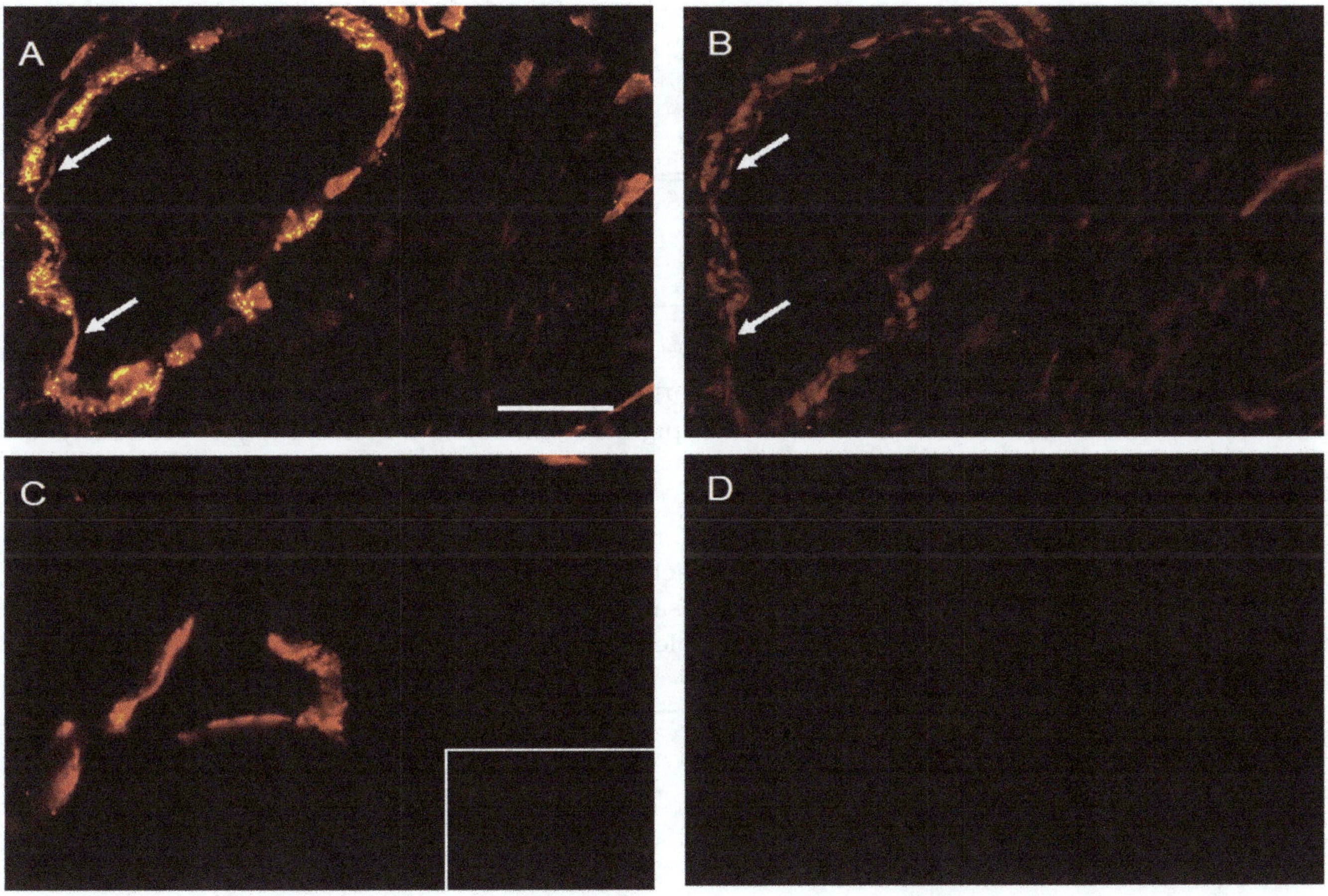

Figure 3. IF staining of infected and non-infected tissue. Stained samples from pig no. 25. **A** and **B** are stains of serial sections from phlegmon/early abscess at the right distal femur. For comparison, **C** and **D** are stains of a non-infected soft tissue sample from an anatomically corresponding position in the left limb of the same animal. (**A**) Staining with anti-VAP-1 and the secondary antibody showed high intracellular and surface expression of VAP-1 in vessels. The scale bar is 50 µm. (**B**) Staining only with the secondary antibody showed VAP-1 surface expression alone and thus indicated that a part of the VAP-1 pool is translocated to the endothelial cell surface (arrow). A signal is also detected on the abluminal side, indicating that the antibody gained access via inter-endothelial junctions. (**C**) Anti-VAP-1 staining followed by the secondary antibody. Negative control staining is shown in the inset. (**D**) Staining only with the secondary antibody showed no VAP-1 surface expression in the non-inflamed tissue.

2.3. *Protein Binding of Radioactivity*

The plasma protein binding results are shown in Figure 4. Overall, protein binding seemed to vary relatively little over the time of scanning (the late measurement in pig no. 10 deviates, but may also have the largest uncertainty due to the low level of radioactivity remaining at the late time point). A constant fraction of protein binding reflects an equilibrium between the protein-bound and non-bound tracer, allowing the plasma to be treated as a single compartment. Partly for this reason, and partly because we lack protein data for the rest of the pigs, we did not include protein binding in further analysis.

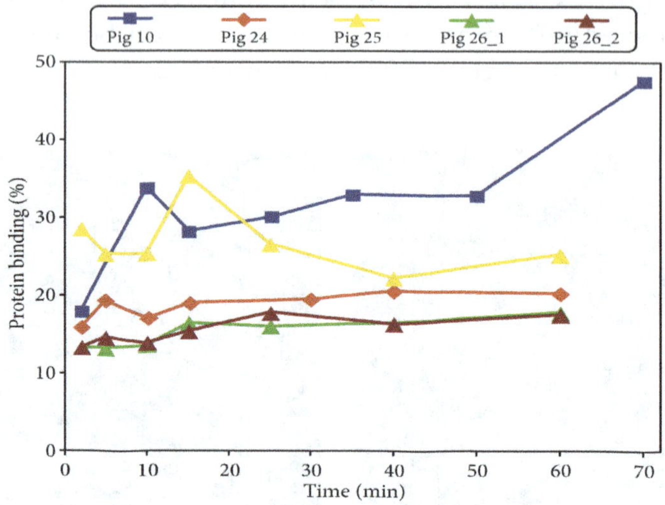

Figure 4. Plasma protein binding of [^{68}Ga]Ga-DOTA-Siglec-9 in the pigs. Percentage of binding as a function of minutes after tracer injection. For pig no. 10, the data are a summary of previously published results [22].

2.4. Analysis of the Parent Tracer Fraction

The parent tracer fraction (fraction of radioactivity originating from [^{68}Ga]Ga-DOTA-Siglec-9) rapidly decreased during the investigated time. A sample fraction curve for the parent tracer is shown in Figure 5. All fraction curves are shown in Supplementary Figure S1.

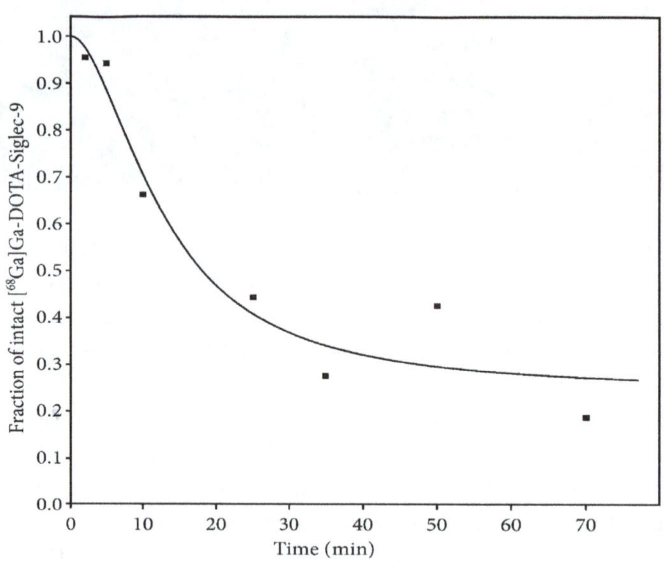

Figure 5. Fraction of radioactivity from intact [^{68}Ga]Ga-DOTA-Siglec-9 (the parent tracer fraction) in arterial plasma as a function of time. Data points and curve fits (Equation (2)) are from pig no. 9 as a representative example.

2.5. VOIs and Model Fits

In the 9 scans, a total of 24 VOI pairs were drawn: 10 VOI pairs were drawn in bone and 14 VOI pairs were drawn in soft tissue positions (counting the VOIs in pig no. 26 twice, as this pig was scanned twice). In pig no. 24, no infectious lesions were identified. In several pigs, bone lesions in the small pedal bones had to be excluded from VOI drawing and analysis, as the resolution of the PET scans would result in a partial volume effect that would be too high for the results to be robust.

The studied lesions are summarized in Tables 2 and 3. The individual VOI volumes (cm^3) can be found in Supplementary Table S1.

Table 2. Investigated osteomyelitis lesions, right hind limb.

Region	Pigs No.
Distal femur	6, 9, 22, 23, 25
Proximal tibia	6, 9, 10, 23
Distal tibia	10

Table 3. Investigated soft tissue infections sites, right hind limb.

Region	Pigs No.
Soft tissue at distal femur	22, 23, 25†
Soft tissue at distal tibia	10
Abscess at calcaneus	9
Soft tissue infection/abscess in the tissue plantar to lateral intermediary phalanxes	10, 25, 26*
Abscess at inoculation site (capsule)	22, 23
Abscess at inoculation site (centre)	22
Abscess in superficial popliteus lymph node	26*

* Pig no. 26 was scanned twice; between the two scans, 5 mg of unlabelled ("cold") DOTA-Siglec-9 peptide was injected into the animal. † See also Figure 3A,B.

For each VOI, the PET data were fitted with the models shown in Figure 6. Using pig no. 9 as an example, the model fits based on uncorrected and corrected input function are shown in Figures 7 and 8, respectively. All model fits are shown in Supplementary Figures S2–S9.

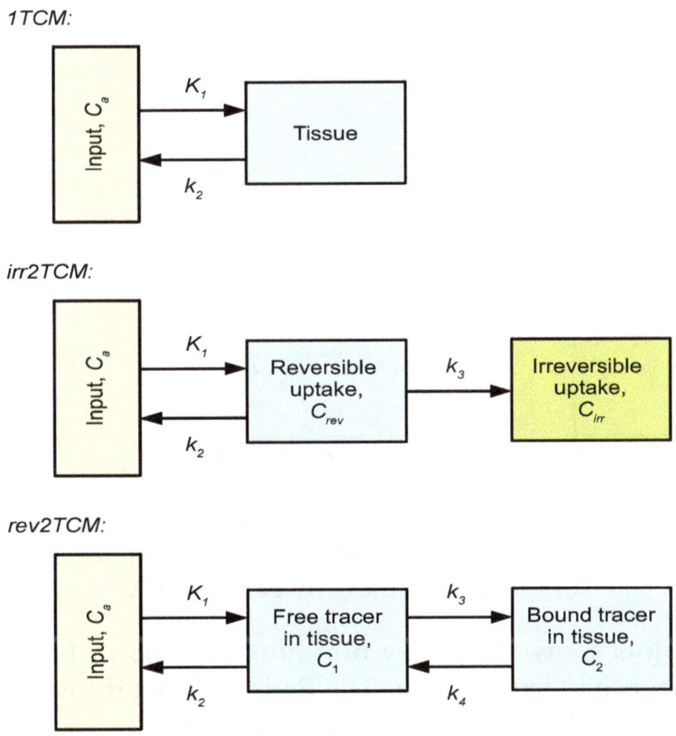

Figure 6. Kinetic models applied for the quantification of [^{68}Ga]Ga-DOTA-Siglec-9 uptake. From top to bottom: 1-tissue compartment model (1TCM), 2-tissue compartment model with irreversible uptake (irr2TCM), and 2TCM with reversible uptake (rev2TCM). The rate constants were fitted as K_1 (unit mL/min/cm^3 or mL/min/100 cm^3), the ratio K_1/k_2 (unit cm^3/mL), k_3 (unit min^{-1}), and the ratio k_3/k_4 (no unit). Additionally, the blood fraction in tissue V_b was fitted.

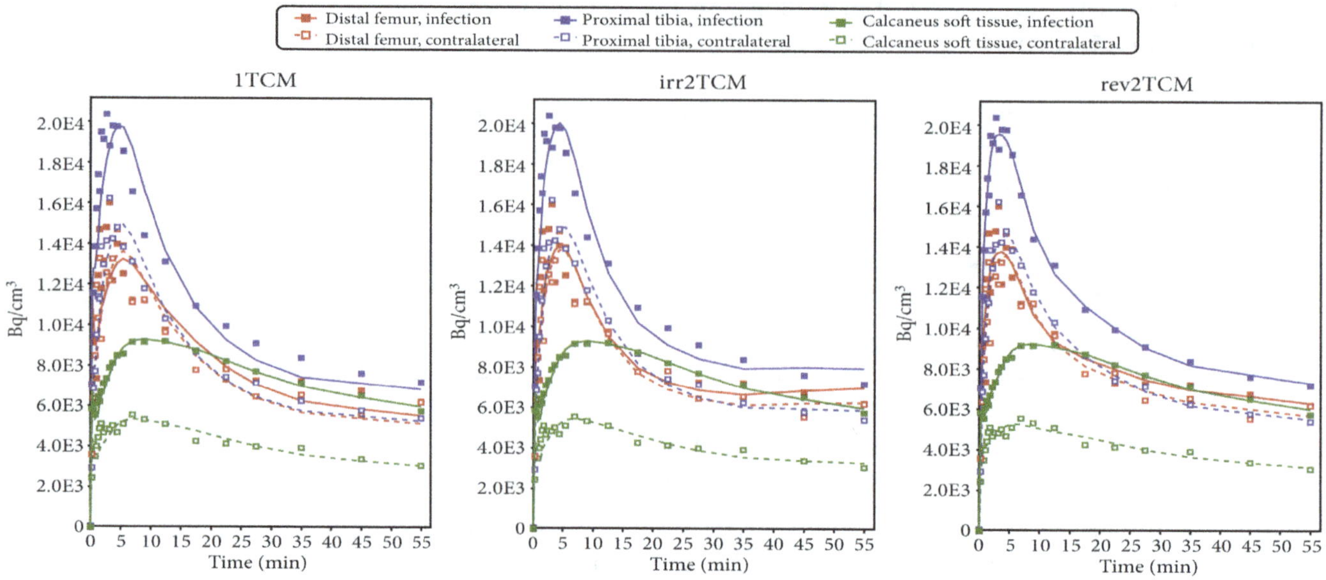

Figure 7. Model fits for pig no. 9 with the *uncorrected* input function. Infection data are from osteomyelitis lesions in the distal femur and proximal tibia and from a soft tissue infection at the calcaneus, all in the animal's right hind limb. Control data are from anatomically corresponding positions in the noninfected left hind limb. All data were modelled with each of the three kinetic models shown in Figure 6.

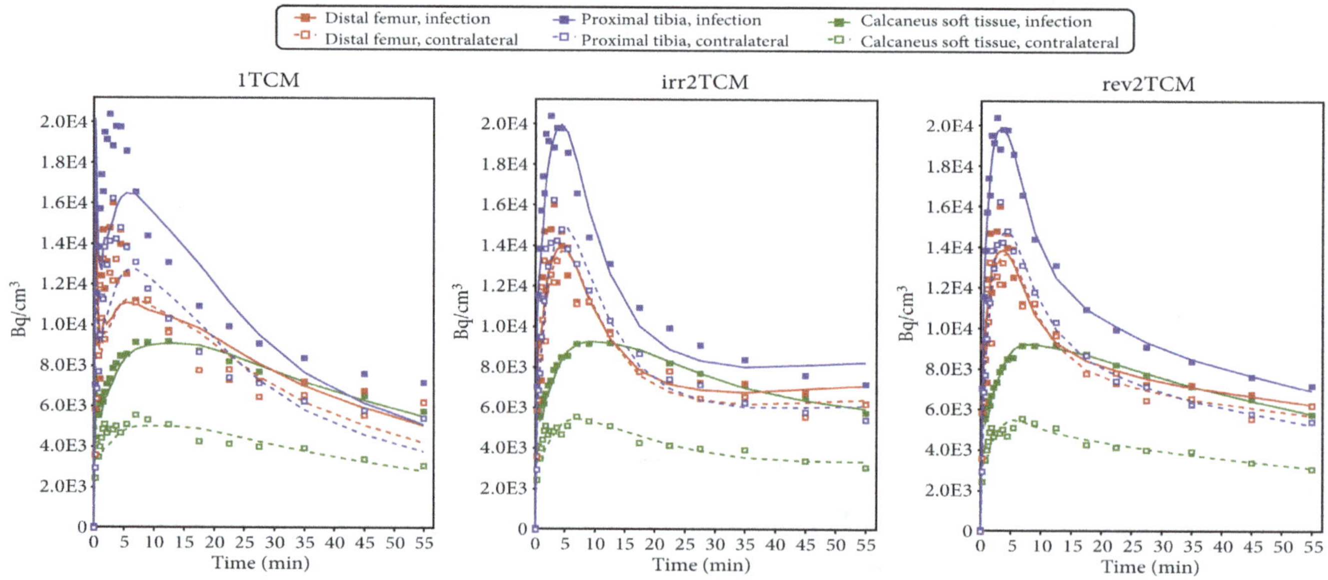

Figure 8. Model fits for pig no. 9 with the *corrected* input function. Same PET data as in Figure 7, different input function. The plots are very similar to those in Figure 7, but not identical; visual differences from Figure 7 are most notable for the early part of 1TCM.

Many of the Patlak plots showed signs of non-linearity and/or horizontal fits, indicating that uptake was reversible rather than irreversible. The Patlak plots for pig no. 9 are shown in Figure 9, and all Patlak plots are shown in Supplementary Figures S2–S9.

Plotting the fitted parameters from the corrected vs. uncorrected input function (plots not shown) revealed that the main difference was a highly elevated ratio k_3/k_4 if the corrected input function was used. A high value of k_3/k_4 indicates that the tracer leaves the second compartment only slowly, i.e., a nearly irreversible uptake. Accordingly, the Patlak plots based on the corrected input function were closer to linearity than the Patlak plots based on the uncorrected input function (cf. Figure 9 and Supplementary Figures S2–S9).

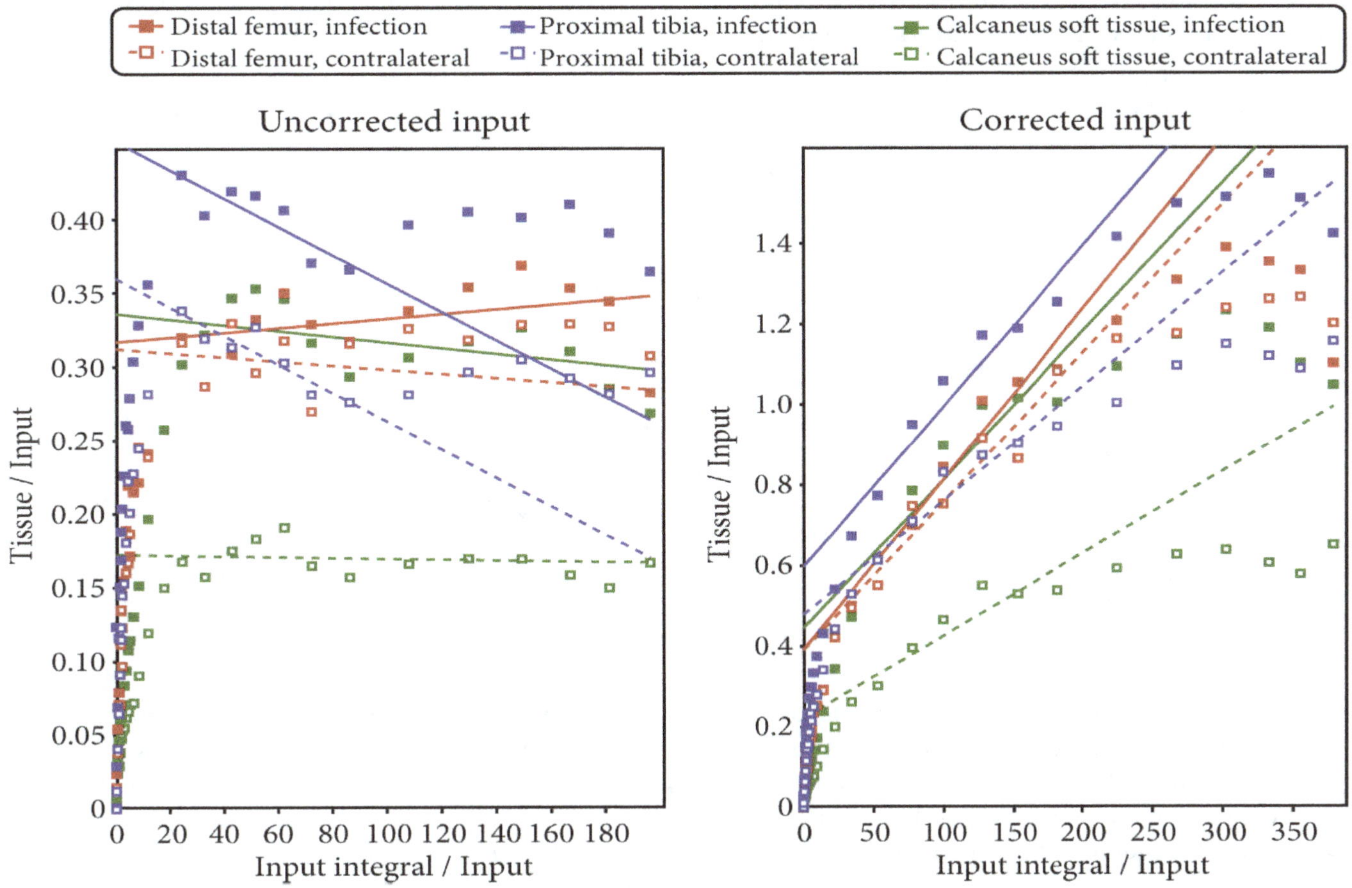

Figure 9. Patlak plots for pig no. 9. **Left**: Based on the uncorrected input function (data as in Figure 7). **Right**: Based on the corrected input function (data as in Figure 8). After the early points, irreversible uptake will be characterized by a linear Patlak plot with a positive slope, while nonlinearity or horizontal slope are signs of reversible uptake.

2.6. The Corrected Akaike Information Criterion (AIC_c)

The AIC_c values favoured the rev2TCM model, whether the input function was the uncorrected or the corrected one. Specifically, when the uncorrected input function was used, rev2TCM gave the lowest AIC_c in 18 of the 24 investigated (18/24) infection VOIs and 17/24 control VOIs. Using the corrected input function, the corresponding numbers were 17/24 and 20/24, respectively. See Supplementary Tables S2 and S3.

2.7. The Volume of Distribution in Tissue (V_T)

Based on the AIC_c results, only the V_T results from the rev2TCM were considered.

The volume of distribution in tissue (V_T) from the VOIs in the infected (right hind limb) and the control (left hind limb) positions are compared in Figure 10. Generally, the V_T results for bone infections (osteomyelitis) were close to the identity line, i.e., similar uptake in infection and control tissue. For the soft tissue infections, most points were above the identity line, indicating higher uptake in the infected soft tissues than in the corresponding control tissues, although this result was less clear when the corrected input function was used.

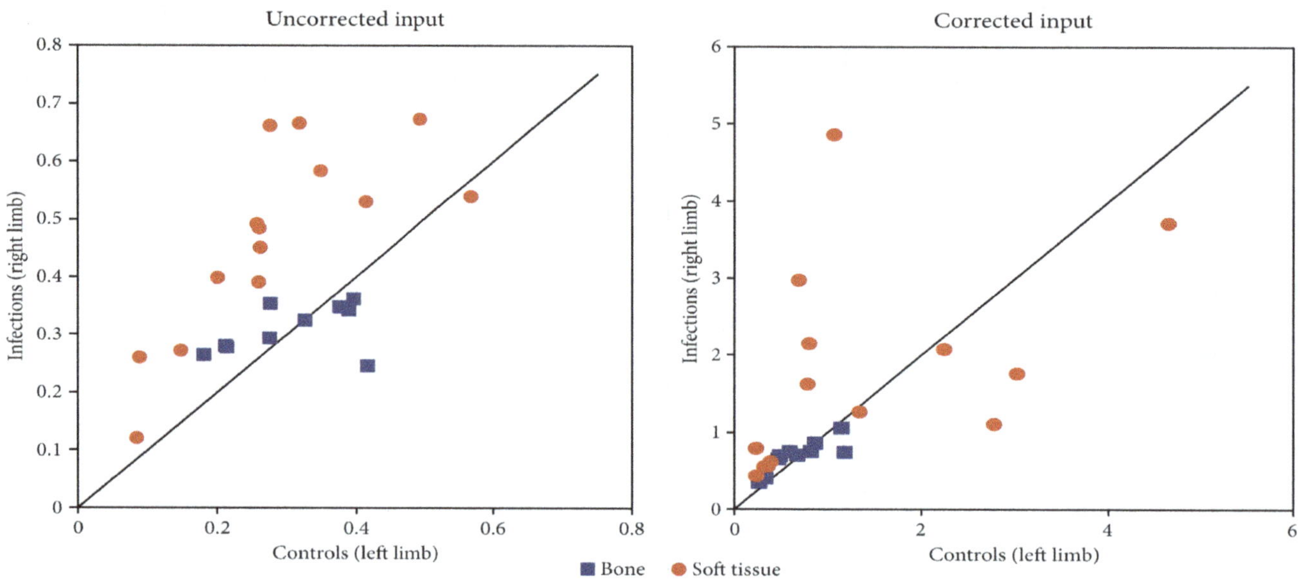

Figure 10. Volume of distribution in infected versus control tissues. Data are the V_T from Equation (6) in infection VOIs and control VOIs. Blue squares are bone VOIs, and red circles are soft tissue VOIs. **Left**: V_T from fit with the uncorrected input function. **Right**: V_T from fit with the corrected input function. Positions on the line correspond to equal values for the infection and control positions. The underlying data of the plots can be found in Supplementary Table S4. See Discussion for a comparison of the scales.

Based on the modelling results from uncorrected input function, the V_T differences between infection VOIs and control VOIs were statistically significant in the soft tissue infections ($p < 0.0001$), but not in the bone infections ($p = 0.83$). More precisely, for soft tissue VOI pairs ($n = 14$), the mean difference $\Delta V_T = V_{T,\text{infection}} - V_{T,\text{control}}$ was 0.18 mL/cm^3, with 95% limits of agreement (LOA) from 0.12 to 0.25 mL/cm^3. For bone VOI pairs ($n = 10$), the mean difference was 0.005 mL/cm^3, with 95% LOA from −0.050 to +0.062 mL/cm^3. No signs of non-normal distributions were found ($p > 0.1$ for both soft tissue and bone infections).

2.8. Correlation Between Standardized Uptake Value (SUV) and V_T

Only V_T values based on the uncorrected input functions were considered. The Pearson correlation coefficient was $r = 0.54$ ($r^2 = 0.29$, $n = 48$, $p < 0.0001$), indicating a moderate correlation. A plot is shown in Supplementary Figure S10.

Often, SUV is not evaluated as an absolute value but relative to a reference tissue. If relative rather than absolute values of V_T and SUV were plotted, then correlation rose to $r = 0.66$ ($r^2 = 0.43$, $n = 24$ pairs, $p = 0.0005$). A plot is shown in Figure 11.

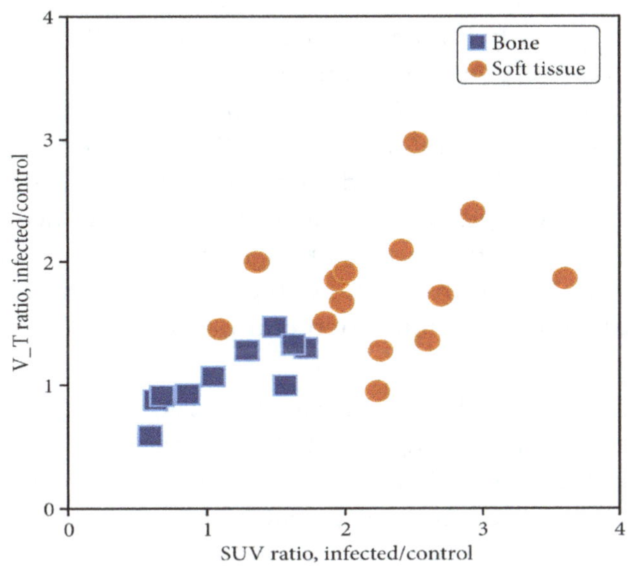

Figure 11. Correlation between relative distribution volume and relative SUV. In the plot $V_{T\text{-ratio}} = V_{T,\text{infected}} / V_{T,\text{control}}$ and $\text{SUV}_{\text{ratio}} = \text{SUV}_{\text{infected}} / \text{SUV}_{\text{control}}$, where for each infection VOI, the control VOI is at the corresponding location in the non-infected limb of the same animal VOI (see main text).

3. Discussion

In this study, we investigated the uptake of [^{68}Ga]Ga-DOTA-Siglec-9 in juvenile pigs with localized *S. aureus* infections, including both bone infection (osteomyelitis) and soft tissue infection.

As in previous studies [10,13], the tracer was found to have an affinity for infected tissues. Siglec-9 is known to bind to VAP-1, and IF staining was consistent with the expression of VAP-1 on cell surfaces in the infected soft tissue.

Kinetic modelling showed that [^{68}Ga]Ga-DOTA-Siglec-9 had reversible uptake kinetics, which could be described with a two-tissue compartment model (i.e., rev2TCM from Figure 6). Visually, the models with fewer parameters provided good fits in many cases (see the 1TCM and irr2TCM curves in Figures 7 and 8); however, the 1TCM curves provided poor fits for the initial part of many curves, and the Patlak plots revealed that models with irreversible uptake such as irr2TCM could not be generally applied (cf. Figure 9). Likewise, the analysis by the AIC_c values (cf. Supplementary Tables S2 and S3) favoured rev2TCM in the large majority of cases.

Based on these results, the following discussion will assume rev2TCM as the chosen model. Physiologically, rev2TCM indicates that the tracer is taken up by the tissue (first compartment), and then the tracer binds to receptors or otherwise changes status in the tissue (second compartment), but with the possibility of unbinding/changing back (reversible model).

3.1. *Using the Corrected or the Uncorrected Input Function*

The radio-HPLC analysis of blood samples revealed a rapid decrease in the parent tracer fraction (Figure 5). However, modelling showed no clear advantage of using a corrected input function. In most fits, the visual difference between using the uncorrected or corrected input function was only minor (compare Figures 7 and 8).

Physiologically, fitting with the uncorrected input function assumes that any radioactive metabolites have the same uptake kinetics as the parent tracer. In contrast, fitting with the corrected input function assumes that the radioactive metabolites have no uptake at all. The real situation is probably somewhere in between.

Mathematically, the inclusion of such a correction has the disadvantage of including a source of uncertainty, which becomes especially important in a case such as the present where the correction in the late part of the scans was considerable (cf. Figure 5).

The volume of distribution (V_T) measures how concentrated the tracer is in tissue relative to plasma (input), cf. Equation (4) in the Material and Methods section. As shown by comparing the scales in Figure 10, the calculated values of V_T depend markedly on the selection of the uncorrected or corrected input function. This dependency is a simple consequence of the math. The corrected input function is by definition only some fraction of the total, uncorrected input function (cf. Figure 5). A given radioactivity concentration in the tissue will be relatively higher when compared to a low number (the corrected input function) than when compared to a higher number (the uncorrected input function).

In summary, our data showed a rapid decrease in the parent tracer (cf. Figure 5), but unfortunately the modelling did not allow us to distinguish between the PET signal from the parent tracer (i.e., [^{68}Ga]Ga-DOTA-Siglec-9) and the PET signal from other radioactive species formed in vivo (i.e., all metabolites containing the ^{68}Ga isotope, possibly including free ^{68}Ga).

Consequently we reason that use of the corrected input function will lead to increased uncertainty of V_T due to possible errors in the measurement of parent tracer fraction. When the uncorrected input function is used, this pitfall is avoided, although at the cost of risking over-simplification. Pragmatically, the following discussion will therefore focus on the results found with the uncorrected input functions, bearing in mind that the physiological reality is likely more complicated than the model. Further studies investigating the nature of the radioactive products of [^{68}Ga]Ga-DOTA-Siglec-9 formed in vivo are warranted.

3.2. *The Volume of Distribution V_T*

The V_T for [^{68}Ga]Ga-DOTA-Siglec-9 in soft tissue infections was found to be higher than that of the corresponding control sites, (red circles in Figure 10, left part). In bone infections (osteomyelitis), however, V_T was not significantly different between the infection and control sites (blue squares in Figure 10, left part).

Retamal et al. [12] used the same tracer to study lung inflammation, also performing kinetic modelling with the model called rev2TCM in our terminology (with no mention of correction for parent tracer fraction), and found that the model described the time–activity curves well. The study also included protein binding, which was found to be constant over time, at a level of approximately 20% in healthy pigs and approximately 50% in the inflamed pigs. Our results (cf. Figure 4) are mostly in accordance with the first of these numbers, which could reflect that from a systemic perspective, a local infection in a single limb is more similar to a healthy pig than to a pig with severe inflammation in both lungs. Retamal et al. found increased uptake of [^{68}Ga]Ga-DOTA-Siglec-9 in inflamed lungs, which is consistent with our results on uptake in soft tissue infection.

In summary, [^{68}Ga]Ga-DOTA-Siglec-9 shows increased uptake in infected (and inflamed) soft tissue compared with control tissue; however, this study fails to demonstrate elevated uptake in infected bone (osteomyelitis). These quantitative results correspond to the visual impression of the sample image in Figure 1, where increased uptake is clear in infected soft tissue but not in the infected bone (cf. with pig no. 25 in Tables 2 and 3). Note, however, that this comparison is partly qualitative. The determination of V_T on a reliable absolute scale will depend on improved knowledge on the nature of the radioactive metabolite products of [^{68}Ga]Ga-DOTA-Siglec-9. The moderate correlation between SUV and V_T indicates that the volume of distribution gives information that is not just a complicated version of the SUV.

In a previous study [18] (in part performed on the same animals), we found only a small increase of blood perfusion in osteomyelitis lesions, while blood perfusion was considerably increased in soft tissue infections. As speculated in that study, an ineffective vascular response to infection may lead to too few leukocytes reaching the infected bone, in part explaining why osteomyelitis is difficult for the body to fight. Similarly, despite the uptake of [^{68}Ga]Ga-DOTA-Siglec-9 in infected tissue, imperfect perfusion can impair effective uptake, which may explain the difference in results for soft tissue infections and osteomyelitis.

3.3. Scan after the Injection of "Cold" DOTA-Siglec-9

Pig no. 26 was scanned twice, and the second scan was performed after the injection of 5 mg of unlabelled DOTA-Siglec-9 peptide, which was intended to block the VAP-1 receptors. The uptake curves for both scans are shown in Supplementary Figures S8 and S9. For the infected lymph node, the bolus passage and initial uptake show differences between the first and the second scan, but otherwise the two sets of curves are very similar. Quantitative distribution volumes are listed in Supplementary Table S4. Rather than the expected decrease from receptor blocking, both lesions in pig no. 26 show an approximately 20% increase in V_T from the first scan to the second when the uncorrected input function is used. With only two lesions in one pig, however, it is difficult to draw conclusions.

Using the corrected input function, Supplementary Table S4 shows pronounced V_T differences (still increases) for the two lesions in pig no. 26, but we are hesitant to draw conclusions from these results, as they may reflect the sensitivity of V_T to the correction (cf. Section 3.1). In addition, pig no. 26 unfortunately showed the lowest parent tracer fractions (cf. Supplementary Figure S1) and therefore had the largest sensitivity to possible errors in the correction of the input function.

3.4. Limitations

A porcine model has the advantage over, e.g., a murine model that the physical sizes involved in both surgery and scans are larger, but the disadvantage is that the cost per animal is higher. Accordingly, this study is limited by a relatively small number of animals.

The non-traumatic osteomyelitis protocol has the advantage that it is a very realistic model of haematogenous osteomyelitis (in humans and animals) and infections were reasonably limited to the right hind limb, but the numbers and locations of infections varied among the animals. However, within the individual pig, the other hind limb could be used as a control, and for soft tissue, the uptake measured as the volume of distribution (V_T) in infected versus control sites showed quite clear differences (Figure 10). As already noted, the study does not claim to report V_T on a robust absolute scale, which would also require data on protein binding in all animals.

A scanner replacement resulted in the last three pigs (no. 24–26) being scanned on a PET/CT scanner of a different brand and a newer generation than the initial scanner, enhancing the spatial resolution of the PET images. This allowed refined VOI drawing in these pigs, as reflected in the generally smaller VOI sizes for these animals (cf. Supplementary Table S1). More precisely drawn VOIs could reduce a possible partial volume effect, in which case uptake would be expected to be more pronounced in pigs no. 24–26 than in the pigs scanned on the initial scanner. However, the results for V_T based on the uncorrected input function (cf. Supplementary Table S4) do not indicate any pronounced effect. Using the corrected input function, pigs no. 25 and 26 do have high V_T values, but these values reflect the pronounced correction for the (possibly artificially low) parent tracer fractions in these pigs (cf. Supplementary Figure S1), while an effect of voxel size should also be reflected in V_T calculated using the uncorrected input function.

Another potential source of error may be that the scans were performed on anaesthetized pigs, as the anaesthetic may affect blood flow and hence the kinetics of the tracer. However, it was not practically feasible to scan awake pigs. Propofol was chosen because it provides relatively uniform and safe anaesthesia over many hours.

The use of penicillin in the animals may have reduced the extent of the studied infections, but has previously been found to provide a better balance between the successful development of osteomyelitis and the avoidance of systemic infections requiring euthanasia of the animal [23]. The use of opioids can have immunosuppressant effects, but so can pain reactions, which are reduced by the pain-killer effect; buprenorphine was chosen because it has shown weaker immune effects than morphine and fentanyl [24]. As the target molecule VAP-1 for the tracer is not related to the infecting agent but is instead part of the natural immune system response, there is no reason to expect direct interference between [^{68}Ga]Ga-DOTA-Siglec-9 and the antibiotic pharmaceuticals (penicillin and buprenorphine).

4. Materials and Methods

4.1. Porcine Infection Protocol

The animal protocol was approved by the Danish Animal Experimental Board, journals no. 2012-15-2934-00123 (original approval) and 2017-15-0201-01239 (renewed approval, no substantial changes to the protocol), and all procedures followed the European Directive 2010/63/EU on the protection of animals used for scientific purposes. The protocol for the haematogenous induction of osteomyelitis in domestic pigs has been detailed elsewhere [23]; for general background, see [14–16].

Briefly, *S. aureus* was inoculated into the right hind limb of juvenile (19–25 kg) Danish Landrace–Yorkshire crossbred female pigs. The pigs were pre-acclimated for at least one week, during which they were housed in groups in boxes with restricted access to food (Dia plus FI, DLG, Copenhagen, Denmark) and *ad libitum* access to tap water. The temperature was 20–24 °C, the humidity was 45–65%, and there were 12 h of darkness and 12 h of light in the stables. The pigs came from a specific pathogen free (SPF) herd and were clinically examined by a veterinarian before inoculation. The pigs were fasted for approximately 16 h before premedication with midazolam and Stresnil and propofol anaesthesia. After inoculation, the pigs were individually housed. The *S. aureus* used was the porcine strain S54F9 [25], and 8000 to 30,000 CFU/kg (colony forming units per kg body weight) were inoculated. To selectively infect the right hind limb, bacteria were injected into the right femoral artery. To further reduce the possibility of systemic infection, the pigs were administered penicillin (10,000 EI/kg) at the onset of the first clinical signs of disease; for such juvenile pigs this dosage has previously been shown to allow the development of osteomyelitis while minimizing cases of systemic infection [23]. To reduce pain in the days until euthanasia, the animals were treated every 8 h with buprenorphine (Temgesic; 0.3 to 0.9 mg intramuscularly, depending on clinical symptoms). Osteomyelitis was allowed to develop for approximately one week, after which the pig was scanned with PET and computed tomography (PET/CT, see below) and euthanized. If a pig reached predefined humane endpoints [23] before this time, it was euthanized (and not scanned).

Although the protocol was originally designed for inducing osteomyelitis [17], several pigs also developed soft tissue infections in the inoculated hind limb, typically related to bone infection or the site of inoculation. This turned out to be an advantage, as it allowed us to compare osteomyelitis and soft tissue infections. Some of the pigs also developed lung abscesses. However, these abscesses were outside the field-of-view of the dynamic PET scans and are therefore not included in this kinetics study.

4.2. Animals and Lesions

This study includes eight pigs dynamically scanned with PET/CT using [^{68}Ga]Ga-DOTA-Siglec-9 (details below). The characteristics of these pigs are summarized in Table 1. These eight pigs are a subset of the animals from the overall osteomyelitis project but represent all pigs in the project scanned with this tracer.

Before euthanasia, each pig was also PET/CT scanned with [^{18}F]FDG; these scans have been reported earlier and found [^{18}F]FDG to be a sensitive (but unspecific) marker of *S. aureus* infection [17,19,26]. Infectious lesions were identified on [^{18}F]FDG PET/CT scans. As part of the post-euthanasia analysis, selected lesions were verified by necropsy to be suppurative and to be caused by the inoculated *S. aureus* strain, S54F9.

For the identified lesions, volumes of interest (VOIs) for PET data analysis were drawn on the [^{68}Ga]Ga-DOTA-Siglec-9 PET/CT scans using Carimas 2.9 software (Turku PET Centre, www.turkupetcentre.fi/carimas). For osteomyelitis lesions, the VOI drawing was based on the CT part of the scan, while for soft tissue lesions the VOI drawing was guided by the PET scan.

For each lesion, a reference VOI was drawn in the anatomically corresponding position in the left, non-infected limb.

4.3. Radiochemistry

The radioactive labelling of DOTA-Siglec-9 has previously been discussed and described in detail [22]. The [^{68}Ga]Ga-DOTA-Siglec-9 radiosynthesis method called method 3 in the reference was applied in this study.

In summary, ^{68}Ga was eluted from a ^{68}Ge/^{68}Ga generator (GalliaPharm, Eckert & Ziegler, Berlin, Germany), trapped on a cation-exchange cartridge (Strata-XC 33 u Polymeric Strong, Phenomenex, Værløse, Denmark), and eluted from the cartridge with an acidified acetone solution. The pH was adjusted using HCl (0.1 M in metal-free water), and acetone was removed by heating. A solution of DOTA-Siglec-9 peptide in metal-free water was added, and ^{68}Ga incorporation took place. Water was added to the mixture, which was then run through a preconditioned C-18 Sep-Pak cartridge to trap [^{68}Ga]Ga-DOTA-Siglec-9. The product [^{68}Ga]Ga-DOTA-Siglec-9 was released from the cartridge with ethanol and diluted with saline. After this process, the product was ready for injection.

After 25 min, a 62% non-decay-corrected (ndc) yield of the product was obtained. The [^{68}Ga]Ga-DOTA-Siglec-9 was found by a radio HPLC system to be more than 98% radiochemically pure, and the specific radioactivity was approximately 35 MBq/nmol. Representative radio-HPLC chromatographs are shown in Supplementary Figure S11.

4.4. Dynamic PET Scans

Before scanning, each pig was anaesthetized with propofol, and catheters were implanted in the jugular vein and carotid artery [17]. After an initial CT scan, the pig was dynamically PET scanned for 60 min in 23 time frames: 8 × 15 s, 4 × 30 s, 2 × 60 s, 2 × 120 s, 4 × 300 s, and 3 × 600 s. The [^{68}Ga]Ga-DOTA-Siglec-9 tracer was injected into the jugular vein at the start of the PET scan. The tracer activities are shown in Table 1. All of these scans were performed at the Department of Nuclear Medicine, Aalborg University Hospital.

Pigs no. 6–23 were scanned on a GE VCT Discovery 64 PET/CT scanner (GE Healthcare, Chicago, IL, USA). The scan field covered 15 cm in the axial direction and was positioned over the pelvis and the hind limbs. The images were reconstructed with an ordered subset expectation maximization (OSEM) algorithm (3D Vue Point, GE). The reconstruction parameters were 2 iterations, 28 subsets, a 128 × 128 matrix in 47 slices, a 5.5 × 5.5 × 3.3 mm^3 voxel size, and a 6 mm Gaussian filter.

Due to scanner replacement, pigs no. 24–26 were scanned on a different scanner than the previous pigs. Pigs no. 24–26 were scanned on a Siemens Biograph mCT (Siemens, Erlangen, Germany) with time-of-flight (TOF) detection. The scan field covered 22 cm in the axial direction, positioned over the pelvis and the hind limbs. The images were reconstructed with an OSEM algorithm without using the resolution recovery option (setting "Iterative + TOF"). The reconstruction parameters were 3 iterations, 21 subsets, a 400 × 400 matrix in 1.02 × 1.02 × 2.03 mm^3 voxels, and a 3 mm Gaussian filter.

On both scanners, image reconstruction included decay-correction to the start of scanning and attenuation-correction based on the CT scan.

4.5. Blood Samples

An arterial blood sample was drawn before the tracer was injected (zero-sample). During the dynamic PET scan, 27 blood samples were drawn. All blood samples were drawn manually from the carotid artery, and the precise time (seconds) of each sample was recorded. Time zero was the time of injection, which was also the scan start time.

In pigs no. 6–10, the blood samples were drawn every 5 s for 50 s (10 samples), at 60, 80, 100, 120, and 150 s post-injection (p.i., 5 samples), and at 3, 4, 5, 6, 8, 10, 15, 20, 30, 40, 55, and 70 min p.i. (12 samples), i.e., 27 blood samples. Samples for analysis of the fraction of radioactivity originating from the parent tracer (rather than from radioactive metabolite products or free gallium) were drawn at 2, 5, 10, 15, 25, 35, 50, and 70 min p.i.

In pigs no. 22–26, the blood sample timing was slightly optimized. Blood samples were drawn every 5 s for 40 s (8 samples), at 50, 60, 80, 100, 120, and 150 s p.i. (6 samples), and at 3, 4, 5, 6, 8, 10, 15, 20, 25, 30, 40, 50, and 60 min p.i. (13 samples), i.e., 27 blood samples. Blood samples for analysis of the parent tracer fraction were drawn at 2, 5, 10, 15, 25, 40, and 60 min p.i.

As noted in Table 1, pig no. 26 was scanned twice, and 5 mg of "cold" (unlabelled) DOTA-Siglec-9 was injected before the second scan. Blood sampling was independently performed for the two scans.

Plasma samples were obtained by collecting the supernatant after the centrifugation of whole blood samples. Aliquots of the samples were counted in a calibrated Wizard 2480 gamma counter (PerkinElmer, Turku, Finland) with an energy window from 450 to 1200 keV. The counting results were converted to decay-corrected radioactivity concentrations (Bq/mL at the time of injection).

The plasma samples for analyses of the parent tracer fraction were denatured by thoroughly mixing 0.5 mL plasma with 0.5 mL acetonitrile, after which the mix was centrifuged (approximately 1 min, 10,000 rpm) to accelerate the precipitation of the plasma proteins. An aliquot was collected for HPLC analysis (see below). The radioactivity of the precipitate was determined with the Wizard 2480 gamma counter. Protein binding was calculated as

$$\text{protein binding} = \frac{\text{precipitate radioactivity}/0.5\ \text{mL}}{\text{plasma radioactivity concentration}} \times 100\%, \tag{1}$$

using decay-corrected activities.

For the determination of parent tracer fractions in a sample, 0.2 mL of the supernatant was diluted with 0.8 mm water; this dilution was run through an HPLC with a fractionation collector. The fraction collector was set up with a 20 s delay to compensate for delays in the system. Twenty fractions of 45 s each were collected and counted in the Wizard 2480 gamma counter.

4.6. Tissue Samples and Immunofluorescence (IF)

As a proof of concept, the surface expression of VAP-1 in infected tissue was tested by an augmented protocol in one pig.

Approximately 10 min before euthanasia, pig no. 25 was administered 10 mg of VAP-1-binding antibody as an intravenous (i.v.) injection (10 mL injected liquid). The antibody was 1B2, a mouse IgM against human VAP-1 that also recognizes porcine VAP-1 [27]. The i.v. injection allowed 1B2 to bind to the VAP-1 expressed on cell surfaces, but not to the VAP-1 within intact cells.

After euthanasia of the pig, soft tissue samples were collected from acutely inflamed areas (phlegmon/early abscess) located peripheral to the osteomyelitis in the distal right femur and from similarly positioned non-inflamed areas in the left hind limb. All samples were embedded in a cryo-compound and frozen in petroleum spirit (VWR, Søborg, Denmark, cat. no. 87125.320) cooled with dry ice. The tissues were stored at −80 °C until use.

Immunofluorescence (IF) analysis was performed on 5 µm thick frozen sections of these samples. The first of two serial sections from the inflamed area (right limb) were stained with anti-VAP-1 mAb (1B2) or a class-matched negative control antibody, 7C7 (10 µg/mL; 1 h at room temperature) and then with a secondary antibody (Alexa 555-goat-anti-mouse IgM 1:100, Southern Biotech 1020-32; 30 min at room temperature), followed by nuclear staining with Hoechst 1:10,000 in PBS for 5 min, Thermo Scientific 6249, Waltham, MA, USA). The combined IF signal thus represented the VAP-1 within the cytoplasm as well as the VAP-1 expressed on cell surfaces. The second section was stained only with the secondary antibody; thus, the IF signal represented only the VAP-1 accessible to the i.v. injected antibody. A pair of sections from the left limb was similarly stained to represent the corresponding signals from non-infected tissue.

4.7. Input Function and Metabolite Correction

For each dynamic PET/CT scan, the decay-corrected plasma samples were used as a basic input function.

For metabolite correction, the parent tracer fraction data were fitted with a Hill-type function:

$$f(t) = 1 - \frac{(1-a)t^b}{c + t^b}, \tag{2}$$

where t is the sampling time (seconds since injection). The function starts at $f(0) = 1$ (thus assuming no metabolism before injection) and has an asymptotic value $f(\infty) = a$. The parameters a, b and c were fitted for each injection of [^{68}Ga]Ga-DOTA-Siglec-9.

In the following text, the *uncorrected input function* denotes the total radioactivity concentration (decay-corrected Bq/mL) from plasma samples, and the *corrected input function* denotes the fraction $f(t)$ multiplied by the uncorrected input function.

As blood samples were taken from the carotid artery (a short distance from the heart), while the PET data were acquired over the hind end of the pig (a longer distance from the heart), the PET data were delayed by some seconds relative to the blood plasma data. To correct for these delays, an offset to the plasma time stamps was determined for each pig using the method described in [19]. The largest of these corrections was 8 s.

4.8. Kinetic Modelling

Data were modelled using the three kinetic models shown in Figure 6. This was performed twice for each model: once with the uncorrected input function and once with the corrected input function. The modelling was performed using software available on the Turku PET Centre website (fit2k for 1TCM, fit3k for irr2TCM, fit4k for rev2TCM) [28].

Data points were weighted based on time frame length (L) and decay:

$$w = L \times \exp(-\lambda t) = L \times 0.5^{t/T} \tag{3}$$

This weighting scheme mirrors the overall count statistics of the decay-corrected PET data. Unlike weights based on counts in a VOI, the weights from Equation (3) do not in themselves contain noise. See reference [19] for a more detailed discussion of this weighting scheme.

For in vivo imaging, the volume of distribution in tissue (V_T) is defined as the ratio of tissue concentration to input concentration at a time when a steady-state has been reached [29], i.e.,

$$V_T = \frac{\text{tissue concentration}}{\text{input concentration}} \text{ (at steady-state)} \tag{4}$$

The measurement of tissue concentration in Bq/cm^3 (from the PET scan) and input concentration in Bq/mL (from plasma samples in the gamma counter) results in mL/cm^3 as the unit of V_T.

For a given model with reversible uptake, the relationship between V_T and the model parameters can be theoretically calculated. In the cases of the 1TCM and the rev2TCM models, these relationships are [29]:

$$\text{1TCM}: \ V_T = \frac{K_1}{k_2} \tag{5}$$

$$\text{rev2CTM}: \ V_T = \frac{K_1}{k_2} \cdot \left(1 + \frac{k_3}{k_4}\right) \tag{6}$$

For models with irreversible uptake, such as irr2TCM, a steady-state is never reached and V_T is not defined. Mathematically, the tracer input concentration will be continually decreasing, while the uptake in the irreversible compartment will monotonically increase, and over time, the fraction in Equation (4) will diverge instead of converging.

The parent tracer fraction appeared to decrease faster in pig no. 26 (both scans) than in the other pigs, and was close to zero after approximately 30 min post-injection (see Supplementary Figure S1). The corrected input function in this case would therefore be close to zero (expectedly with high percentage errors) at late time points, which could lead to unreliable estimation of V_T = tissue concentration/input concentration. For these reasons, modelling of pig no. 26 with the corrected input function was performed using only the data within the interval 0–30 min rather than the full interval 0–60 min.

4.9. Evaluation

In addition to visual inspections of the fits, the three models were compared using the corrected Akaike information criterion (AIC_c), which favours a good fit, but penalizes the use of excessive fitting parameters [30,31]. The absolute value of AIC_c depends on both the data and the model, but for a given data set, the lowest value of AIC_c indicates the most favourable model.

Furthermore, Patlak plots [32,33] were calculated to help determine whether uptake was reversible or irreversible. A linear Patlak plot (after an equilibration time) is a sign of irreversible uptake, while a system with only reversible uptake will result in a non-linear Patlak plot that eventually approaches a constant value. The Patlak plot is directly calculated from the data, without the assumption of any specific uptake model. The Patlak plots were based on the data from 10 to 60 min (10–30 min in pig no. 26 with corrected input function).

As a measure not requiring modelling, standardized uptake values (SUV) were also calculated, and the correlation between SUV and the volume of distribution V_T was determined. The SUV calculation was based on the time interval 10 to 30 min, chosen as a time interval after the passage of the bolus peak, but not so late that a considerable part of the tracer with reversible binding (i.e., tracer not remaining in the tissue indefinitely) would have left the tissue yet.

4.10. Statistics

To compare the infected and control VOIs (i.e., right vs. left), a two-tailed paired t-test was used, with a significance level of $p < 0.05$. The normality of the differences was tested with the Shapiro–Wilk W test. The correlation between the volume of distribution V_T and SUV was defined using Pearson analysis. Statistics were calculated with StatsDirect version 3.1.14 (www.statsdirect.com).

5. Conclusions

Using the VAP-1-targeted leukocyte ligand Siglec-9, the immunofluorescence analysis of infected tissue samples indicated that VAP-1 was expressed on the cell surfaces in infected tissue, while surface VAP-1 was not observed in non-infected tissue.

The uptake kinetics of [^{68}Ga]Ga-DOTA-Siglec-9 with localized infection in pigs were found to be well described with a reversible 2-tissue compartment model, similar to the model used by Retamal et al. [12] in a study of severe lung inflammation, also in anaesthetized pigs.

We found that the parent tracer fraction decreased relatively rapidly, but despite this finding, we were unable to demonstrate an advantage of taking tracer metabolism into account in the analysis. More detailed analyses of the radioactive species occurring after the i.v. injection of [^{68}Ga]Ga-DOTA-Siglec-9 in the body are warranted.

The [^{68}Ga]Ga-DOTA-Siglec-9 uptake, evaluated as the volume of distribution, showed affinity to infection in soft tissue; however, no increased uptake in bone infections (osteomyelitis) could be demonstrated. This difference may be related to a previous report that found infected soft tissue to be more highly perfused than infected bone tissue (osteomyelitis).

Author Contributions: Conceptualization, L.J., A.R., S.J., S.B.H., P.A., A.K.O.A., O.L.N., S.B.J.; Methodology, L.J., P.A, A.K.O.A., O.L.N., S.B.J.; Software, L.J. and V.O; Validation, L.J. and S.B.H.; Formal Analysis, L.J. and S.B.H.; Investigation, S.J., P.A., A.K.O.A., O.L.N. and S.B.J.; Resources, A.R., S.J., P.A., A.K.O.A. and S.B.J.; Data Curation, L.J. and V.O.; Writing—Original Draft Preparation, L.J.; Writing—Review & Editing, L.J., A.R., V.O., S.J., S.B.H., P.A., A.K.O.A., O.L.N., S.B.J.; Visualization, L.J. and A.R.; Supervision, P.A., O.L.N. and S.B.J.; Project Administration, P.A., A.K.O.A., O.L.N. and S.B.J.; Funding Acquisition, A.R., A.K.O.A., O.L.N. and S.B.J.

Acknowledgments: The authors thank Timo Kattelus for technical assistance on the graphics. Part of the material in this paper has been presented at the European Conference on Medical Physics, Copenhagen 2018 [34].

References

1. Jamar, F.; Buscombe, J.; Chiti, A.; Christian, P.E.; Delbeke, D.; Donohoe, K.J.; Israel, O.; Martin-Comin, J.; Signore, A. EANM/SNMMI Guideline for ^{18}F-FDG Use in Inflammation and Infection. *J. Nucl. Med.* **2013**, *54*, 647–658. [CrossRef] [PubMed]
2. Signore, A.; Jamar, F.; Israel, O.; Buscombe, J.; Martin-Comin, J.; Lazzeri, E. Clinical indications, image acquisition and data interpretation for white blood cells and anti-granulocyte monoclonal antibody scintigraphy: An EANM procedural guideline. *Eur. J. Nucl. Med. Mol. Imaging* **2018**, *45*, 1816–1831. [CrossRef] [PubMed]
3. Palestro, C.J. Radionuclide imaging of osteomyelitis. *Semin. Nucl. Med.* **2015**, *45*, 32–46. [CrossRef] [PubMed]
4. Miñana, E.; Roldán, M.; Chivato, T.; Martínez, T.; Fuente, T. Quantification of the chromosomal radiation damage induced by labelling of leukocytes with [18F]FDG. *Nucl. Med. Biol.* **2015**, *42*, 720–723. [CrossRef]
5. Salmi, M.; Jalkanen, S. VAP-1: An adhesin and an enzyme. *Trends Immunol.* **2001**, *22*, 211–216. [CrossRef]
6. Jalkanen, S.; Salmi, M. VAP-1 and CD73, endothelial cell surface enzymes in leukocyte extravasation. *Arterioscler. Thromb. Vasc. Biol.* **2008**, *28*, 18–26. [CrossRef]
7. Roivainen, A.; Jalkanen, S.; Nanni, C. Gallium-labelled peptides for imaging of inflammation. *Eur. J. Nucl. Med. Mol. Imaging* **2012**, *39*, 68–77. [CrossRef]
8. Aalto, K.; Autio, A.; Kiss, E.A.; Elima, K.; Nymalm, Y.; Veres, T.Z.; Marttila-Ichihara, F.; Elovaara, H.; Saanijoki, T.; Crocker, P.R.; et al. Siglec-9 is a novel leukocyte ligand for vascular adhesion protein-1 and can be used in PET imaging of inflammation and cancer. *Blood* **2011**, *118*, 3725–3733. [CrossRef]
9. Salmi, M.; Jalkanen, S. Vascular adhesion protein-1: A cell surface amine oxidase in translation. *Antioxid. Redox Signal.* **2019**, *30*, 314–332. [CrossRef]
10. Ahtinen, H.; Kulkova, J.; Lindholm, L.; Eerola, E.; Hakanen, A.J.; Moritz, N.; Söderström, M.; Saanijoki, T.; Jalkanen, S.; Roivainen, A.; et al. ^{68}Ga-DOTA-Siglec-9 PET/CT imaging of peri-implant tissue responses and staphylococcal infections. *EJNMMI Res.* **2014**, *4*, 45. [CrossRef]
11. Siitonen, R.; Pietikäinen, A.; Liljenbäck, H.; Käkelä, M.; Söderström, M.; Jalkanen, S.; Hytönen, J.; Roivainen, A. Targeting of vascular adhesion protein-1 by positron emission tomography visualizes sites of inflammation in *Borrelia burgdorferi*-infected mice. *Arthritis Res. Ther.* **2017**, *19*, 254. [CrossRef]
12. Retamal, J.; Sörensen, J.; Lubberink, M.; Suarez-Sipmann, F.; Borges, J.B.; Feinstein, R.; Jalkanen, S.; Antoni, G.; Hedenstierna, G.; Roivainen, A.; et al. Feasibility of ^{68}Ga-labeled Siglec-9 peptide for the imaging of acute lung inflammation: A pilot study in a porcine model of acute respiratory distress syndrome. *Am. J. Nucl. Med. Mol. Imaging* **2016**, *6*, 18–31. [PubMed]
13. Virtanen, H.; Silvola, J.M.U.; Autio, A.; Li, X.-G.; Liljenbäck, H.; Hellberg, S.; Siitonen, R.; Ståhle, M.; Käkelä, M.; Airaksinen, A.J.; et al. Comparison of ^{68}Ga-DOTA-Siglec-9 and ^{18}F-fluorodeoxyribose-Siglec-9: Inflammation imaging and radiation dosimetry. *Contrast Media Mol. Imaging* **2017**, *2017*, 7645070. [CrossRef] [PubMed]
14. Johansen, L.K.; Svalastoga, E.L.; Frees, D.; Aalbæk, B.; Koch, J.; Iburg, T.M.; Nielsen, O.L.; Leifsson, P.S.; Jensen, H.E. A new technique for modeling of hematogenous osteomyelitis in pigs: Inoculation into femoral artery. *J. Invest. Surg.* **2013**, *26*, 149–153. [CrossRef] [PubMed]

15. Jensen, H.E.; Nielsen, O.L.; Agerholm, J.S.; Iburg, T.; Johansen, L.K.; Johannesson, E.; Møller, M.; Jahn, L.; Munk, L.; Aalbaek, B.; et al. A non-traumatic *Staphylococcus aureus* osteomyelitis model in pigs. *In Vivo* **2010**, *24*, 257–264.
16. Johansen, L.K.; Koch, J.; Frees, D.; Aalbæk, B.; Nielsen, O.L.; Leifsson, P.S.; Iburg, T.M.; Svalastoga, E.; Buelund, L.E.; Bjarnsholt, T.; et al. Pathology and biofilm formation in a porcine model of staphylococcal osteomyelitis. *J. Comp. Pathol.* **2012**, *147*, 343–353. [CrossRef]
17. Nielsen, O.L.; Afzelius, P.; Bender, D.; Schønheyder, H.C.; Leifsson, P.S.; Nielsen, K.M.; Larsen, J.O.; Jensen, S.B.; Alstrup, A.K.O. Comparison of autologous ^{111}In-leukocytes, ^{18}F-FDG, ^{11}C-methionine, ^{11}C-PK11195 and ^{68}Ga-citrate for diagnostic nuclear imaging in a juvenile porcine haematogenous staphylococcus aureus osteomyelitis model. *Am. J. Nucl. Med. Mol. Imaging* **2015**, *5*, 169–182.
18. Jødal, L.; Nielsen, O.L.; Afzelius, P.; Alstrup, A.K.O.; Hansen, S.B. Blood perfusion in osteomyelitis studied with [^{15}O] water PET in a juvenile porcine model. *EJNMMI Res.* **2017**, *7*, 4. [CrossRef]
19. Jødal, L.; Jensen, S.B.; Nielsen, O.L.; Afzelius, P.; Borghammer, P.; Alstrup, A.K.O.; Hansen, S.B. Kinetic modelling of infection tracers [^{18}F]FDG, [^{68}Ga]Ga-citrate, [^{11}C]methionine, and [^{11}C]donepezil in a porcine osteomyelitis model. *Contrast Media Mol. Imaging* **2017**, *2017*, 9256858. [CrossRef]
20. Afzelius, P.; Alstrup, A.K.O.; Schønheyder, H.C.; Borghammer, P.; Bender, D.; Jensen, S.B.; Nielsen, O.L. Utility of ^{11}C-methionine and ^{11}C-donepezil for imaging of *Staphylococcus aureus* induced osteomyelitis in a juvenile porcine model: Comparison to autologous ^{111}In-labelled leukocytes, ^{99m}Tc-DPD, and ^{18}F-FDG. *Am. J. Nucl. Med. Mol. Imaging* **2016**, *6*, 286–300.
21. Afzelius, P.; Nielsen, O.L.; Schønheyder, H.C.; Alstrup, A.K.O.; Hansen, S.B. An untapped potential for imaging of peripheral osteomyelitis in paediatrics using [^{18}F] FDG PET/CT—The inference from a juvenile porcine model. *EJNMMI Res.* **2019**, *9*, 29. [CrossRef] [PubMed]
22. Jensen, S.B.; Käkelä, M.; Jødal, L.; Moisio, O.; Alstrup, A.K.O.; Jalkanen, S.; Roivainen, A. Exploring the radiosynthesis and *in vitro* characteristics of [^{68}Ga]Ga-DOTA-Siglec-9. *J. Label. Compd. Radiopharm.* **2017**, *60*, 439–449. [CrossRef] [PubMed]
23. Alstrup, A.K.O.; Nielsen, K.M.; Schønheyder, H.C.; Jensen, S.B.; Afzelius, P.; Leifsson, P.S.; Nielsen, O.L. Refinement of a hematogenous localized osteomyelitis model in pigs. *Scand. J. Lab. Anim. Sci.* **2016**, *42*, 1–4.
24. Sacerdote, P. Opioid-induced immunosuppression. *Curr. Opin. Support. Palliat. Care* **2008**, *2*, 14–18. [CrossRef]
25. Aalbæk, B.; Jensen, L.K.; Jensen, H.E.; Olsen, J.E.; Christensen, H. Whole-genome sequence of *Staphylococcus aureus* S54F9 isolated from a chronic disseminated porcine lung abscess and used in human infection models. *Genome Announc.* **2015**, *3*, e01207-15. [CrossRef]
26. Afzelius, P.; Nielsen, O.L.; Alstrup, A.K.O.; Bender, D.; Leifsson, P.S.; Jensen, S.B.; Schønheyder, H.C. Biodistribution of the radionuclides ^{18}F-FDG, ^{11}C-methionine, ^{11}C-PK11195, and ^{68}Ga-citrate in domestic juvenile female pigs and morphological and molecular imaging of the tracers in hematogenously disseminated *Staphylococcus aureus* lesions. *Am. J. Nucl. Med. Mol. Imaging* **2016**, *6*, 42–58.
27. Jaakkola, K.; Nikula, T.; Holopainen, R.; Vähäsilta, T.; Matikainen, M.-T.; Laukkanen, M.-L.; Huupponen, R.; Halkola, L.; Nieminen, L.; Hiltunen, J.; et al. In vivo detection of vascular adhesion protein-1 in experimental inflammation. *Am. J. Pathol.* **2000**, *157*, 463–471. [CrossRef]
28. TPC List of Applications in TPCCLIB. Available online: http://www.turkupetcentre.net/programs/doc/index.html (accessed on 19 February 2019).
29. Innis, R.B.; Cunningham, V.J.; Delforge, J.; Fujita, M.; Gjedde, A.; Gunn, R.N.; Holden, J.; Houle, S.; Huang, S.-C.; Ichise, M.; et al. Consensus nomenclature for in vivo imaging of reversibly binding radioligands. *J. Cereb. Blood Flow Metab.* **2007**, *27*, 1533–1539. [CrossRef]
30. Akaike, H. A new look at the statistical model identification. *IEEE Trans. Autom. Control* **1974**, *19*, 716–723. [CrossRef]
31. Burnham, K.P.; Anderson, D.R. Multimodel inference: Understanding AIC and BIC in model selection. *Sociol. Methods Res.* **2004**, *33*, 261–304. [CrossRef]
32. Patlak, C.S.; Blasberg, R.G.; Fenstermacher, J.D. Graphical evaluation of blood-to-brain transfer constants from multiple-time uptake data. *J. Cereb. Blood Flow Metab.* **1983**, *3*, 1–7. [CrossRef] [PubMed]

33. Patlak, C.S.; Blasberg, R.G. Graphical evaluation of blood-to-brain transfer constants from multiple-time uptake data. Generalizations. *J. Cereb. Blood Flow Metab.* **1985**, *5*, 584–590. [CrossRef] [PubMed]
34. Jødal, L.; Roivainen, A.; Oikonen, V.; Jalkanen, S.; Hansen, S.B.; Afzelius, P.; Alstrup, A.K.O.; Nielsen, O.L.; Jensen, S.B. [P083] Kinetic modelling of [68Ga]Ga-DOTA-Siglec-9 in a porcine infection model. *Phys. Med.* **2018**, *52*, 124–125. [CrossRef]

4

PET Imaging of the Adenosine A_{2A} Receptor in the Rotenone-Based Mouse Model of Parkinson's Disease with [18F]FESCH Synthesized by a Simplified Two-Step One-Pot Radiolabeling Strategy

Susann Schröder [1,*], Thu Hang Lai [2], Magali Toussaint [2], Mathias Kranz [3,4], Alexandra Chovsepian [5], Qi Shang [6,7], Sladjana Dukić-Stefanović [2], Winnie Deuther-Conrad [2], Rodrigo Teodoro [2], Barbara Wenzel [2], Rareş-Petru Moldovan [2], Francisco Pan-Montojo [5,6] and Peter Brust [2]

1 ROTOP Pharmaka Ltd., Department of Research and Development, Dresden 01328, Germany
2 Helmholtz-Zentrum Dresden-Rossendorf (HZDR), Department of Neuroradiopharmaceuticals, Institute of Radiopharmaceutical Cancer Research, Research Site Leipzig, Leipzig 04318, Germany; t.lai@hzdr.de (T.H.L.); m.toussaint@hzdr.de (M.T.); s.dukic-stefanovic@hzdr.de (S.D.-S.); w.deuther-conrad@hzdr.de (W.D.-C.); r.teodoro@hzdr.de (R.T.); b.wenzel@hzdr.de (B.W.); r.moldovan@hzdr.de (R.-P.M.); p.brust@HZDR.de (P.B.)
3 PET Imaging Center, University Hospital of North Norway (UNN), Tromsø 9009, Norway; mathias.kranz@uit.no
4 Nuclear Medicine and Radiation Biology Research Group, The Arctic University of Norway, Tromsø 9009, Norway
5 University Hospital Munich, Department of Psychiatry, Ludwig-Maximilians-Universität (LMU) Munich, Munich 80336, Germany; alexandra.chovsepian@med.uni-muenchen.de (A.C.); Francisco.Pan-Montojo@med.uni-muenchen.de (F.P.-M.)
6 University Hospital Munich, Department of Neurology, Ludwig-Maximilians-Universität (LMU) Munich, Munich 81377, Germany; shangqi0911@gmail.com
7 University Hospital Carl Gustav Carus, Clinic of Neurology, Technische Universität Dresden (TUD), Dresden 01307, Germany
* Correspondence: s.schroeder@hzdr.de

Abstract: The adenosine A_{2A} receptor ($A_{2A}R$) is regarded as a particularly appropriate target for non-dopaminergic treatment of Parkinson's disease (PD). An increased $A_{2A}R$ availability has been found in the human striatum at early stages of PD and in patients with PD and dyskinesias. The aim of this small animal positron emission tomography/magnetic resonance (PET/MR) imaging study was to investigate whether rotenone-treated mice reflect the aspect of striatal $A_{2A}R$ upregulation in PD. For that purpose, we selected the known $A_{2A}R$-specific radiotracer [^{18}F]**FESCH** and developed a simplified two-step one-pot radiosynthesis. PET images showed a high uptake of [^{18}F]**FESCH** in the mouse striatum. Concomitantly, metabolism studies with [^{18}F]**FESCH** revealed the presence of a brain-penetrant radiometabolite. In rotenone-treated mice, a slightly higher striatal $A_{2A}R$ binding of [^{18}F]**FESCH** was found. Nonetheless, the correlation between the increased $A_{2A}R$ levels within the proposed PD animal model remains to be further investigated.

Keywords: adenosine A_{2A} receptor; Parkinson's disease; rotenone-based mouse model; PET imaging; [^{18}F]**FESCH**; two-step one-pot radiosynthesis

---

1. Introduction

Parkinson's disease (PD) is characterized by the degeneration of dopaminergic neurons in the brain, especially in the substantia nigra, resulting in a decreased dopamine level in the striatum.

Consequently, stimulation of the dopamine D_2 receptor (D_2R) is reduced and, further, the morphology of striatal neurons and synaptic connections is changing. These effects lead to motor dysfunctions like bradykinesia, tremor, rigor, and postural instability [1,2]. The standard therapy of PD is based on the pharmacological increase of dopamine levels either by administration of L-DOPA as metabolic precursor of dopamine or by dopamine agonists. Further strategies to raise or maintain the dopamine levels are based on inhibitors for dopamine reuptake and dopamine-degrading enzymes (e.g., monoamine oxidase B, catechol-*O*-methyl transferase) [2]. These dopamine- increasing drugs have only a positive effect on motor functions at short-term treatment but cause undesirable side effects at long-term treatment like dyskinesia, nausea, and hallucinations. Due to these limitations, the medicinal research is currently focusing on non-dopaminergic therapies of PD [2,3].

The adenosine A_{2A} receptor ($A_{2A}R$) is a G-protein coupled receptor that is highly expressed in the basal ganglia of the brain, mainly in striatopallidal GABAergic neurons. Furthermore, in this brain area the $A_{2A}R$ and the D_2R are co-localized and form heteromeric receptor complexes while showing contradictory effects on motor functions [2]. For example, an L-DOPA-induced increase of dopamine stimulates the D_2R leading to enhanced motor activity. Activation of the $A_{2A}R$ by adenosine or appropriate agonists results in the inhibition of the D_2R and, thus, in reduced dopamine binding [2,4,5]. Pharmacological inhibition of the $A_{2A}R$ amplifies the D_2R-dependent signaling cascade and improves motor symptoms [2,3,5,6]. Since the $A_{2A}R$ modulates the dopamine binding affinity of the D_2R, selective $A_{2A}R$ antagonists have great potential as appropriate non-dopaminergic PD therapeutics [2,3,6]. In clinical phase II and III trials, the $A_{2A}R$ antagonists **istradefylline, preladenant**, and **tozadenant** improved motor symptoms in PD patients [7–9]. Out of these, **istradefylline** (Nourianz®) has already been approved in Japan [10] and currently by the U.S. Food and Drug Administration (FDA) as an adjunctive treatment to L-DOPA.

Furthermore, a comparative neuropathological postmortem study on brain slices from healthy subjects and PD patients showed a 2.5-fold increased striatal $A_{2A}R$ protein level already at early PD stages pointing out that $A_{2A}R$ upregulation is an initial event in the pathogenesis of the disease [11]. Though, it remains unclear whether there is a correlation between altered $A_{2A}R$ expression and motor symptoms in PD.

Molecular imaging of the $A_{2A}R$ with positron emission tomography (PET) enables the non-invasive investigation of pathological changes of the receptor level in the human brain [12].

A clinical PET study using [^{11}C]**SCH442416** (Figure 1) revealed a 70–80% increased $A_{2A}R$ availability in the striatum of PD patients with L-DOPA-induced dyskinesia [13]. This strongly indicates a key role of $A_{2A}R$ not only in the development of PD [11] but also in the progression of the disease and in association with the dopaminergic standard therapy [2,13]. Hence, $A_{2A}R$-PET is considered as an appropriate tool for early diagnosis and staging of PD as well as evaluation of potential $A_{2A}R$ antagonists for PD treatment by means of receptor occupancy studies. The main disadvantage of ^{11}C-labeled radiotracers for clinical routine applications is the short half-life of the nuclide ($t_{1/2}$ = 20.3 min). To date, there is only one ^{18}F-labeled ($t_{1/2}$ = 109.7 min) $A_{2A}R$ radiotracer, [^{18}F]**MNI-444** [14,15] (Figure 1), that has already been evaluated in a clinical PET study. In healthy volunteers [15], a high uptake of activity in the striatum has been observed. However, no follow-up studies have been published since 2015 and further data of [^{18}F]**MNI-444** regarding specificity of $A_{2A}R$ binding in humans or selectivity over the adenosine A_1 receptor (A_1R), which is also highly expressed in the brain [16,17], are not yet available. For that reason, we selected the well-studied and highly $A_{2A}R$-selective radiotracer [^{18}F]**FESCH** [18–21] ($K_i(hA_{2A}R)$ = 12.4 nM, $K_i(hA_1R) \sim 10$ μM, former [^{18}F]**MRS5425** [18]) for our purposes, which is the [^{18}F]fluoroethoxy analog of [^{11}C]**SCH442416** (Figure 1). [^{18}F]**FESCH** has been evaluated in healthy rats and in rats with unilateral PD symptoms by PET showing an $A_{2A}R$-specific binding in the striatum and a significantly increased $A_{2A}R$-mediated uptake in the 6-hydroxydopamine-lesioned hemisphere of 9–12% [19,21]. Therefore, [^{18}F]**FESCH** has been stated as the most suitable radiotracer for quantification of the $A_{2A}R$ in the brain with PET [21].

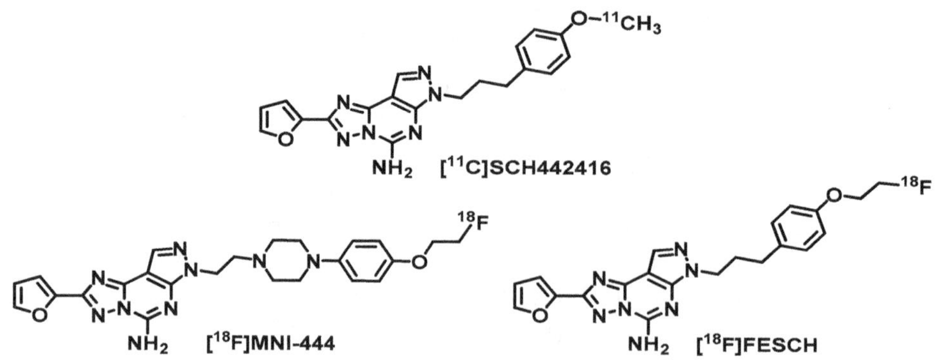

Figure 1. Molecular structures of the herein discussed radiotracers for positron emission tomography (PET) imaging of the adenosine A_{2A} receptor ($A_{2A}R$).

The rotenone-based mouse model has been well established for pre-clinical investigations of PD [22–24]. Chronic administration of the neurotoxin rotenone to mice leads to relapse of dopaminergic neurons and changes in motor functions similar to the symptoms in PD patients [24–26]. In this small animal PET/MR imaging study with [^{18}F]**FESCH**, we aimed to validate if rotenone-treated mice reflect the aspect of striatal $A_{2A}R$ upregulation in PD. In addition, we investigated [^{18}F]**FESCH** by in vitro autoradiography on mouse brain slices and in vivo metabolism as well as baseline and blocking PET studies in healthy CD-1 mice.

2. Results and Discussion

The $A_{2A}R$ antagonist **FESCH** and the required known phenol precursor desmethyl SCH442416 for ^{18}F-labeling were synthesized in three or two steps, respectively, from commercially available 2-(furan-2-yl)-7*H*-pyrazolo[4,3-*e*][1,2,4]triazolo[1,5-*c*]pyrimidine-5-amin and 1-(3-bromopropyl)-4-methoxybenzene according to procedures described in the literature [18,27,28]. Evaluation of **FESCH** in an established binding assay revealed high $A_{2A}R$ affinity ($K_i(hA_{2A}R) = 0.6 \pm 0.1$ nM, n = 4) and good A_1R selectivity ($K_i(hA_1R) = 203 \pm 40$ nM, n = 4).

The initially published radiosynthesis of [^{18}F]**FESCH** comprises a two-step two-pot procedure [19,20]. Briefly, the respective [^{18}F]fluoroethyl intermediate from the ^{18}F-labeling step was isolated either by semi-preparative HPLC [19] or solid-phase extraction on a cartridge [20] and, only then, reacted with the phenol precursor desmethyl SCH442416. To simplify the radiosynthesis and avoid loss of activity through purification of the [^{18}F]fluoroethyl intermediate, we developed a two-step one-pot strategy for the production of [^{18}F]**FESCH** [29] (see Scheme 1). First, ethane-1,2-diol bis(4-methylbenzenesulfonate) was ^{18}F-labeled via nucleophilic substitution of one tosylate group using anhydrous K^+/[^{18}F]F^-/K_{222}-carbonate complex in acetonitrile. Notably, desmethyl SCH442416 was pre-treated with aqueous tetrabutylammonium hydroxide (TBAOH) in acetonitrile to generate the activated phenolate which was directly reacted with the non-isolated 2-[^{18}F]fluoroethyl tosylate. Besides, further bases and solvents were tested for the [^{18}F]fluoroethylation of desmethyl SCH442416 resulting in decreased yields of [^{18}F]**FESCH** mainly due to partial decomposition of the phenol precursor under these conditions. Preliminary experiments using potassium carbonate or cesium carbonate (1.5–2.5 eq.) for activation of desmethyl SCH442416 (1–2 mg) and either acetonitrile or a 1:1 mixture of acetonitrile and *N,N*-dimethylformamide or *tert*-butanol as solvents revealed labeling yields of 4–14% based on TLC analysis of the reaction mixtures after 10 min at 120 °C, respectively. Replacement of the base by TBAOH (2.5 eq.) and the use of acetonitrile only resulted in a significantly increased labeling yield of 25%. Final optimization was achieved by increasing the amount of the phenol precursor to 2.5 mg leading to $46.4 \pm 8.5\%$ (n = 9) of non-isolated [^{18}F]**FESCH**.

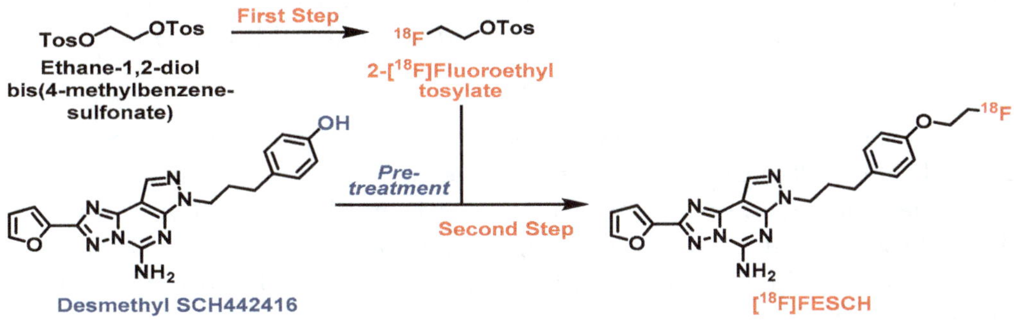

Scheme 1. Simplified two-step one-pot radiosynthesis of [^{18}F]**FESCH**. Reagents and conditions: (First step) 2 mg ethane-1,2-diol bis(4-methylbenzenesulfonate) in 100 µL MeCN, ~ 3 GBq azeotropically dried K^+/[^{18}F]F^-/K_{222}-carbonate complex in 400 µL MeCN, 90 °C, 10 min; (Second step) 2.5 mg desmethyl SCH442416 pre-treated with 10 µL $TBAOH_{aq.}$ (40%) in 490 µL MeCN at 90 °C for 10 min, directly added to 2-[^{18}F]fluoroethyl tosylate, 120 °C, 10 min.

[^{18}F]**FESCH** was purified by semi-preparative HPLC (see Figure 2) and concentrated via solid-phase extraction on a pre-conditioned reversed-phase cartridge followed by elution with absolute ethanol. After evaporation of the solvent, the radiotracer was finally formulated in sterile isotonic saline with a maximum ethanol content of 10% for better solubility. The identity of [^{18}F]**FESCH** was confirmed by analytical HPLC using an aliquot of the final product spiked with the non-radioactive reference compound (Figure 2).

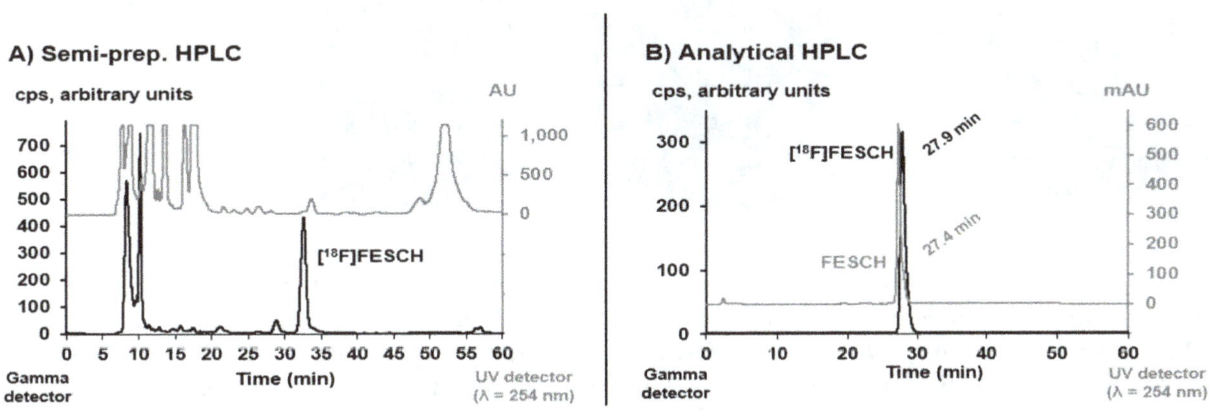

Figure 2. (**A**) Semi-preparative HPLC profile of the crude reaction mixture for isolation of [^{18}F]**FESCH** (column: Reprosil-Pur 120 C18-AQ, 250 × 10 mm, particle size: 10 µm, eluent: 50% MeCN/20 mM $NH_4OAc_{aq.}$, flow: 7 mL/min). (**B**) Analytical HPLC profile of the formulated radiotracer [^{18}F]**FESCH** spiked with the non-radioactive reference **FESCH** (column: Reprosil-Pur 120 C18-AQ, 250 × 4.6 mm, particle size: 5 µm; eluent: 26-90-26% MeCN/20 mM $NH_4OAc_{aq.}$, flow: 1 mL/min).

The herein described one-pot radiolabeling strategy provided [^{18}F]**FESCH** with a high molar activity of 116 ± 18.5 GBq/µmol (n = 7, end of synthesis) and an overall radiochemical yield of 16.1 ± 1.5% (n = 9, end of bombardment), which is a significant improvement compared to the published two-pot procedure (7 ± 2% [20]). The required total synthesis time of 114 ± 6 min and the achieved radiochemical purity of ≥ 98% were very similar for both methods.

In vitro stability of [^{18}F]**FESCH** was examined in isotonic saline and pig plasma. Samples of each medium were analyzed by radio-HPLC after 60 min incubation at 37 °C and no degradation or defluorination of the radiotracer was observed. This result is contradictory to the published stability of [^{18}F]**FESCH** especially in saline where only 85–90% of intact radiotracer have been detected by radio-TLC while multiple spots were observed [20]. Thus, Khanapur et al. [20] formulated [^{18}F]**FESCH** in phosphate-buffered saline, but Bhattacharjee et al. [19] used a saline solution of [^{18}F]**FESCH** for biological investigations. At present, we have no explanation for that and as we detected only the intact radiotracer in isotonic saline (see Figure 2), formulation of [^{18}F]**FESCH** in another medium was not required.

The distribution coefficient of [^{18}F]**FESCH** was determined by partitioning between *n*-octanol and phosphate-buffered saline (PBS, pH = 7.4) at ambient temperature using the conventional shake-flask method. The obtained log$D_{7.4}$ value of 1.97 ± 0.17 (n = 4) emphasizes the lipophilic character of the radiotracer which allows a passive diffusion through the blood–brain barrier [30–32]. However, there is a discrepancy compared to the published logD value of 3.16 ± 0.03 [20] which might be caused by different experimental setups.

In vitro autoradiography studies were accomplished by incubating sections of mouse brain with [^{18}F]**FESCH**. Non-specific binding was assessed by co-incubation with an excess of either **FESCH** or **ZM241385**, respectively. The images demonstrated an A_{2A}R-specific accumulation of [^{18}F]**FESCH** in the striatum (Figure 3), which is characterized by the binding parameters K_D = 4.69 ± 1.17 nM and B_{max} = 497 ± 97 fmol/mg wet weight consistent with the literature [33].

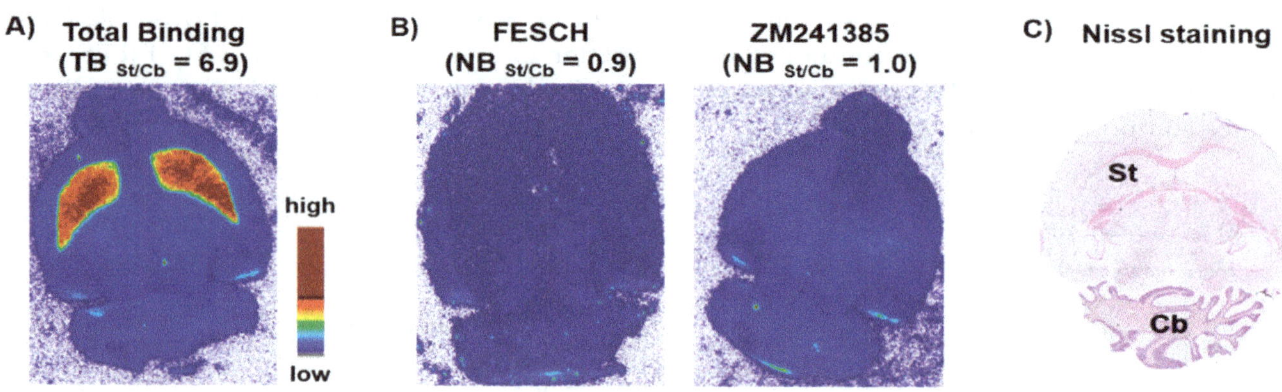

Figure 3. Representative autoradiographic images of transversal CD-1 mouse brain slices. (**A**) In vitro distribution of activity after incubation with 0.2 MBq/mL of [^{18}F]**FESCH** (TB = total binding). (**B**) Non-specific binding (NB) of [^{18}F]**FESCH** determined in the presence of 1 μM of **FESCH** or **ZM241385**, respectively, as blocking agents. (**C**) Nissl staining, St = Striatum, Cb = Cerebellum.

For in vivo imaging investigations in healthy CD-1 mice (n = 12, 10 weeks, 30–35 g), [^{18}F]**FESCH** was injected intravenously (baseline: 2.8 ± 2 MBq, vehicle: 5.8 ± 2 MBq, blocking: 6.4 ± 2.5 MBq with n = 4, respectively) and whole body scans were performed for 60 min in listmode with a Mediso nanoScan® PET/MR scanner followed by dynamic reconstruction. Time-activity curves (TACs) were generated for regions of interest such as striatum and cerebellum as reference region. The obtained PET images showed a high striatal uptake of [^{18}F]**FESCH** with a standardized uptake value ratio (SUVR) for striatum over cerebellum of > 5 (9–30 min post injection (p.i.)). In vivo selectivity for the A_{2A}R was highlighted by the significant reduction of the SUVR by 29–42% (9–30 min p.i. with $p < 0.05$) after pre-injection of **tozadenant** as blocking agent (Figure 4). The highest achievable dose of **tozadenant** was 2.5 mg/kg with respect to solubility and volume of injection as well as the concentrations of DMSO and Kolliphor® EL suitable for in vivo application in mice. The herein observed blocking effect is in accordance with the estimated A_{2A}R occupancy for **tozadenant** in rhesus monkey of about 72% at 5 mg/kg [14]. These results indicate that [^{18}F]**FESCH** is a promising radiotracer for molecular imaging of the A_{2A}R in the brain.

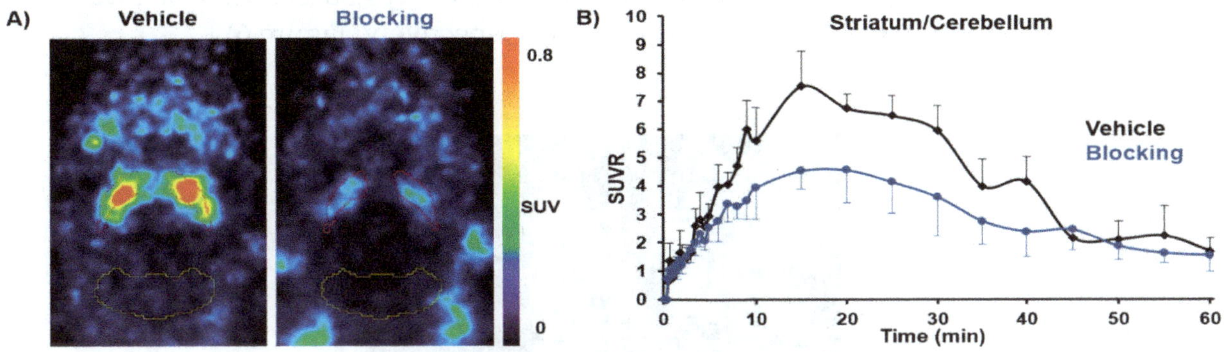

Figure 4. (**A**) Representative horizontal PET images of [^{18}F]**FESCH** uptake (average 10–30 min) in the brain of healthy CD-1 mice under vehicle (15 min pre-injection of DMSO:Kolliphor® EL:0.9% NaCl, 1:2:7, 5 μL/g) and blocking conditions (15 min pre-injection of **tozadenant** 2.5 mg/kg in DMSO:Kolliphor® EL:0.9% NaCl, 1:2:7, 5 μL/g; red = striatum; yellow = cerebellum). (**B**) Averaged TACs of [^{18}F]**FESCH** for vehicle (n = 4) and **tozadenant** pre-injected mice (n = 4) with SUVRs for striatum over cerebellum.

However, a representative metabolism study revealed only moderate in vivo stability of [^{18}F]**FESCH**. Analytical radio-HPLC (Figure 5) of the extracted mouse plasma sample showed 41% of intact radiotracer at 15 min p.i. (recovery of total activity = 84%). In the analyzed brain sample, one polar radiometabolite ([^{18}F]**M1**) was detected accounting for 29% of the total extracted activity at 15 min p.i. (recovery = 98%).

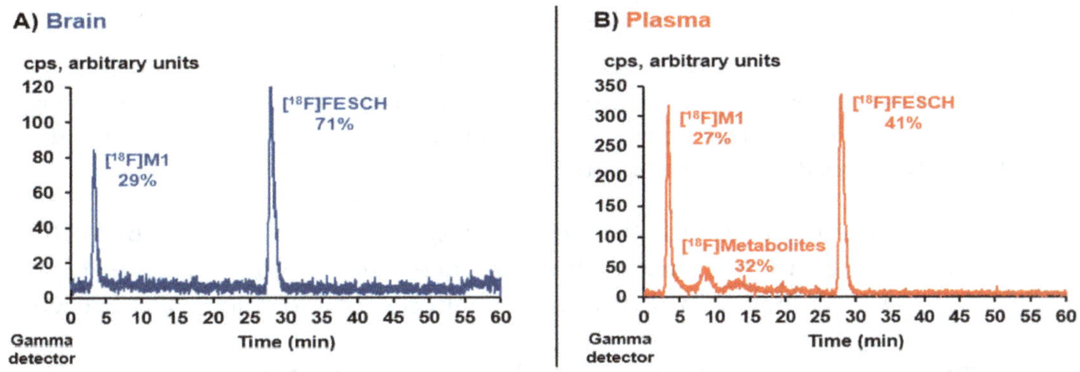

Figure 5. Representative in vivo metabolism study of CD-1 mouse plasma and brain samples at 15 min p.i. of [^{18}F]**FESCH** (~ 17 MBq): Analytical radio-HPLC profiles of extracted (**A**) brain and (**B**) plasma sample (column: Reprosil-Pur 120 C18-AQ, 250 × 4.6 mm, particle size: 5 μm; eluent: 26-90-26% MeCN/20 mM $NH_4OAc_{aq.}$, flow: 1 mL/min).

Compared to the published study in Wistar-Unilever rats (46% intact radiotracer in plasma at 60 min p.i. [20]) the in vivo degradation of [^{18}F]**FESCH** appears to be somewhat faster in mice. Notably and to the best of our knowledge, the formation of brain-penetrating radiometabolites of [^{18}F]**FESCH** has not been regarded before. Based on our experiences with radiotracers bearing a [^{18}F]fluoroethoxy moiety [34,35], the herein observed radiometabolite [^{18}F]**M1** is proposed to be 2-[^{18}F]fluoroethanol or the oxidized 2-[^{18}F]fluoroacetaldehyde and 2-[^{18}F]fluoroacetate, resulting from a cytochrome P450 enzyme-induced metabolic degradation [36,37], which are able to cross the blood–brain barrier [38–41].

For PET/MR studies with [^{18}F]**FESCH** in the rotenone-based mouse model of PD, the radiotracer (9.7 ± 1.3 MBq) was administrated to C57BL/6JRj mice (control: n = 5; rotenone-treated: n = 7; 16 months, 28–35 g) followed by the same imaging protocol used for the baseline and blocking studies in CD-1 mice. Although statistically not significant, the averaged TACs between 2 and 61 min p.i. revealed a slightly higher uptake of [^{18}F]**FESCH** in the striatum of rotenone-treated mice compared to controls.

An increase of the SUVR for striatum over cerebellum by 15–33% was observed, which was caused by the elevated SUV for striatum of 11–27% (21–61 min p.i., respectively; Figure 6).

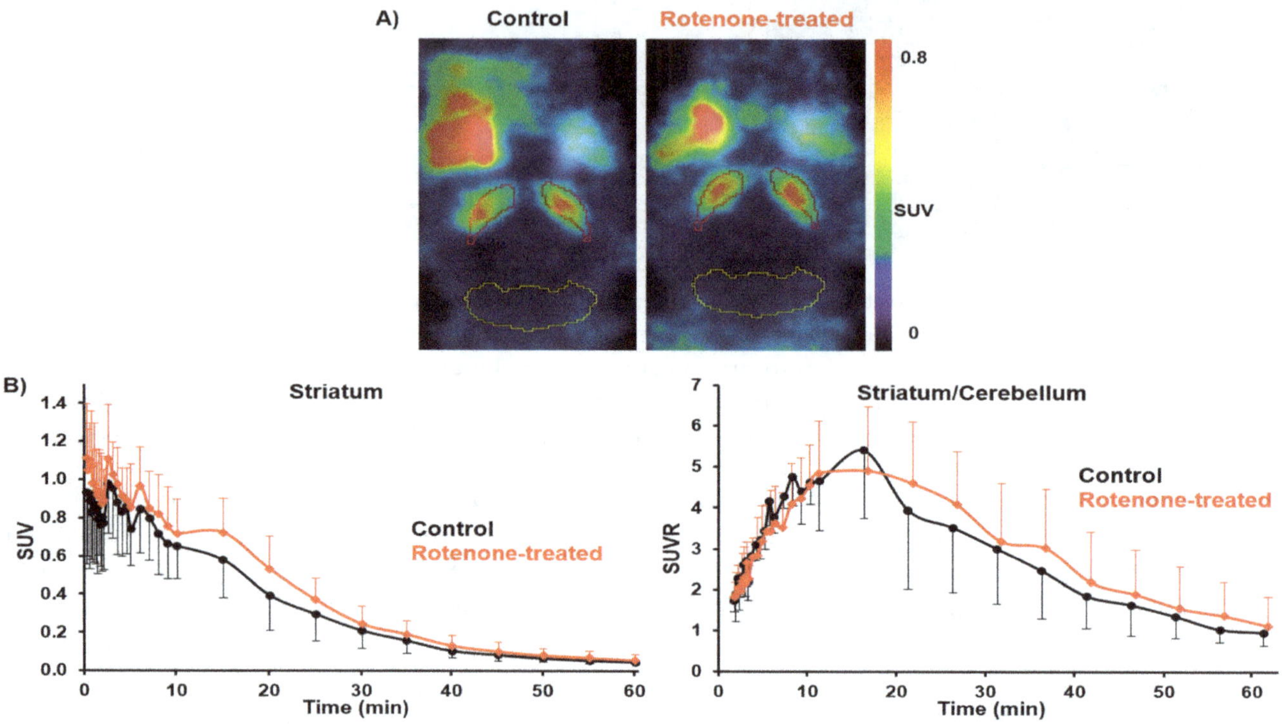

Figure 6. (**A**) Representative horizontal PET images of [^{18}F]**FESCH** uptake (average 2–61 min) in the brain of control and rotenone-treated C57BL/6JRj mice (red = striatum; yellow = cerebellum). (**B**) Averaged TACs of [^{18}F]**FESCH** for control (n = 5) and rotenone-treated mice (n = 7) with SUVs for striatum and SUVRs for striatum over cerebellum.

These results are in accordance with the determined $A_{2A}R$ levels on C57BL/6JRj mouse brain sections from a comparative in vitro immunofluorescence study. No significant difference in the fluorescence signal of the $A_{2A}R$ between control and rotenone-treated mice was observed (Figure 7).

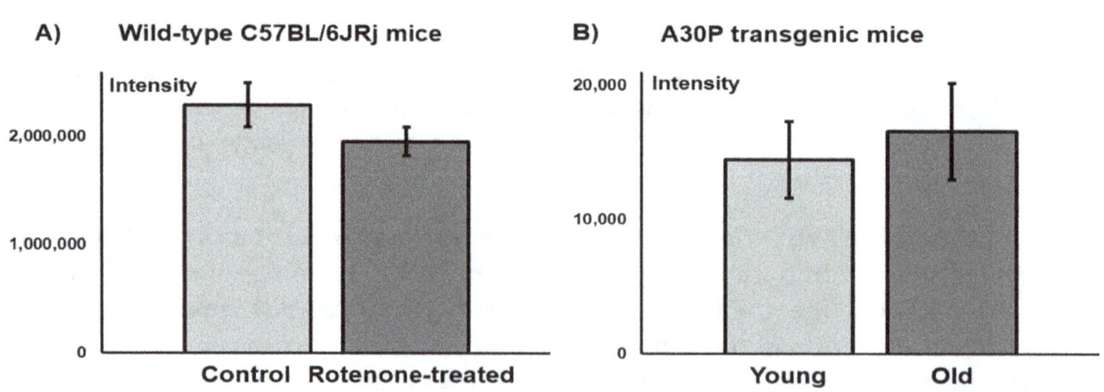

Figure 7. Mean fluorescence intensity of $A_{2A}R$ staining on the striatum of coronal C57BL/6JRj mouse brain sections: (**A**) Control vs. rotenone-treated wild-type mice (n = 3, respectively); (**B**) Young (39 weeks) vs. old (71–76 weeks) A30P transgenic mice (n = 3, respectively).

The increased $A_{2A}R$ availability in the striatum of PD patients appears to be related to L-DOPA-induced dyskinesia. In the rotenone-treated mice, we did not identify any signs of dyskinesia and, thus, it is not surprising that in this PD mouse model no significant increase in the $A_{2A}R$ density was detected either by PET imaging or by immunofluorescence staining. With regard to dyskinesia, the rotenone model is comparable to another neurotoxin-based PD mouse model using 1-methyl-4-phenyl-1,2,3,6-tetrahydropyridine (MPTP), where only weak signs of dyskinesia were observed and this exclusively under L-DOPA treatment [42]. To date, unilateral injection of 6-hydroxydopamine (6-OHDA) is the only effective neurotoxin-related approach to replicate evidently some forms of dyskinesia in rats and mice. In the 6-OHDA mouse model, dyskinesia is detected as abnormal involuntary movements (AIMs) with a more simplified range than in rats, presenting more prominent rotational locomotion with less dystonic features, i.e., axial AIMs [42]. None of the above-mentioned AIMs were detected in the rotenone-treated mice. Consequently, it remains to be examined whether treatment with L-DOPA would lead to dyskinesia in the rotenone model as shown for the MPTP model and if this would cause a quantifiable increase in striatal $A_{2A}R$ levels.

In contrast to the above-discussed neurotoxin-based PD animal models, the A30P mouse line represents a transgenic model of PD. This mouse line overexpresses the human A30P mutation in the α-synuclein gene, where the 30th amino acid residue alanine is replaced by proline, in all neurons. The A30P mutation is associated with rare familial cases of PD. Since α-synuclein is a main constituent of Lewy bodies, the A30P transgenic mice are characterized by Lewy body formation in neuronal cell bodies and neurites throughout the brain [43]. The α-synuclein pathology and PD-associated symptoms become prominent at about 69 weeks of age [43,44]. In an ongoing study, we detected slightly, but due to the rather small and highly variable data set statistically non-significant, higher striatal mean fluorescence intensities of the $A_{2A}R$ signal in older symptomatic A30P transgenic mice compared to younger ones without symptoms (see Figure 7). We will further investigate this PD mouse model by small animal PET/MR imaging studies using a novel derivative of [^{18}F]**FESCH** currently under development.

3. Summary and Conclusions

In this study, we investigated the suitability of the known radiotracer [^{18}F]**FESCH** for in vitro and in vivo imaging of the $A_{2A}R$ in the mouse brain by autoradiography and small animal PET/MR. Contrary to previous estimations, the herein observed brain-penetrating radiometabolite might limit the applicability of [^{18}F]**FESCH** for valid quantification of $A_{2A}R$ levels in the striatum with PET. One promising strategy to decelerate the degradation of ^{18}F-labeled radiotracers is the deuterium-hydrogen exchange at the metabolic labile position in the molecular structure of the compound [45]. Thus, our recent efforts are focused on a deuterated derivative of [^{18}F]**FESCH** with enhanced in vivo stability particularly at the [^{18}F]fluoroethoxy side chain.

In the investigated rotenone-based mouse model of PD, no significant difference in the striatal $A_{2A}R$ density between rotenone-treated mice and controls was detectable by PET imaging or immunofluorescence staining. These results indicate that the rotenone model does not reflect upregulation of striatal $A_{2A}R$ in PD, which appears to be related to dyskinesia. Therefore, it remains to be further examined whether treatment with L-DOPA could cause a detectable increase in $A_{2A}R$ levels in the striatum, which would induce observable dyskinesia in this PD model. In a parallel and ongoing study to characterize the A30P mouse model, initial findings reveal that this transgenic model might be more suitable with regard to displaying PD-like pathological changes in $A_{2A}R$ availability.

4. Materials and Methods

4.1. General Information

Chemicals and solvents were purchased from standard commercial sources in analytical grade and were used without further purification. Radio-TLCs were performed on pre-coated silica gel plates (Alugram® Xtra SIL G/UV_{254}, Polygram® SIL G/UV_{254}; Carl Roth, Karlsruhe, Germany). The compounds were localized at 254 nm (UV lamp). Radio-TLC was recorded using a bioimaging analyzer system (BAS-1800 II, Fuji Photo Film, Co. Ltd., Tokyo, Japan) and images were evaluated with Aida 2.31 software (raytest Isotopenmessgeräte GmbH, Straubenhardt, Germany). Column chromatography was conducted on silica gel (0.06–0.20 mm; Carl Roth, Karlsruhe, Germany). HPLC separations were performed on JASCO systems equipped with UV detectors from JASCO Deutschland GmbH (Pfungstadt, Germany) and activity detectors from raytest Isotopenmessgeräte GmbH (GABI Star, Straubenhardt, Germany).

Semi-preparative HPLC conditions were: Column: Reprosil-Pur C18-AQ, 250 × 10 mm; particle size: 10 μm; eluent: 50% MeCN/20 mM $NH_4OAc_{aq.}$; flow: 7 mL/min; ambient temperature; UV detection at 254 nm.

Analytical HPLC conditions were: Column: Reprosil-Pur C18-AQ, 250 × 4.6 mm; particle size: 5 μm; gradient: 0–10 min: 26% MeCN, 10–35 min: 26% → 90% MeCN, 35–45 min: 90% MeCN, 45–50 min: 90% → 26% MeCN, 50–60 min: 26% MeCN/20 mM $NH_4OAc_{aq.}$; isocratic: 40% MeCN/20 mM $NH_4OAc_{aq.}$; flow: 1 mL/min; ambient temperature; UV detection at 254 nm. Molar activity was determined on the base of a calibration curve (0.05–2.0 μg **FESCH**) carried out under isocratic HPLC conditions (36% MeCN/20 mM $NH_4OAc_{aq.}$) using chromatograms obtained at 264 nm as the maximum of UV absorbance.

No-carrier-added (n.c.a.) [^{18}F]fluoride ($t_{1/2}$ = 109.8 min) was produced via the [^{18}O(p,n)^{18}F] nuclear reaction by irradiation of [^{18}O]H_2O (Hyox 18 enriched water, Rotem Industries Ltd, Arava, Israel) on a Cyclone®18/9 (IBA RadioPharma Solutions, Louvain-la-Neuve, Belgium) with fixed energy proton beam using Nirta® [^{18}F]fluoride XL target.

4.2. Radiosynthesis

The aqueous solution of no-carrier-added [^{18}F]fluoride (~ 3 GBq) was trapped on a Chromafix® 30 PS-HCO_3^- cartridge (MACHEREY-NAGEL GmbH & Co. KG, Düren, Germany). The activity was eluted with 300 μL of an aqueous K_2CO_3-solution (1.78 mg, 12.9 μmol) into a 4-mL V-vial containing Kryptofix 2.2.2 ($K_{2.2.2}$, 5.6 mg, 14.9 μmol) in 1 mL MeCN. The K^+/[^{18}F]F^-/$K_{2.2.2}$-carbonate complex was azeotropically dried under vacuum and argon flow within 7–10 min using a Discover PETwave Microwave CEM® (75 W, 50–60 °C, power cycling mode, CEM GmbH, Kamp-Lintfort, Germany). Two aliquots of MeCN (2 × 1 mL) were added during the drying procedure and the final complex was dissolved in 400 μL MeCN ready for radiolabeling.

The aliphatic radiolabeling of ethane-1,2-diol bis(4-methylbenzenesulfonate) (Sigma-Aldrich, Munich, Germany; 2 mg in 100 μL MeCN) was performed under conventional heating at 90 °C for 10 min. After pre-heating of the phenol precursor desmethyl SCH442416 (2.5 mg in 490 μL MeCN) with 10 μL $TBAOH_{aq.}$ (40%) at 90 °C for 10 min, this solution was directly added to the crude 2-[^{18}F]fluoroethyl tosylate and the reaction mixture was stirred for 10 min at 120 °C. Aliquots of the reaction mixtures from both steps were analyzed by radio-TLC (EtOAc/petroleum ether; first step = 1:1; second step = 6:1) or radio-HPLC (isocratic mode, see General Information) to determine the radiochemical yields of crude 2-[^{18}F]fluoroethyl tosylate (R_f = 0.7, 87.0 ± 2.3%; n = 9) and [^{18}F]**FESCH** (R_f = 0.5, 46.4 ± 8.5%; t_R = 29.4 min, 34.4 ± 4.1%, decay corrected for t_R = 0 min; n = 9), respectively.

After dilution with water (1:1), the crude reaction mixture was applied to an isocratic semi-preparative HPLC (see General Information) for isolation of the desired radiotracer [^{18}F]**FESCH** (t_R = 32–33 min). The collected fractions were diluted with water (total volume = 40 mL), passed through a Sep-Pak® C18 Plus cartridge (Waters, Milford, MA, USA; pre-conditioned with 5 mL of absolute EtOH and 60 mL water), and eluted with 1.5 mL of absolute EtOH. Evaporation of the solvent at 70 °C under a gentle argon stream and subsequent formulation of the radiotracer in sterile isotonic saline containing 10% EtOH afforded a [^{18}F]**FESCH** solution usable for biological investigations.

The identity of the radiotracer was proved by analytical radio-HPLC (see General Information) of samples of [^{18}F]**FESCH** spiked with the non-radioactive reference compound **FESCH** using a gradient and an isocratic mode.

4.3. *Investigation of In Vitro Stability and Lipophilicity ($logD_{7.4}$)*

The in vitro stability of [^{18}F]**FESCH** (4–6 MBq) was studied by incubation in isotonic saline and pig plasma (500 µL each) at 37 °C. Samples were taken at 60 min and analyzed by radio-HPLC (see General Information).

The lipophilicity of [^{18}F]**FESCH** was examined by partitioning between *n*-octanol and phosphate-buffered saline (PBS, pH = 7.4) at ambient temperature using the conventional shake-flask method. The radiotracer (65 µL, ~ 8 MBq) was added to a tube containing the *n*-octanol/PBS-mixture (6 mL, 1:1, four-fold determination). The tubes were shaken for 20 min using a mechanical shaker (HS250 basic, IKA Labortechnik GmbH & Co. KG, Staufen, Germany) followed by centrifugation (5500 rpm for 5 min) and separation of the phases. Aliquots were taken from the organic and the aqueous phase (1 mL each) and activity was measured with an automated gamma counter (1480 WIZARD, Fa. Perkin Elmer, Waltham, MA, USA). The distribution coefficient ($D_{7.4}$) was calculated as [activity (cpm/mL) in *n*-octanol]/[activity (cpm/mL) in PBS, pH = 7.4] stated as the decade logarithm ($logD_{7.4}$).

4.4. *Binding Assay*

Membrane homogenates prepared from stably transfected CHO-K1 cells (Chinese hamster ovary cells, clone K1) with the human A_1R or $A_{2A}R$, provided by Prof. Klotz, University of Würzburg, Würzburg, Germany, were used for the binding experiments. The following radioligands were employed: [^{3}H]**ZM241385** for the $A_{2A}R$ and [^{3}H]**DPCPX** for the A_1R. For the determination of $A_{2A}R$ and A_1R binding affinity of reference compound, frozen cell suspensions were thawed, homogenized by a 27-gauge needle, and diluted with 50 mM TRIS-HCl buffer (pH = 7.4, 100 mM NaCl, 5 mM $MgCl_2$, 1 mM EDTA) containing 1 µU/mL adenosine deaminase (ADA). Membrane suspension was incubated with 1.5 nM [^{3}H]**ZM241385** or 1 nM [^{3}H]**DPCPX** and various concentrations of the test compound. Non-specific binding was determined by co-incubation with 10 µM **ZM241385** or 1 µM **DPCPX**. The incubation was performed at room temperature for 90 min and terminated by rapid filtration using Whatman GF/B glass-fiber filters, pre-soaked in 0.3% polyethyleneimine and a 48-channel harvester (Biomedical Research and Development Laboratories, Gaithersburg, MD, USA) followed by washing four times with ice-cold TRIS-HCl buffer. Filter-bound radioactivity was quantified by liquid scintillation counting. At least two separate experiments were performed for determination of K_i values. All data were analyzed with GraphPad Prism, Version 4.1 (GraphPad Inc., La Jolla, CA, USA), according to the Cheng–Prusoff equation.

4.5. *Animal Experiments*

All experimental work including animals was conducted in accordance with the national legislation on the use of animals for research (Tierschutzgesetz (TierSchG), Tierschutz-Versuchstierverordnung (TierSchVersV)) and was approved by the responsible animal care committees of the Free State of Bavaria and the Free State of Saxony (TVV 08/13, 24-9168.11/18/8, June 12th, 2013 and TVV 18/18, DD24.1-5131/446/19, June 20th, 2018; Landesdirektion Sachsen). Female CD-1 mice, 10–12 weeks, were obtained from the Medizinisch-Experimentelles Zentrum at University of Leipzig, Leipzig, Germany.

4.5.1. In Vitro Autoradiography

Cryosections of brains obtained from female CD-1 mice (10–12 weeks) were thawed, dried in a stream of cold air, and pre-incubated in 50 mM TRIS-HCl buffer (pH = 7.4, 100 mM NaCl, 5 mM $MgCl_2$, 1 mM EDTA) containing 1 µU/mL adenosine deaminase (ADA) for 15 min at ambient temperature. Afterwards, brain sections were incubated with 0.1–0.2 MBq/mL [^{18}F]**FESCH** in buffer for 90 min at room temperature. Non-specific binding was determined in the presence of 1 µM of **FESCH** or **ZM241385**, respectively. Subsequently, the sections were washed twice for 5 min in ice-cold TRIS-HCl buffer, and dipped for 5 s in ice-cold deionized water. The sections were rapidly dried in a stream of cold air before being exposed overnight on an imaging plate (Fujifilm Corporation, Tokyo, Japan). Developed autoradiographs were analyzed in a phosphor imager (HD-CR 35, Duerr NDT GmbH, Bietigheim Bissingen, Germany). The quantification was performed by using 2D-densitometric analysis (AIDA 2.31 software, raytest Isotopenmessgeräte GmbH, Straubenhardt, Germany). Further data analysis was performed with GraphPad Prism, Version 4.1 (GraphPad Inc., La Jolla, CA, USA).

4.5.2. Rotenone-Based and A30P Transgenic Mouse Models of Parkinson's Disease

Animal Housing

Male wild-type C57BL/6JRj mice (Janvier Labs, Le Genest-Saint-Isle, France) and male (Thy1)-*h*[A30P]α-syn transgenic C57BL/6JRj mice (generated according to the protocol by Kahle et al. [43], hereafter "A30P transgenic mice") were housed at room temperature under a 12:12 h dark:light cycle. Food and water was provided ad libidum.

Oral Rotenone Administration

Wild-type C57BL/6JRj mice (12 months) were divided into two groups and treated 5 days a week for 4 months. A 1.2 mm × 60 mm gavage (Unimed, Lausanne, Switzerland) was used to administer 0.01 mL/g animal weight of rotenone (Sigma-Aldrich, Munich, Germany) solution corresponding to a 5 mg/kg dose. Controls were treated only with the vehicle solution (2% carboxymethyl cellulose (Sigma-Aldrich, Munich, Germany) and 1.25% chloroform (Carl Roth, Karlsruhe, Germany)).

4.5.3. Immunofluorescence Staining and Imaging

Immunostaining

Cryosections of brains obtained from wild-type C57BL/6JRj mice (16 months, vehicle and rotenone-treated) or A30P transgenic mice (young group = 39 weeks; old group = 71–76 weeks) were immunostained using the free-floating technique and all procedures took place in a well of a 12-well plate. Briefly, brain sections were washed with PBS (pH = 7.4) for 10 min, then blocked with blocking solution (PBS, 0.02% Triton-X and 5% donkey serum) for 1 h, and incubated in the first antibody (1:100, rabbit anti-adenosine receptor A_{2A}, ab3461, Abcam, Cambridge, UK) in blocking solution at 4 °C overnight. On the next day, sections were washed in PBS (4 × 15 min) and incubated with the secondary antibody (1:500, donkey Alexa® 555 anti-rabbit, Invitrogen/Thermo Fisher Scientific Inc., Waltham, MA, USA) for three hours at room temperature. Sections were washed in PBS (4 × 15 min), transferred to the slide, and mounted with Mowiol mounting medium (50% PBS, 25% ethylenglycol and 25% glycerol).

Microscopy and Image Analysis

Images were obtained with an Apotome.2 fluorescence microscope (Carl Zeiss Microscopy GmbH, Jena, Germany). Mean fluorescence intensity (MFI) in the striatum was measured using Fiji-ImageJ, a free-software for image analysis (ImageJ v1.52p, National Institutes of Health (NIH), Bethesda, MD, USA). MFI values were normalized to background signal.

4.5.4. Small Animal PET/MR Studies

For the time of the experiments, female CD-1 mice (n = 12; age = 10 weeks; weight = 30–35 g) and male C57BL/6JRj mice (control with n = 5; rotenone-treated with n = 7; age = 16 months; weight = 28–35 g) were kept in a dedicated climatic chamber with free access to water and food under a 12:12 h dark:light cycle at a constant temperature of 24 °C. The animals received an injection of $[^{18}F]$**FESCH** into the tail vein (5.0 ± 2.5 MBq for CD-1 mice) or retro-orbital (9.7 ± 1.3 MBq for C57BL/6JRj mice) followed by a 60-min PET/MR scan (Mediso nanoScan®, Budapest, Hungary). Each PET image was corrected for random coincidences, dead time, scatter, and attenuation (AC), based on a whole body (WB) MR scan. The reconstruction parameters for the list mode data were the following: 3D-ordered subset expectation maximization (OSEM), 4 iterations, 6 subsets, energy window = 400–600 keV, coincidence mode = 1–5, ring difference = 81. The mice were positioned prone in a special mouse bed (heated up to 37 °C), with the head fixed to a mouth piece for the anesthetic gas supply with isoflurane in 40% air and 60% oxygen (anesthesia unit: U-410, Agnthos, Lidingö, Sweden; gas blender: MCQ, Rome, Italy). The PET data were collected by a continuous WB scan during the entire investigation. Following the 60-min PET scan, a T1-weighted WB gradient echo sequence (GRE, repetition time = 20 ms, echo time = 6.4 ms) was performed for AC and anatomical orientation. Image registration and evaluation of the region of interest (ROI) were done with PMOD (PMOD Technologies LLC, v. 3.9, Zurich, Switzerland).

The respective brain regions were identified using the mouse brain atlas template Ma–Benveniste–Mirrione–FDG. The activity data are expressed as mean standardized uptake value (SUV) of the overall ROI.

4.5.5. In Vivo Metabolism Study

The radiotracer [^{18}F]**FESCH** (~ 17 MBq in 150 μL isotonic saline) was injected into a female CD-1 mouse via the tail vein. Brain and blood samples were obtained at 15 min p.i., plasma separated by centrifugation (14,000 × *g*, 1 min), and brain homogenized in ~ 1 mL isotonic saline on ice (10 strokes of a polytetrafluoroethylene (Teflon®) plunger at 1000 rpm in a borosilicate glass cylinder; Potter S Homogenizer, B. Braun Melsungen AG, Melsungen, Germany).

Two consecutive extractions were performed as duplicate (plasma) or triplicate (brain) determinations. Plasma (50 μL) and brain samples (250 μL) were added to an ice-cold acetone/water mixture (4:1; plasma or brain sample/organic solvent = 1:4). The samples were vortexed for 1 min, incubated on ice for 10 min (first extraction) or 5 min (second extraction) and centrifuged at 10,000 rpm for 5 min. Supernatants were collected and the precipitates were re-dissolved in 100 μL of the ice-cold acetone/water mixture (4:1) for the second extraction. Activity of aliquots from supernatants of each extraction step and of the precipitates was quantified using an automated gamma counter (1480 WIZARD, Fa. Perkin Elmer). The supernatants from both extractions were combined, concentrated at 70 °C under argon stream, and analyzed by radio-HPLC (gradient mode, see General Information). By this protocol, [^{18}F]**FESCH** was quantitatively extracted from the biological material as proven by in vitro incubation of the radiotracer in pig plasma.

Author Contributions: S.S., T.H.L., and R.-P.M. designed and performed organic syntheses; S.S., T.H.L., R.T., and B.W. designed and performed radiosyntheses; S.S., T.H.L., A.C., S.D.-S., W.D.-C., F.P.-M., and P.B. designed and performed in vitro and in vivo studies; M.T., M.K., Q.S., W.D.-C., and P.B. designed and performed PET/MR studies; S.S., T.H.L., M.T., M.K., A.C., Q.S., S.D.-S., W.D.-C., F.P.-M., and P.B. analyzed the data. All authors read and approved the final manuscript.

Acknowledgments: We thank Karsten Franke and Steffen Fischer, HZDR, for providing [^{18}F]fluoride.

References

1. Gerlach, M.; Reichmann, H.; Riederer, P. *Die Parkinson-Krankheit: Grundlagen, Klinik, Therapie*; Springer: Wien, Austria; New York, NY, USA, 2007; p. 453.
2. De Lera Ruiz, M.; Lim, Y.-H.; Zheng, J. Adenosine A_{2A} receptor as a drug discovery target. *J. Med. Chem.* **2014**, *57*, 3623–3650. [CrossRef] [PubMed]
3. Jorg, M.; Scammells, P.J.; Capuano, B. The dopamine D_2 and adenosine A_{2A} receptors: Past, present and future trends for the treatment of Parkinson's disease. *Curr. Med. Chem.* **2014**, *21*, 3188–3210. [CrossRef] [PubMed]

4. Ferre, S.; von Euler, G.; Johansson, B.; Fredholm, B.B.; Fuxe, K. Stimulation of high-affinity adenosine A_2 receptors decreases the affinity of dopamine D_2 receptors in rat striatal membranes. *Proc. Natl. Acad. Sci. USA* **1991**, *88*, 7238–7241. [CrossRef] [PubMed]
5. Ferré, S.; Bonaventura, J.; Tomasi, D.; Navarro, G.; Moreno, E.; Cortés, A.; Lluís, C.; Casadó, V.; Volkow, N.D. Allosteric mechanisms within the adenosine A_{2A}–dopamine D_2 receptor heterotetramer. *Neuropharmacology* **2016**, *104*, 154–160. [CrossRef]
6. Nazario, L.R.; da Silva, R.S.; Bonan, C.D. Targeting adenosine signaling in Parkinson's disease: From pharmacological to non-pharmacological approaches. *Front. Neurosci.* **2017**, *11*, 658. [CrossRef]
7. LeWitt, P.A.; Guttman, M.; Tetrud, J.W.; Tuite, P.J.; Mori, A.; Chaikin, P.; Sussman, N.M.; Group, U.S.S. Adenosine A_{2A} receptor antagonist istradefylline (KW-6002) reduces "off" time in Parkinson's disease: A double-blind, randomized, multicenter clinical trial (6002-US-005). *Ann. Neurol.* **2008**, *63*, 295–302. [CrossRef]
8. Hauser, R.A.; Cantillon, M.; Pourcher, E.; Micheli, F.; Mok, V.; Onofrj, M.; Huyck, S.; Wolski, K. Preladenant in patients with Parkinson's disease and motor fluctuations: A phase 2, double-blind, randomised trial. *Lancet Neurol.* **2011**, *10*, 221–229. [CrossRef]
9. Hauser, R.A.; Olanow, C.W.; Kieburtz, K.D.; Pourcher, E.; Docu-Axelerad, A.; Lew, M.; Kozyolkin, O.; Neale, A.; Resburg, C.; Meya, U.; et al. Tozadenant (SYN115) in patients with Parkinson's disease who have motor fluctuations on levodopa: A phase 2b, double-blind, randomised trial. *Lancet Neurol.* **2014**, *13*, 767–776. [CrossRef]
10. Dungo, R.; Deeks, E.D. Istradefylline: First global approval. *Drugs* **2013**, *73*, 875–882. [CrossRef]
11. Villar-Menéndez, I.; Porta, S.; Buira, S.P.; Pereira-Veiga, T.; Díaz-Sánchez, S.; Albasanz, J.L.; Ferrer, I.; Martín, M.; Barrachina, M. Increased striatal adenosine A_{2A} receptor levels is an early event in Parkinson's disease-related pathology and it is potentially regulated by miR-34b. *Neurobiol. Dis.* **2014**, *69*, 206–214. [CrossRef]
12. Khanapur, S.; Waarde, A.V.; Ishiwata, K.; Leenders, K.L.; Dierckx, R.A.J.O.; Elsinga, P.H. Adenosine A_{2A} receptor antagonists as positron emission tomography (PET) tracers. *Curr. Med. Chem.* **2014**, *21*, 312–328. [CrossRef]
13. Ramlackhansingh, A.F.; Bose, S.K.; Ahmed, I.; Turkheimer, F.E.; Pavese, N.; Brooks, D.J. Adenosine 2A receptor availability in dyskinetic and nondyskinetic patients with Parkinson disease. *Neurology* **2011**, *76*, 1811–1816. [CrossRef]
14. Barret, O.; Hannestad, J.; Alagille, D.; Vala, C.; Tavares, A.; Papin, C.; Morley, T.; Fowles, K.; Lee, H.; Seibyl, J.; et al. Adenosine 2A receptor occupancy by tozadenant and preladenant in rhesus monkeys. *J. Nucl. Med.* **2014**, *55*, 1712–1718. [CrossRef]
15. Barret, O.; Hannestad, J.; Vala, C.; Alagille, D.; Tavares, A.; Laruelle, M.; Jennings, D.; Marek, K.; Russell, D.; Seibyl, J.; et al. Characterization in humans of ^{18}F-MNI-444, a novel PET radiotracer for brain adenosine A_{2A} receptors. *J. Nucl. Med.* **2015**, *56*, 586–591. [CrossRef]
16. Chen, J.-F.; Eltzschig, H.K.; Fredholm, B.B. Adenosine receptors as drug targets—What are the challenges? *Nat. Rev. Drug Discov.* **2013**, *12*, 265–286. [CrossRef] [PubMed]
17. Svenningsson, P.; Hall, H.; Sedvall, G.; Fredholm, B.B. Distribution of adenosine receptors in the postmortem human brain: An extended autoradiographic study. *Synapse* **1997**, *27*, 322–335. [CrossRef]
18. Shinkre, B.A.; Kumar, T.S.; Gao, Z.-G.; Deflorian, F.; Jacobson, K.A.; Trenkle, W.C. Synthesis and evaluation of 1,2,4-triazolo[1,5-*c*]pyrimidine derivatives as A_{2A} receptor-selective antagonists. *Bioorg. Med. Chem. Lett.* **2010**, *20*, 5690–5694. [CrossRef] [PubMed]
19. Bhattacharjee, A.K.; Lang, L.; Jacobson, O.; Shinkre, B.; Ma, Y.; Niu, G.; Trenkle, W.C.; Jacobson, K.A.; Chen, X.; Kiesewetter, D.O. Striatal adenosine A_{2A} receptor-mediated positron emission tomographic imaging in 6-hydroxydopamine-lesioned rats using [^{18}F]-MRS5425. *Nucl. Med. Biol.* **2011**, *38*, 897–906. [CrossRef]
20. Khanapur, S.; Paul, S.; Shah, A.; Vatakuti, S.; Koole, M.J.B.; Zijlma, R.; Dierckx, R.A.J.O.; Luurtsema, G.; Garg, P.; van Waarde, A.; et al. Development of [^{18}F]-labeled pyrazolo[4,3-*e*]-1,2,4- triazolo[1,5-*c*]pyrimidine (SCH442416) analogs for the imaging of cerebral adenosine A_{2A} receptors with positron emission tomography. *J. Med. Chem.* **2014**, *57*, 6765–6780. [CrossRef]
21. Khanapur, S.; van Waarde, A.; Dierckx, R.A.; Elsinga, P.H.; Koole, M.J. Preclinical evaluation and quantification of ^{18}F-fluoroethyl and ^{18}F-fluoropropyl analogs of SCH442416 as radioligands for PET imaging of the adenosine A_{2A} receptor in rat brain. *J. Nucl. Med.* **2017**, *58*, 466–472. [CrossRef]

22. Pan-Montojo, F.; Anichtchik, O.; Dening, Y.; Knels, L.; Pursche, S.; Jung, R.; Jackson, S.; Gille, G.; Spillantini, M.G.; Reichmann, H.; et al. Progression of Parkinson's disease pathology is reproduced by intragastric administration of rotenone in mice. *PLoS ONE* **2010**, *5*, e8762. [CrossRef] [PubMed]
23. Arnhold, M.; Dening, Y.; Chopin, M.; Arévalo, E.; Schwarz, M.; Reichmann, H.; Gille, G.; Funk, R.H.W.; Pan-Montojo, F. Changes in the sympathetic innervation of the gut in rotenone-treated mice as possible early biomarker for Parkinson's disease. *Clin. Auton. Res.* **2016**, *26*, 211–222. [CrossRef]
24. Pan-Montojo, F.; Schwarz, M.; Winkler, C.; Arnhold, M.; O'Sullivan, G.A.; Pal, A.; Said, J.; Marsico, G.; Verbavatz, J.M.; Rodrigo-Angulo, M.; et al. Environmental toxins trigger PD-like progression via increased alpha-synuclein release from enteric neurons in mice. *Sci. Rep.* **2012**, *2*, 898. [CrossRef] [PubMed]
25. Moon, Y.; Lee, K.H.; Park, J.-H.; Geum, D.; Kim, K. Mitochondrial membrane depolarization and the selective death of dopaminergic neurons by rotenone: Protective effect of coenzyme Q10. *J. Neurochem.* **2005**, *93*, 1199–1208. [CrossRef] [PubMed]
26. Betarbet, R.; Sherer, T.B.; MacKenzie, G.; Garcia-Osuna, M.; Panov, A.V.; Greenamyre, J.T. Chronic systemic pesticide exposure reproduces features of Parkinson's disease. *Nat. Neurosci.* **2000**, *3*, 1301–1306. [CrossRef] [PubMed]
27. Baraldi, P.G.; Cacciari, B.; Romagnoli, R.; Spalluto, G.; Monopoli, A.; Ongini, E.; Varani, K.; Borea, P.A. 7-Substituted 5-amino-2-(2-furyl)pyrazolo[4,3-*e*]-1,2,4-triazolo[1,5-*c*]pyrimidines as A_{2A} adenosine receptor antagonists: A study on the importance of modifications at the side chain on the activity and solubility. *J. Med. Chem.* **2002**, *45*, 115–126. [CrossRef]
28. Damont, A.; Hinnen, F.; Kuhnast, B.; Schöllhorn-Peyronneau, M.-A.; James, M.; Luus, C.; Tavitian, B.; Kassiou, M.; Dollé, F. Radiosynthesis of [^{18}F]DPA-714, a selective radioligand for imaging the translocator protein (18 kDa) with PET. *J. Label. Compd. Rad.* **2008**, *51*, 286–292. [CrossRef]
29. Schröder, S.; Lai, T.H.; Kranz, M.; Toussaint, M.; Shang, Q.; Dukic-Stefanovic, S.; Pan-Montojo, F.; Brust, P. Investigation of [^{18}F]FESCH for PET imaging of the adenosine A_{2A} receptor in a rotenone-based mouse model of Parkinson´s disease and development of a two-step one-pot radiolabeling strategy. *J. Label. Compd. Rad.* **2019**, *62*, S183.
30. Tavares, A.A.S.; Lewsey, J.; Dewar, D.; Pimlott, S.L. Radiotracer properties determined by high performance liquid chromatography: A potential tool for brain radiotracer discovery. *Nucl. Med. Biol.* **2012**, *39*, 127–135. [CrossRef]
31. Clark, D.E. *In silico* prediction of blood–brain barrier permeation. *Drug Discov. Today* **2003**, *8*, 927–933. [CrossRef]
32. Waterhouse, R.N. Determination of lipophilicity and its use as a predictor of blood–brain barrier penetration of molecular imaging agents. *Mol. Imaging Biol.* **2003**, *5*, 376–389. [CrossRef] [PubMed]
33. Sihver, W.; Schulze, A.; Wutz, W.; Stusgen, S.; Olsson, R.A.; Bier, D.; Holschbach, M.H. Autoradiographic comparison of *in vitro* binding characteristics of various tritiated adenosine A_{2A} receptor ligands in rat, mouse and pig brain and first *ex vivo* results. *Eur. J. Pharmacol.* **2009**, *616*, 107–114. [CrossRef] [PubMed]
34. Schröder, S.; Wenzel, B.; Deuther-Conrad, W.; Teodoro, R.; Kranz, M.; Scheunemann, M.; Egerland, U.; Höfgen, N.; Briel, D.; Steinbach, J.; et al. Investigation of an ^{18}F-labelled imidazopyridotriazine for molecular imaging of cyclic nucleotide phosphodiesterase 2A. *Molecules* **2018**, *23*, 556. [CrossRef] [PubMed]
35. Liu, J.; Wenzel, B.; Dukic-Stefanovic, S.; Teodoro, R.; Ludwig, F.-A.; Deuther-Conrad, W.; Schröder, S.; Chezal, J.-M.; Moreau, E.; Brust, P.; et al. Development of a new radiofluorinated quinoline analog for PET imaging of phosphodiesterase 5 (PDE5) in brain. *Pharmaceuticals* **2016**, *9*, 22. [CrossRef] [PubMed]
36. Zoghbi, S.S.; Shetty, H.U.; Ichise, M.; Fujita, M.; Imaizumi, M.; Liow, J.-S.; Shah, J.; Musachio, J.L.; Pike, V.W.; Innis, R.B. PET imaging of the dopamine transporter with [^{18}F]FECNT: A polar radiometabolite confounds brain radioligand measurements. *J. Nucl. Med.* **2006**, *47*, 520–527.
37. Evens, N.; Vandeputte, C.; Muccioli, G.G.; Lambert, D.M.; Baekelandt, V.; Verbruggen, A.M.; Debyser, Z.; Van Laere, K.; Bormans, G.M. Synthesis, *in vitro* and *in vivo* evaluation of fluorine-18 labelled FE-GW405833 as a PET tracer for type 2 cannabinoid receptor imaging. *Bioorgan. Med. Chem.* **2011**, *19*, 4499–4505. [CrossRef]
38. Lear, J.L.; Ackermann, R.F. Evaluation of radiolabeled acetate and fluoroacetate as potential tracers of cerebral oxidative metabolism. *Metab. Brain Dis.* **1990**, *5*, 45–56. [CrossRef]
39. Mori, T.; Sun, L.-Q.; Kobayashi, M.; Kiyono, Y.; Okazawa, H.; Furukawa, T.; Kawashima, H.; Welch, M.J.; Fujibayashi, Y. Preparation and evaluation of ethyl[^{18}F]fluoroacetate as a proradiotracer of [^{18}F]fluoroacetate for the measurement of glial metabolism by PET. *Nucl. Med. Biol.* **2009**, *36*, 155–162. [CrossRef]

40. Muir, D.; Berl, S.; Clarke, D.D. Acetate and fluoroacetate as possible markers for glial metabolism *in vivo*. *Brain Res.* **1986**, *380*, 336–340. [CrossRef]
41. Ponde, D.E.; Dence, C.S.; Oyama, N.; Kim, J.; Tai, Y.-C.; Laforest, R.; Siegel, B.A.; Welch, M.J. ^{18}F-Fluoroacetate: A potential acetate analog for prostate tumor imaging—*In vivo* evaluation of ^{18}F-fluoroacetate versus ^{11}C-acetate. *J. Nucl. Med.* **2007**, *48*, 420–428.
42. Peng, Q.; Zhong, S.; Tan, Y.; Zeng, W.; Wang, J.; Cheng, C.; Yang, X.; Wu, Y.; Cao, X.; Xu, Y. The rodent models of dyskinesia and their behavioral assessment. *Front. Neurol.* **2019**, *10*, 1016. [CrossRef] [PubMed]
43. Kahle, P.J.; Neumann, M.; Ozmen, L.; Müller, V.; Jacobsen, H.; Schindzielorz, A.; Okochi, M.; Leimer, U.; van der Putten, H.; Probst, A.; et al. Subcellular localization of wild-type and Parkinson's disease-associated mutant α-synuclein in human and transgenic mouse brain. *J. Neurosci.* **2000**, *20*, 6365–6373. [CrossRef] [PubMed]
44. Wagner, J.; Ryazanov, S.; Leonov, A.; Levin, J.; Shi, S.; Schmidt, F.; Prix, C.; Pan-Montojo, F.; Bertsch, U.; Mitteregger-Kretzschmar, G.; et al. Anle138b: A novel oligomer modulator for disease-modifying therapy of neurodegenerative diseases such as prion and Parkinson's disease. *Acta Neuropathol.* **2013**, *125*, 795–813. [CrossRef] [PubMed]
45. Kuchar, M.; Mamat, C. Methods to increase the metabolic stability of ^{18}F-radiotracers. *Molecules* **2015**, *20*, 16186–16220. [CrossRef]

5

Development of Novel Analogs of the Monocarboxylate Transporter Ligand FACH and Biological Validation of One Potential Radiotracer for Positron Emission Tomography (PET) Imaging

Masoud Sadeghzadeh [1,*], Barbara Wenzel [1], Daniel Gündel [1], Winnie Deuther-Conrad [1], Magali Toussaint [1], Rareş-Petru Moldovan [1], Steffen Fischer [1], Friedrich-Alexander Ludwig [1], Rodrigo Teodoro [1], Shirisha Jonnalagadda [2], Sravan K. Jonnalagadda [2], Gerrit Schüürmann [3,4], Venkatram R. Mereddy [2], Lester R. Drewes [5] and Peter Brust [1]

[1] Department of Neuroradiopharmaceuticals, Institute of Radiopharmaceutical Cancer Research, Helmholtz-Zentrum Dresden-Rossendorf, Permoserstraße 15, 04318 Leipzig, Germany; b.wenzel@hzdr.de (B.W.); d.guendel@hzdr.de (D.G.); w.deuther-conrad@hzdr.de (W.D.-C.); m.toussaint@hzdr.de (M.T.); r.moldovan@hzdr.de (R.-P.M.); s.fischer@hzdr.de (S.F.); f.ludwig@hzdr.de (F.-A.L.); r.teodoro@hzdr.de (R.T.); p.brust@hzdr.de (P.B.)

[2] Department of Chemistry and Biochemistry, Department of Pharmacy Practice & Pharmaceutical Sciences, University of Minnesota, Duluth, MN 55812, USA; sgurrapu@d.umn.edu (S.J.); skjonnal@d.umn.edu (S.K.J.); vmereddy@d.umn.edu (V.R.M.)

[3] UFZ Department of Ecological Chemistry, Helmholtz Centre for Environmental Research, Permoserstraße 15, 04318 Leipzig, Germany; gerrit.schuurmann@ufz.de

[4] Institute of Organic Chemistry, Technical University Bergakademie Freiberg, Leipziger Straße 29, 09599 Freiberg, Germany

[5] Department of Biomedical Sciences, University of Minnesota Medical School Duluth, 251 SMed, 1035 University Drive, Duluth, MN 55812, USA; ldrewes@d.umn.edu

* Correspondence: m.sadeghzadeh@hzdr.de

Academic Editors: Anne Roivainen and Xiang-Guo Li

Abstract: Monocarboxylate transporters 1-4 (MCT1-4) are involved in several metabolism-related diseases, especially cancer, providing the chance to be considered as relevant targets for diagnosis and therapy. [^{18}F]FACH was recently developed and showed very promising preclinical results as a potential positron emission tomography (PET) radiotracer for imaging of MCTs. Given that [^{18}F]FACH did not show high blood-brain barrier permeability, the current work is aimed to investigate whether more lipophilic analogs of FACH could improve brain uptake for imaging of gliomas, while retaining binding to MCTs. The 2-fluoropyridinyl-substituted analogs **1** and **2** were synthesized and their MCT1 inhibition was estimated by [^{14}C]lactate uptake assay on rat brain endothelial-4 (RBE4) cells. While compounds **1** and **2** showed lower MCT1 inhibitory potencies than FACH (IC_{50} = 11 nM) by factors of 11 and 25, respectively, **1** (IC_{50} = 118 nM) could still be a suitable PET candidate. Therefore, **1** was selected for radiosynthesis of [^{18}F]**1** and subsequent biological evaluation for imaging of the MCT expression in mouse brain. Regarding lipophilicity, the experimental log $D_{7.4}$ result for [^{18}F]**1** agrees pretty well with its predicted value. In vivo and in vitro studies revealed high uptake of the new radiotracer in kidney and other peripheral MCT-expressing organs together with significant reduction by using specific MCT1 inhibitor α-cyano-4-hydroxycinnamic acid. Despite a higher lipophilicity of [^{18}F]**1** compared to [^{18}F]FACH, the in vivo brain uptake of [^{18}F]**1** was in a similar range, which is reflected by calculated BBB permeabilities as well through similar transport rates by MCTs on RBE4 cells. Further investigation is needed to clarify the MCT-mediated transport mechanism of these radiotracers in brain.

Keywords: monocarboxylate transporters (MCTs); FACH; ^{18}F-labeled analog of FACH; α-CCA; blood-brain barrier (BBB); positron emission tomography (PET) imaging

1. Introduction

Monocarboxylate transporters (MCTs), comprising 14 isoforms, are dedicated to the solute carrier 16 (*SLC16*) gene family [1,2]. Of all the MCT isoforms, MCT1-4 are well characterized and known as membrane-bound carriers that bidirectionally transport short-chain monocarboxylic acids, most notably L-lactate, pyruvate, and ketone bodies along with protons across the plasma membrane of mammalian cells [2]. The tissue distribution of the MCT isoforms is quite variable. Although MCT1 is ubiquitously distributed in the muscles, it is additionally expressed along with MCT4 in the brain and other peripheral organs like small intestine, liver, heart, kidney, and blood cells [1,3]. Aberrant expression such as, upregulation of MCT1 and MCT4 has been reported in a large number of tumors (e.g., neuroblastomas, high-grade gliomas, carcinomas of renal cells, breast epithelium, colorectal and squamous tissues, and cervical and lung cancers) where expression is correlated to poor outcomes. In these tissues, the MCTs serve to facilitate the shuttling of lactate between cells with different metabolic requirements [4–6]. Due to the metabolic reprogramming, considered as a hallmark of cancer, tumor cells indeed switch from glucose to lactate as a crucial energy supply, hence, their metabolism heavily relies on glycolysis and consequently the lactate efflux through MCT1 and MCT4 in order to prevent their own acidosis and to regenerate NAD^+ [7]. Accordingly, both transporters are attractive therapeutic and even diagnostic targets for the treatment and detection of human cancers [4,7,8].

Positron emission tomography (PET) is known as a powerful tool for non-invasive molecular detection of early metabolic changes in cancer progression [9]. [^{18}F]Fluorodeoxyglucose ([^{18}F]FDG), a radiolabeled glucose analog, is well known as a standard PET tracer used for diagnosis, staging and treatment monitoring in clinical oncology [10,11]. Considering the lack of specificity and sensitivity of [^{18}F]FDG for several types of tumors [10], there is still an unmet clinical need for cancer detection and therapy. Thus, the complementary concept based on components of the aerobic glycolysis and metabolism by malignant cells is more intriguing and potentially rewarding [2,12–14]. In this regard, [^{18}F]DASA-23, recently developed as a potent radiotracer for imaging tumor glycolysis by targeting pyruvate kinase M2, is currently in phase I clinical trials (ClinicalTrials.gov, NCT03539731) [15]. Because the metabolic reprogramming in cancer cells may also result in the overexpression of MCT1/MCT4 in many cancers [4,7], MCT-targeting PET studies provide an opportunity to achieve more accurate and useful understanding of certain aspects of the tumor-specific metabolism [8,16].

During the last decade, only a few ^{11}C- or ^{18}F-labeled substrates of MCTs such as [^{11}C]lactate, [^{11}C]pyruvate as well as their ^{18}F-labeled analogs were investigated for imaging of MCTs by PET [17–20]. To the best of our knowledge, only limited examples of the MCTs inhibitors were investigated as PET radiotracers for in vivo applications [21]. Although one of the best characterized inhibitors, α-cyano-4-hydroxycinnamic acid (α-CCA), possesses a 10-fold selectivity for MCT1 compared to other subtypes (Figure 1) [22], it also shows significant inhibitory potency towards the mitochondrial pyruvate carrier in isolated mitochondria [23]. Accordingly, very potent and more specific MCT1/MCT4 inhibitors have been developed based on a comprehensive structure-activity relationship study on a series of α-CCA derivatives [24,25]. Based on this approach, we recently developed and evaluated [^{18}F]FACH as the first ^{18}F-labeled inhibitor of MCTs (Figure 1) [26]. Along with a high inhibitory potency towards MCT1 (11.0 nM) and MCT4 (6.5 nM) [26], [^{18}F]FACH showed very promising pharmacokinetics in healthy mice, in particular in the kidneys, as organ with a high physiological expression of MCT1 [1,3,27].

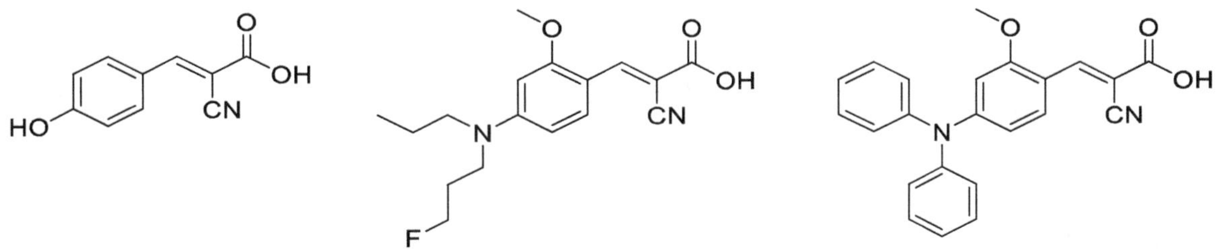

	α-CCA	FACH	Compound A
IC_{50} (MCT1)[a]:	150 μM	11 nM	8.0 nM
IC_{50} (MCT4)[a]:	—	6.5 nM	23.0 nM

Figure 1. Chemical structures of α-CCA and its novel derivatives as potent monocarboxylate transporters 1/4 (MCT1/MCT4) inhibitors; [a] Inhibition of [^{14}C]lactate uptake was determined in RBE4 cells (for MCT1) and in MDA-MB-231 cells (for MCT4) by measuring intracellular radioactivity after 60 min incubation without and with the respective inhibitor at 37 °C [25].

Nonetheless, [^{18}F]FACH showed only moderate brain uptake, which might be related to the rather hydrophilic features (log $D_{7.4}$ = 0.42) [28], assuming that [^{18}F]FACH could only passively enter the brain. This assumption would be in accordance with the fact that for the structural analog α-CCA, the site of its MCT inhibition has been demonstrated to be the extracellular surface [29,30]. Moreover, it is well established that MCT1 is also the prominent monocarboxylic acid transporter in the cerebral microvascular endothelium, facilitating the bidirectional transport of lactate through brain endothelial cells and the blood-brain barrier (BBB) [31]. Many brain tumors, such as gliomas and neuroblastomas, produce high amounts of lactic acid and consequently up-regulate MCT1, thus, inducing acidosis in the tumor microenvironment [5]. MCT1 is therefore proposed as a most likely therapeutic target for neuroblastomas and gliomas, and α-CCA has been able to suppress tumor growth via inhibition of MCT1 [5,32,33]. Accordingly, the development of MCT1-targeting radiotracers possessing sufficiently high brain permeability would be an important step forward toward brain imaging.

Although α-CCA as well as its new analog FACH (Figure 1) contain a Michael acceptor unit, their highly predominating carboxylate form under physiological conditions (ACD-calculated $pK_a < 1$ vs. pH 7.4; see Table 1 below) masks a respective electrophilic reactivity. This implies that these compounds are most likely not active as protein-attacking electrophiles. Moreover and as mentioned above, α-CCA has been reported to remain extracellular, inhibiting MCT from the outside in a competitive manner and without adverse effects under therapeutic concentrations [29,30].

In this context, it is interesting that for all respective cinnamic acid derivatives, the electron-withdrawing α-CN substituent is required for their MCT inhibition potency, which holds also for FACH [26]. As a possible explanation, we hypothesize that their non-covalent interaction with the MCT protein at the cellular surface may include an electrostatic Arg-carboxylate binding motif as primary anchor. This may facilitate a further complex stabilization through approaching a Cys-thiol by the Michael acceptor β-carbon that is activated further through the α-CN substitution (Figure 2, left). To balance the carboxylate anionic charge, a separate extracellular proton, required for the MCT action as respective symporter, could be attached temporarily at a His-nitrogen (not shown in Figure 2). In case of a successful carboxylate transport such as for the lactate efflux, a respective (additional) His-proton could be liberated to the interstitial compartment.

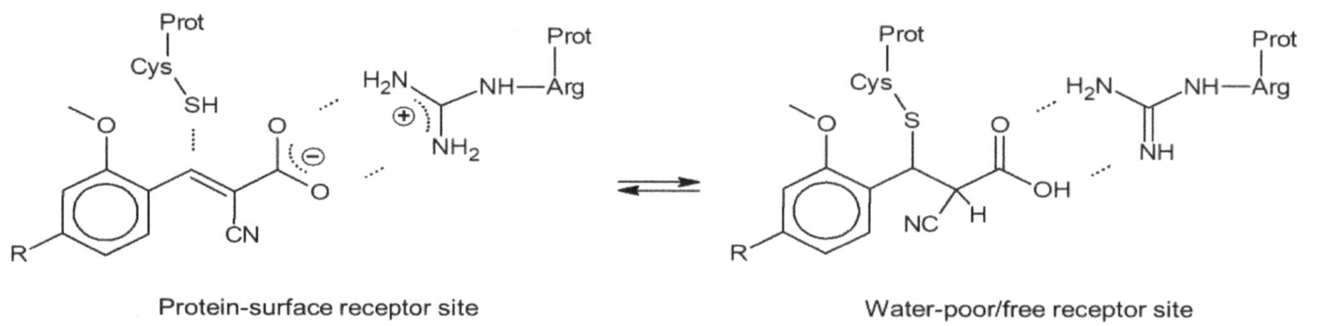

Figure 2. Hypothetical MCT-inhibitor binding at the extracellular surface (left) and at an interior protein site with no aqueous solvation (right). Michael addition may become active for the neutral carboxylic acid form (right), but would be reversible due to the α-CN substitution that enhances the retro-Michael reaction significantly (see, e.g., [34,35]).

In case the Arg-carboxylate interaction would result in a charge compensation sufficient to unmask the Michael acceptor reactivity, the Cys-thiol might add to the α,β-unsaturated unit, possibly following a proton transfer from Arg to the carboxylate (right part of Figure 2). In this case, however, the α-CN substituent enhances both the Michael and the retro-Michael reactivity, making this covalent reaction reversible through stabilization of the carbanion intermediate [34,35]. In conclusion, we hypothesize that despite the Michael acceptor unit common to all cinnamic acid derivatives, their mode of action is probably non-covalent or under water-poor/free conditions at least only temporarily covalent, with a correspondingly negligible risk to form permanent covalent bonds to nucleophilic protein sites. Results from a respective toxicity study will be reported in due course.

With the goal to improve the brain uptake by passive diffusion, we designed new analogs of FACH by replacing the less lipophilic propyl groups with more lipophilic aryl and heteroaryl moieties (Figure 3). Notably, the structurally modified analogs yet need to retain an acceptable inhibitory potency towards MCT1. On the basis of compound A, which was reported to exhibit high MCT1 inhibition (IC_{50} = 8.0 nM, Figure 1) [25], two fluorinated analogs were developed by introducing 2-fluoropyridinyl and phenyl groups (compounds **1** and **2**, Figure 3). Herein we describe the organic synthesis of the new compounds and their inhibitory potency for MCT1-mediated lactate transport. Furthermore, radiofluorination of **1** was performed and the resulting new radiotracer [^{18}F]**1** was investigated in mice to assess the impact of higher lipophilicity on the in vivo features compared to [^{18}F]FACH for imaging of MCT1 in mouse brain.

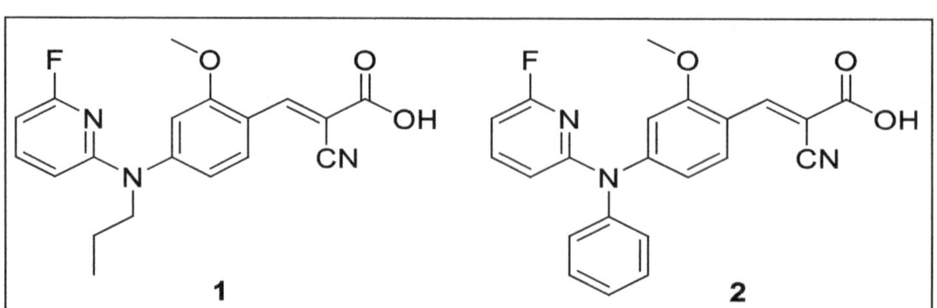

Figure 3. New analogs of FACH investigated in the current study.

2. Results and Discussion

2.1. Organic Chemistry and Monocarboxylate Transporter Inhibition

For developing the compounds **1** and **2**, the di-arylamine intermediate **5** was synthesized via the Buchwald-Hartwig aryl amination according to the previously reported procedures (Scheme 1) [36,37].

Alkylation of 6-fluoro-*N*-(3-methoxyphenyl)pyridin-2-amine **5** using 1-iodopropane and sodium hydride afforded **6** in 95% yield [38]. Compound **7** was obtained via a second Buchwald–Hartwig amination of **5** with phenyl bromide in negligible yield (< 10%). However, a stepwise addition of the palladium (Pd) catalyst and the phosphine ligand together with a longer reaction time led to the formation of **7** in moderate yield (46%). This might be related to the decreased electron density of the nitrogen atom due to the 2-fluoropyridinyl substituent and/or the steric hindrance effect. Both **6** and **7** were afterwards subjected to Vilsmeier–Haack formylation [39] to afford **8** and **9** with yields of 57% and 68%, respectively. Finally, Knoevenagel condensation of aldehydes **8** and **9** with cyanoacetic acid generated **1** and **2** in nearly quantitative yields (Scheme 1) [26].

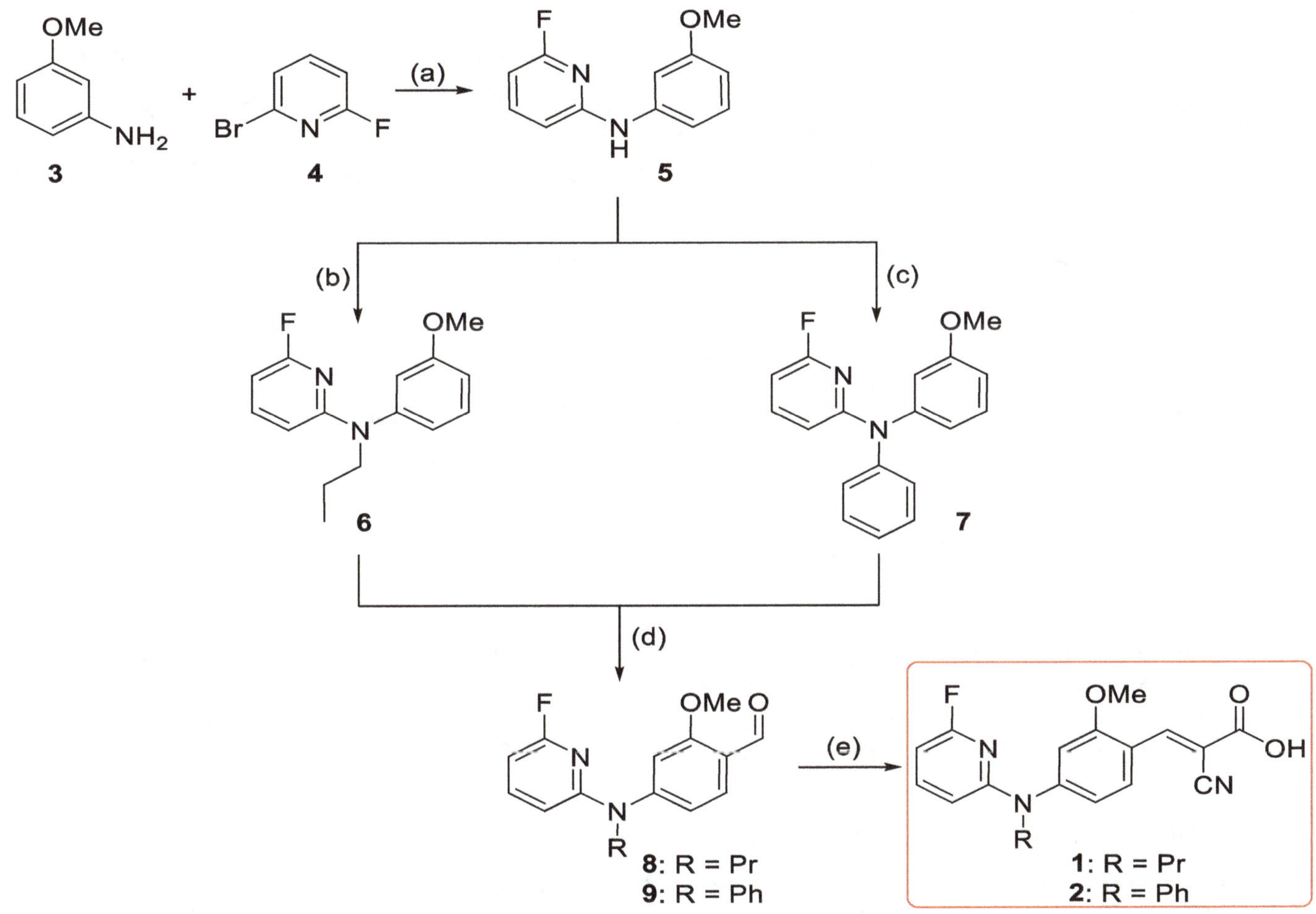

Scheme 1. Synthesis of **1** and **2**; reagents and reaction conditions: (a) $Pd(OAc)_2$ (5 mol %), Xantphos (5 mol %), Cs_2CO_3, 1,4-dioxane, Ar, 105 °C, 50 min, 96%; (b) 1-iodopropane, NaH (60% oil dispersion), DMF, Ar, r.t., 1.5 h, 95%; (c) PhBr, $Pd(OAc)_2$ (15 mol %), Xantphos (15 mol %), Cs_2CO_3, 1,4-dioxane, Ar, 105 °C, 24 h, 46%; (d) $POCl_3$, DMF, Ar, 80 °C, 2–4 h, 57% (for **8**) and 68% (for **9**); (e) *i.* cyanoacetic acid, piperidine, ACN, reflux; *ii.* HCl (6 M), r.t. 30 min, 95% (for **1**) and 98% (for **2**).

Inhibition of MCT1-mediated lactate transport of **1** and **2** was investigated by [^{14}C]lactate uptake assays using immortalized rat brain endothelial-4 cells (RBE4) [40] which express mainly MCT1 [24,25]. Both compounds dose-dependently inhibited the lactate uptake, with IC_{50} values of 118 nM (**1**) and 274 nM (**2**). Accordingly, replacing the 1-fluoropropyl group of FACH by a 2-fluoropyridinyl group in **1** resulted in a 10-fold decrease of the inhibitory potency. When comparing **2** with compound A, the substitution of the phenyl ring by a 2-fluoropyridinyl ring in **2** (Figure 1) caused an even stronger reduction of the inhibitory potency [25]. We therefore decided to proceed with **1** for radiofluorination and biological evaluation.

In order to develop the new MCT1-targeting radiotracer [^{18}F]**1**, a precursor including a suitable leaving group was required for the nucleophilic aromatic substitution (S_NAr) with [^{18}F]fluoride. A nitro precursor (**15**) with an unprotected carboxylic acid function (Scheme 2) was synthesized considering the good results obtained for the aliphatic nucleophilic substitution with unprotected precursor in the one-step radiosynthesis of [^{18}F]FACH [28]. Initial Buchwald–Hartwig aryl amination between 2-amino-6-nitropyridine and 3-bromoanisole provided the *N*-substituted anisidine **12** in 80% yield (Scheme 2) [36]. Alkylation of **12** under basic condition provided **13** with a yield of 93% [38]. Vilsmeier–Haack formylation of **13** gave aldehyde **14** in 92% yield [39]. It was followed by Knoevenagel condensation with cyanoacetic acid to provide **15** in 67% overall yield [26]. The chemical purity of the precursor **15** was > 98%, according to NMR and HPLC analyses.

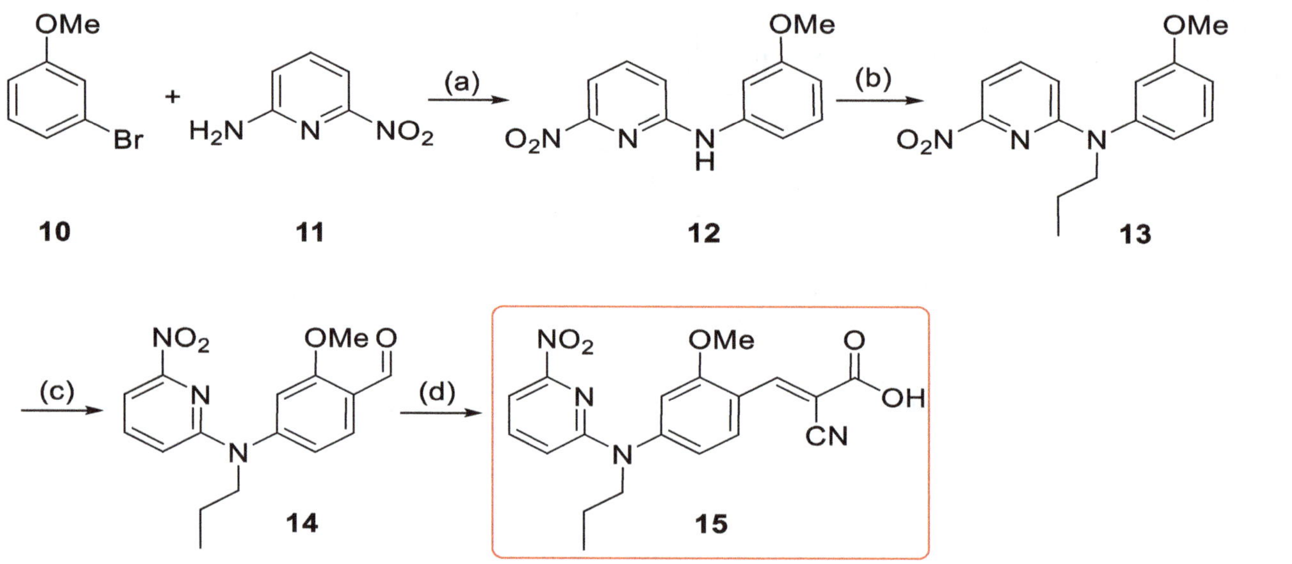

Scheme 2. Synthesis of the nitro precursor (**15**): Reagents and reaction conditions: (a) $Pd(OAc)_2$ (5 mol %), Xantphos (5 mol %), Cs_2CO_3, 1,4-dioxane, Ar, 105 °C, 2 h, 80%; (b) 1-iodopropane, NaH (60% oil dispersion), DMF, Ar, r.t., 1.5 h, 93%; (c) $POCl_3$, DMF, Ar, 80 °C, 1.5 h, 92%; (d) i. cyanoacetic acid, piperidine, ACN, reflux, 5 h; ii. HCl (6 M), r.t. 30 min, above 98%.

2.2. *Radiosynthesis, Stability, and Determination of log $D_{7.4}$*

As shown in Scheme 3, [^{18}F]**1** was synthesized on the basis of an S_NAr reaction via substitution of the NO_2 leaving group of **15** by [^{18}F]fluoride in the presence of Kryptofix® ($K_{2.2.2}$) and K_2CO_3. In dimethylsulfoxide (DMSO), the S_NAr reaction proceeded smoothly and resulted in high radiochemical yields of 73 ± 12% (n = 4, non-isolated, radio-HPLC) for [^{18}F]**1** after 15 min conventional heating at 130 °C. Besides unreacted [^{18}F]F^-, radioactive by-products accounted for less than 5%. [^{18}F]**1** was isolated by semi-preparative HPLC (Supplementary Data, Figure S1A), trapped on a pre-conditioned Sep-Pak C18 light cartridge, eluted with ethanol, and formulated in isotonic saline containing 10% of EtOH (*v*/*v*) for better solubility. Analytical radio- and UV-HPLC analyses of the final product co-eluted with the reference **1**, confirmed the identity of the radiotracer (Supplementary Data, Figure S1B). Finally, [^{18}F]**1** was obtained with radiochemical yields of 51 ± 11% (n = 3, decay-corrected to the end of the bombardment) in a total radiosynthesis time of about 90 min, at a radiochemical purity of ≥ 98% and with molar activities in the range of 180–200 GBq/μmol (n = 3, end of synthesis) using starting activities of 2–3 GBq.

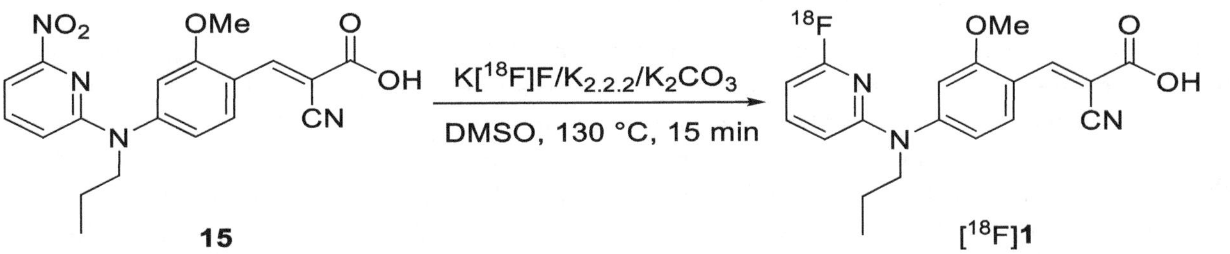

Scheme 3. Radiosynthesis of [^{18}F]**1**.

The stability of the radiotracer was investigated by incubation of [^{18}F]**1** in *n*-octanol, saline, phosphate-buffered saline (PBS) and ethanol. Samples were analyzed by radio-thin-layer chromatography (TLC) and radio-HPLC and no degradation or defluorination was observed in any of the solvents after 60 min incubation at 40 °C.

A variety of physicochemical parameters affects the brain permeability of different brain-targeting radiotracers [41]. Lipophilicity, often, but not necessarily, correlates with the ability to cross the BBB, and is considered as an important physicochemical property. In Table 1, calculated bioavailability-related parameters are listed for α-CCA, FACH and selected structural analogs. Accordingly, the new derivatives **1** and **2** show the desired higher hydrophobicity (log K_{OW} = logarithmic *n*-octanol/water partition coefficient [42], log $D_{7.4}$ = log K_{OW} corrected for ionization at pH 7.4 [43,44]) as compared to FACH. Nevertheless, Table 1 also shows that the predicted brain-blood partition coefficients (log K_{BB} [43]) of **1** (–0.49) and **2** (–1.05) are below the one of FACH (–0.10).

Table 1. Calculated physicochemical parameters of our drug candidates and structurally related compounds.[1]

Compound	log K_{OW}	log $D_{7.4}$	f_u	pK_a	log K_{BB}
FACH	4.43	0.69	4.5×10^{-8}	0.05	−0.10
Compound A	5.41	1.66	2.5×10^{-7}	0.80	−0.57
1	4.83	1.08	7.4×10^{-8}	0.27	−0.49
2	5.07	1.32	2.1×10^{-7}	0.73	−1.05
Cinnamic acid	2.07	−0.91	8.7×10^{-4}	4.34	−0.14
α-CN cinnamic acid	2.27	−1.48	1.6×10^{-7}	0.60	−0.54
α-CCA	1.79	−1.96	2.8×10^{-7}	0.85	−0.45

[1] The decadic logarithms of the *n*-octanol/water partition coefficient (log K_{OW}) have been calculated with EPI Suite [42], and these values have been employed for predicting the pK_a-pH-corrected *n*-octanol/water distribution coefficients, log $D_{7.4}$. For the latter, the ACD approach log K_{OW} (ionized) = log K_{OW} (unionized) − 3.75 (applicable for the relevant range of log K_{OW} data) [43,44] with $D_{7.4} = f_u \times K_{OW} + (1 - f_u) \times K_{OW}$ (ionized) has been employed (see also [44]). Note that the ACD-calculated log K_{OW} data are lower by 0.5–1.5 log units except for a slightly larger value for cinnamic acid, resulting in correspondingly lower calculated log $D_{7.4}$ data. Moreover, f_u denotes the compound fraction unionized at pH 7.4 according to the Henderson-Hasselbalch relationship, and pK_a as well as the brain-blood partition coefficient (K_{BB}) have been calculated with the ACD software.

Note further that FACH is both more lipophilic and more BBB-permeable than α-CCA. Regarding the Michael-acceptor unit mentioned above, comparison of cinnamic acid and its α-CN derivative shows that the α-CN substitution decreases the pK_a value by 3.7 units, most likely because of its combined inductive and mesomeric electron-withdrawing effect. Accordingly, all α-CCA derivatives are significantly acidic with pK_a values below 1, indicating for all of them that the dissociated carboxylate form is prevalent under physiological conditions. Experimental investigation of the lipophilicity of [^{18}F]**1** through employing the shake-flask method using *n*-octanol and PBS (pH 7.4) resulted in a log $D_{7.4}$ value of 0.820 ± 0.003 (n = 4). This value agrees pretty well with its calculated counterpart of 1.08 (Table 1), which holds correspondingly for the FACH log $D_{7.4}$ value (0.42 experimental [28] vs. 0.69 calculated) as well as for the respective difference in log $D_{7.4}$ values.

2.3. *In Vitro and In Vivo Biological Validation of [^{18}F]**1***

It is well demonstrated that several members of the MCT family are highly expressed in mammalian kidney, where over 95% of the lactate reabsorption takes place [1,3,45,46]. MCT1 mRNA and protein have clearly been detected on both the human kidney derived cell line HK-2 and human kidney cortex. In HK-2 cells it was found exclusively on the basal membrane [45]. Therefore, the specific binding of [^{18}F]**1** to MCTs was initially proven by in vitro autoradiography using cryosections of the mouse kidney. As reflected by the autoradiographic images presented in Figure 4, co-incubation of ~1 nM [^{18}F]**1** with 10 µM α-CCA-Na resulted in significantly lower binding of the radiotracer. Therefore, the binding of [^{18}F]**1** in mouse kidney in vitro is highly specific.

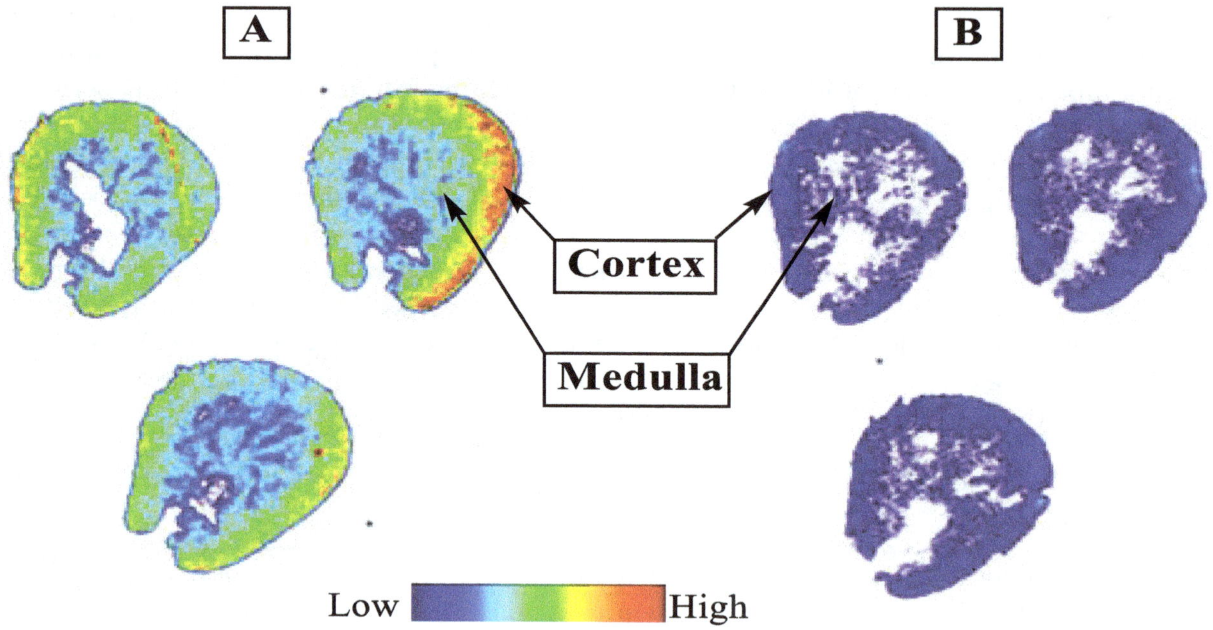

Figure 4. In vitro autoradiography of [^{18}F]**1** in transversal cryosections of the mouse kidney. Total (**A**) and non-specific (**B**) binding of ~1 nM [^{18}F]**1** obtained without and with co-incubation with 10 µM α-CCA-Na.

To investigate the stability of [^{18}F]**1** in vivo, samples of plasma and brain homogenates obtained from CD-1 mice at 30 min after intravenous injection of the radiotracer were analyzed for radiometabolites by using reversed-phase and micellar (MLC) radio-HPLC. MLC allows a direct injection of the samples into the HPLC system without the elimination of the tissue matrix as already described [47,48]. In general, the results obtained with both methods are comparable and the analyses revealed solely intact radiotracer and no detectable radiometabolites in plasma (Figure 5A–B) and brain (Supplementary Data, Figure S2) samples. Notably, in both samples two peaks a/b were detected by analytical HPLC (Figure 5/Figure S2) which are supposed to represent the neutral and deprotonated form of the radiotracer ([^{18}F]**1a/b**). This finding suggests that the analytical HPLC conditions do not reflect the physiological milieu at which the neutral compound fraction would be negligible according to the Henderson–Hasselbalch equation. Research into the speciation of **1** under analytical-chemical conditions is subject to a future investigation.

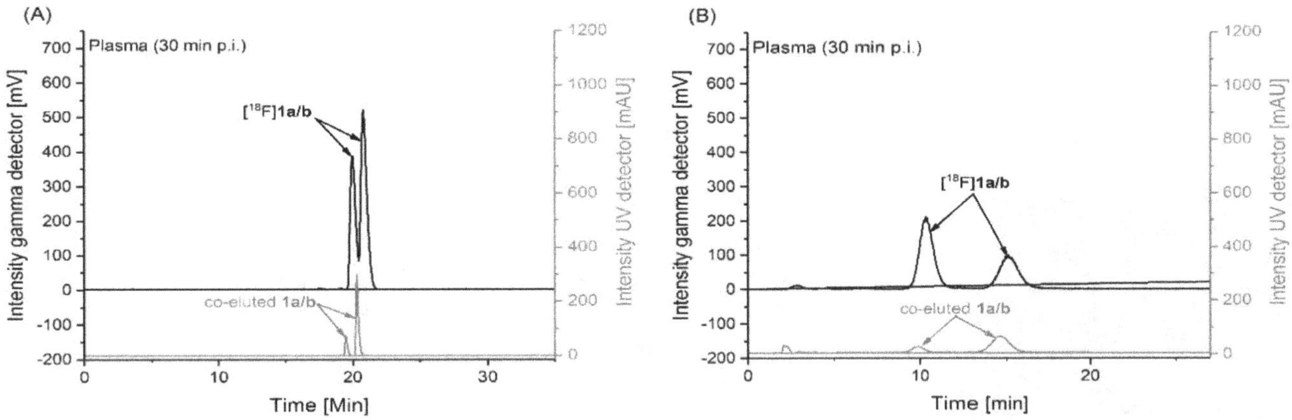

Figure 5. Analytical UV- and radio-HPLC chromatograms representing two peaks a/b which are supposed to reflect the neutral and deprotonated form of the radiotracer ([^{18}F]**1a/b**) in mouse plasma at 30 min p.i. measured under: (**A**) reversed phase (Reprosil-Pur C18-AQ, 250 × 4.6 mm, gradient with an eluent mixture of ACN/20 mM NH_4OAc (aq.), 370 nm, 1.0 mL/min), and (**B**) micellar conditions (Reprosil-Pur C18-AQ, 250 × 4.6 mm, isocratic mode with water containing 50 mM sodium dodecyl sulfate/10 mM $NaHPO_4$, 1.0 mL/min).

Pharmacokinetic studies of [^{18}F]**1** were performed by dynamic PET imaging in mouse using a dedicated small animal PET/MR camera. The target-specificity of [^{18}F]**1** was investigated by pre-administration of the blocking compound α-CCA-Na. Maximum intensity projections of PET studies from a representative control and α-CCA-Na treated animals and time-activity curves (TACs) from tissues of interest are presented in Figure 6. [^{18}F]**1** cleared rapidly from the blood with an initial TAC peak standardized uptake value (SUV) of 7.3 and a SUV of 1.5 after 10 min followed by a slow blood clearance to a SUV of 0.9 after 60 min in the control group (Figure 6B). Pre-administration of the MCT inhibitor α-CCA-Na resulted in an initial TAC peak SUV of 6.9 which was comparable to the control group, whereas a higher SUV of 3.5 after 10 min and a SUV of 1.5 was reached after 60 min p.i., reflecting higher availability of the radiotracer in the blood (Figure 6B). This is expected to be caused by blocking the uptake of [^{18}F]**1** in peripheral organs in vivo. In comparison to the control conditions, the pre-administration of α-CCA-Na significantly reduced the activity accumulation in the MCT1-expressing renal cortex [46] throughout the whole imaging period, which is shown by the SUV ratio (SUVR) of kidney cortex-to-blood (Figure 6D). Furthermore, the displacement study revealed 39.2% drop of the SUV, 20 min after i.v. injection of α-CCA-Na (Figure 6E), which implicates a reversible tissue uptake of [^{18}F]**1** in the kidney cortex. Nevertheless, further studies are needed to clarify the exact mechanism of the radiotracer uptake. Regarding liver, where the highly expressed MCT1 transports L-lactate into the parenchymal cells for gluconeogenesis [1], a constantly increasing accumulation of activity can be observed under both control and blocking conditions, although at lower values under pre-administration of α-CCA-Na (Figure 6C).

Taking into consideration the high activity concentrations persistently accumulated in the kidney and liver, the blocking effect of α-CCA-Na in both tissues will result in a strong increase in the fraction of available tracer in blood as reflected by the higher SUV in blood observed in the blocking experiments (Area Under the Curve $(AUC)_{0-60\ min}$ = 140 SUV × minutes) compared to the control experiments ($AUC_{0-60\ min}$ = 75 SUV × minutes).

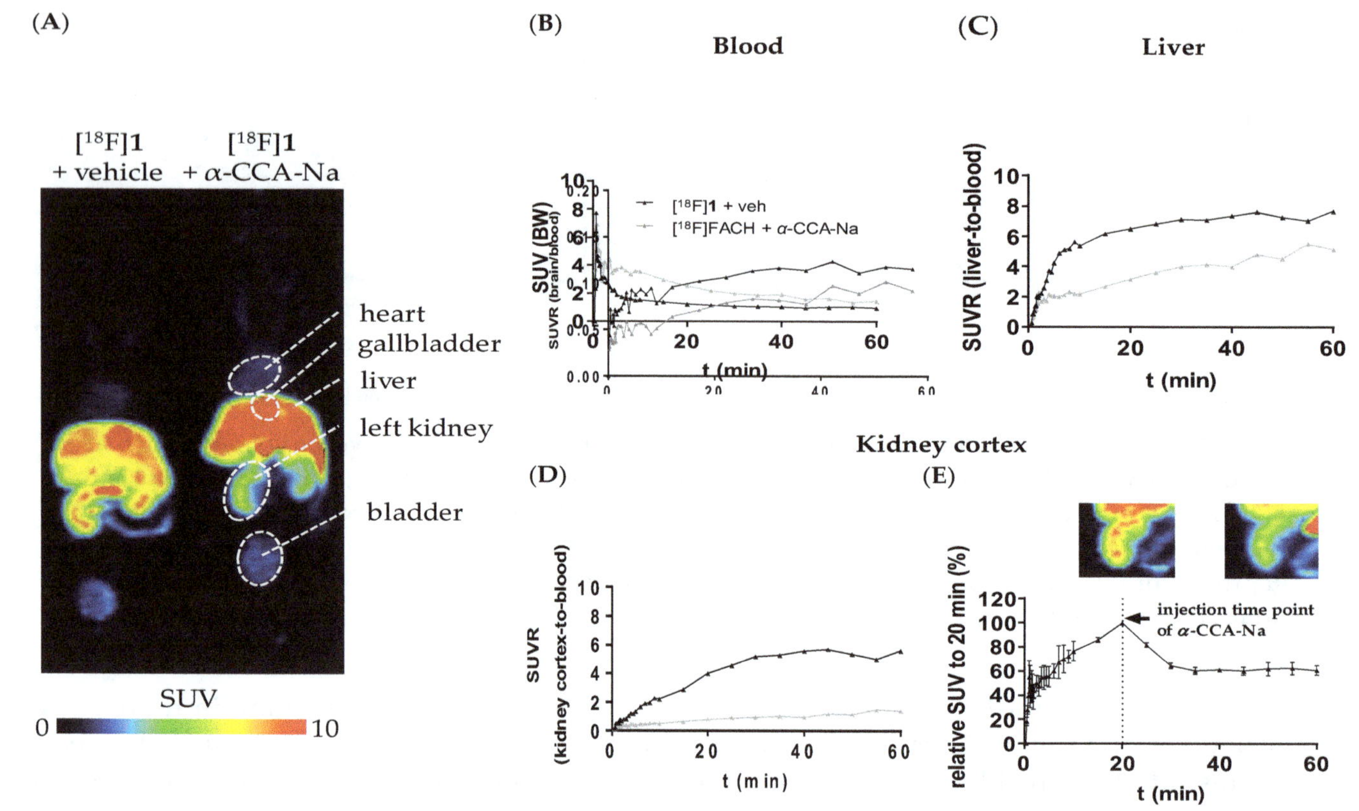

Figure 6. (**A**) Maximum intensity projections (MIPs) of small animal positron emission tomography (PET) images (45–60 min p.i., n = 1) of female CD-1 mice depicting the differential distribution of [^{18}F]**1** in peripheral organs without and with pre-administration of α-CCA-Na; (**B**–**D**) Time-activity curves representing the SUV of blood, as well as the standardized uptake value (SUV) ratio (SUVR) from liver-to-blood and kidney cortex-to-blood; (**E**) displacement study: i.v. application of α-CCA-Na 20 min after tracer injection (n = 2), MIPs of the left kidney (left: 15–20 min p.i. and right: 45–60 min p.i.).

According to Figure 7A, [^{18}F]**1** shows a similar brain uptake as [^{18}F]FACH despite a somewhat higher lipophilicity. Note, however, that this is in accordance with our ACD predictions regarding both log $D_{7.4}$ and log K_{BB} values (Table 1). The slightly higher lipophilicity (log K_{ow} and log $D_{7.4}$) of **1** is accompanied by a slightly lower BBB penetration (log K_{BB}), demonstrating further that passive brain uptake is not governed alone by log $D_{7.4}$. Moreover, a selective uptake into a particular brain region could not be verified for both radiotracers (Figure 7, C and D). The SUVR (brain-to-blood) of [^{18}F]**1** was reduced by α-CCA-Na by only 25% compared to the control animal (Figure 7B), which is much less than the reduction of kidney uptake and indicates that the uptake of [^{18}F]**1** into the brain is partially mediated by MCT1 expressed at the endothelial cells of the BBB [49,50], and partly by non-specific diffusion mediated by lipophilicity.

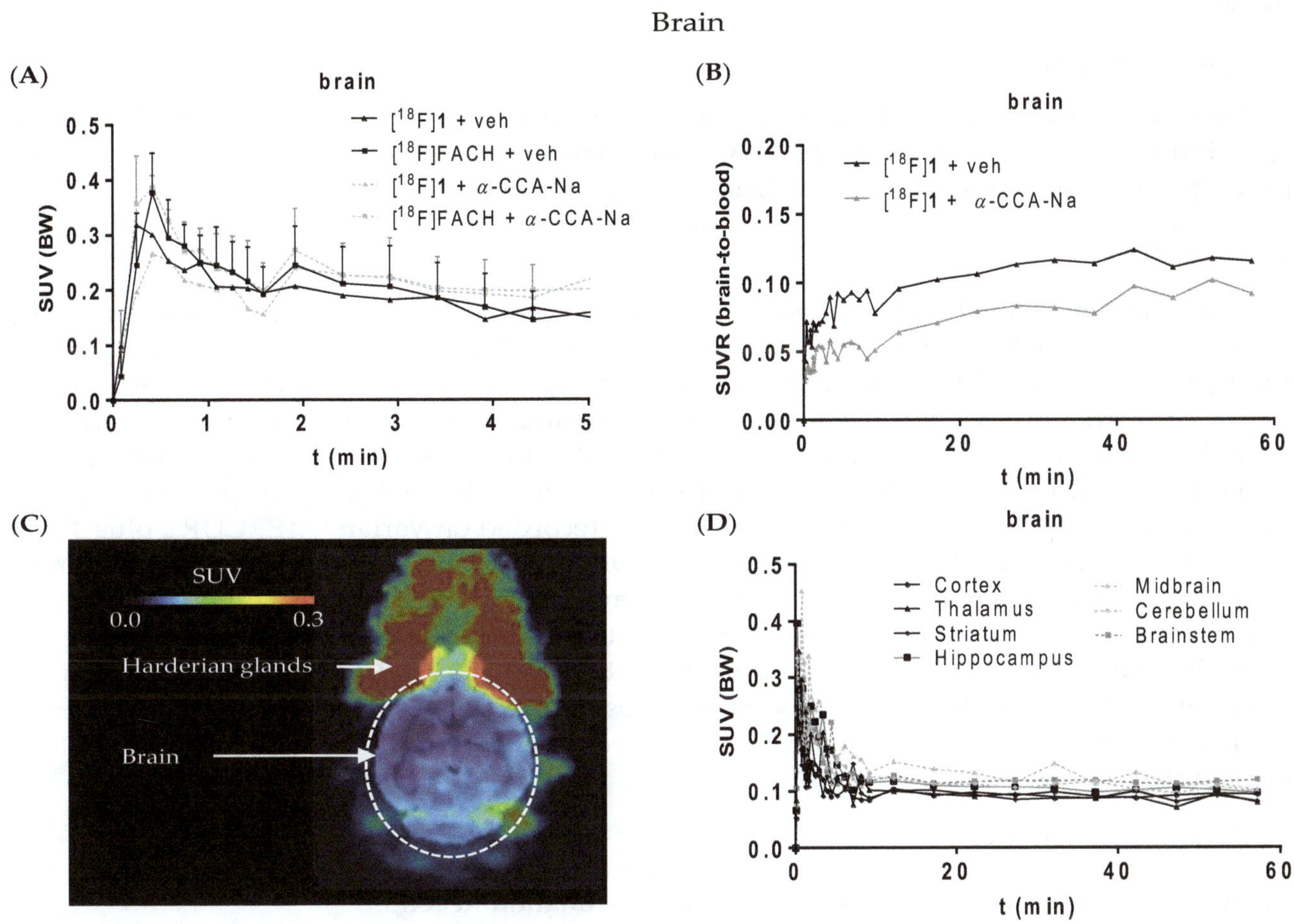

Figure 7. (**A**) Time-activity curve of [^{18}F]**1** (n = 1) and [^{18}F]FACH (n = 3) representing the SUVs without and with pre-administration of α-CCA-Na; (**B**) The SUVR of [^{18}F]**1** showing the brain to blood uptake ratio (n = 1); (**C**) horizontal section of representative PET image (averaged time frames from 0–60 min p.i.) of mouse head; (**D**) SUVs of different brain regions over time after injection of [^{18}F]**1**.

Brain capillary endothelial cells are tightly bound to each other and constitute the permeability barrier of the BBB/Neurovascular Unit (NVU), which serves to restrict the transport of compounds into the brain. The permeation of compounds across the BBB/NVU is determined not only by lipophilicity, ionic feature and molecular size, but also by various transporters expressed on the endothelial cell membrane [51]. For example, the radiotracer [^{11}C]choline has initially been demonstrated a comparably low brain accumulation with 0.08% of injected dose/g brain (%ID/g) 10 min after injection in mice [52] and 0.15% ID/g at 15 min after injection in rats [53]. This low uptake of [^{11}C]choline from blood is mediated by a choline-specific transport system of brain endothelial cell membranes [54]. Despite the low BBB/NVU permeability of [^{11}C]choline, it is a clinically relevant radiopharmaceutical for brain tumor imaging with high and specific accumulation in proliferating cancer cells [55,56]. Notably, in our control experiment using the MCT radioligand [^{18}F]**1,** a moderate brain accumulation of 0.4% ID/g at 10 min after injection was observed. It has been shown that MCT1 is expressed along with MCT4 in the cerebral microvascular endothelium cells suggesting a key role in transporting endogenous monocarboxylates into and out of the brain [50,57,58]. Together with the important role of MCT1 and MCT4 for glioma metabolism [5,32,33,59], it provides evidence that [^{18}F]FACH and/or [^{18}F]**1** might be suitable for brain tumor imaging.

3. Materials and Methods

3.1. Organic Synthesis

The syntheses of **1**, **2** and **15** (nitro precursor) were implemented by slight modifications of the previously reported procedures [26,36–39]. All final compounds described here meet the purity requirements determined by HPLC, NMR, and HR-MS analyses.

3.1.1. General Information

Unless otherwise noted, moisture-sensitive reactions were conducted under dry nitrogen or argon. $Pd(OAc)_2$, Xantphos (4,5-bis(diphenylphosphino)-9,9-dimethylxanthene), and Cs_2CO_3 were purchased from Sigma-Aldrich (SIGMA-ALDRICH Chemie GmbH, Schnelldorf, Germany). Other chemicals and reagents were purchased from commercial sources and were used without further purification. For thin-layer chromatography (TLC), Silica gel 60 F254 plates (Merck KGaA, Darmstadt, Germany) were used. Flash chromatography (fc) was performed using Silica gel 60, 40–64 μm (Merck). Room temperature was 21 °C. ^{1}H, ^{13}C, and ^{19}F spectra were recorded on Varian "MERCURY plus 300/400" (Varian, Palo Alto, CA, USA) and Bruker Advance DRX-400 (Bruker, Billerica, MA, USA); δ in ppm related to tetramethylsilane; coupling constants (*J*) are given with 0.1 Hz resolution. Multiplicities of NMR signals are indicated as follows: s (singlet), d (doublet), t (triplet), q (quartet), m (multiplet), dd (doublet of doublets), ddd (doublet of doublet of doublets), td (triplet of doublets), dq (doublet of quartets) and h (hexet (sextet)). High-resolution mass spectra (HR-MS) were recorded on an FT-ICR APEX II spectrometer (Bruker Daltonics; Bruker Corporation, Billerica, MA, USA) using electrospray ionization (ESI) in positive ion mode.

3.1.2. General Procedures

General Procedure A: The Buchwald-Hartwig Aryl Amination Reaction.

Substituted halide (2.5 mmol, 1.0 eq.) was dissolved in dry dioxane (10 mL) in a dry Schlenk tube, under an argon atmosphere. $Pd(OAc)_2$ (28 mg, 0.125 mmol, 0.05 eq.), Xantphos (72 mg, 0.125 mmol, 0.05 eq.), and Cs_2CO_3 (2.04 g, 6.25 mmol, 2.5 eq.) were added afterwards and the mixture was stirred at 75 °C. After 20 min, amine (3.0 mmol, 1.2 eq.) was added, and the reaction mixture was conducted at 105 °C under an argon atmosphere. The reaction monitored by TLC and it was completed in 30 min. After cooling to room temperature, the reaction mixture was diluted with diethyl ether (Et_2O), the solids were filtered and washed by Et_2O. The solvents were evaporated under *vacuum* and the oily residue was then purified by column chromatography.

General Procedure B

To a solution of substituted amine (2.0 mmol, 1.0 eq.) in *N,N*-dimethylformamide (DMF, 10 mL), NaH (26.0 mmol of a 60% dispersion in mineral oil, 13.0 eq.) was added in small portions under argon. 1-Iodopropane (0.488 mL, 5.0 mmol, 2.5 eq.) was thereafter added to the mixture. After stirring for 1 h at room temperature, the mixture was slowly poured on an ice-water mixture and stirred for 5 min. The mixture was extracted with ethyl acetate (EtOAc, 2 × 25 mL), the extracts were combined, dried with anhydrous $MgSO_4$, and concentrated by evaporation of the solvents under vacuum. The residue was then purified by column chromatography.

General Procedure C

$POCl_3$ (1.03 mL, 11.0 mmol, 1.1 eq.) was added dropwise to DMF (4.6 mL, 60.0 mmol, 6.0 eq.) at 0 °C and the mixture was stirred 30 min at room temperature. To this solution, *N,N*-disubstituted aniline (10.0 mmol, 1.0 eq.) was added and the reaction mixture was heated up to 80 °C. After 2–4 h, the reaction was quenched by addition of a mixture of ice water, stirred for additional 5 min. The pH was thereafter adjusted to 6–7 by using aqueous 1 M NaOH. The residue was extracted with chloroform

($CHCl_3$, 3 × 15 mL), and the organic phases were combined, washed with H_2O and brine. The extracts were dried with anhydrous $MgSO_4$ and the corresponding *N,N*-disubstituted benzaldehyde was purified by column chromatography after evaporation of the solvents.

To a solution of the substituted benzaldehyde (5.0 mmol, 1.0 eq.) in 20 mL acetonitrile (ACN), cyanoacetic acid (0.991 mL, 15.0 mmol, 3.0 eq.) and piperidine (0.494 mL, 5.0 mmol, 1.0 eq.) were added and refluxed overnight at 85 °C. Upon the completion of the reaction, as judged by TLC, the above solution was poured into a mixture of 3M HCl (10 mL) on ice. The solution was stirred for 30 min and the solids were filtered using a Büchner funnel and washed with ice-cold ACN. The solid was afterwards poured into adequate amount of *n*-hexane and stirred for 15 min to remove the remaining aldehyde. The final compounds were obtained in pure form after filtration of the solids and consequent washing with *n*-hexane.

6-Fluoro-N-(3-methoxyphenyl)pyridin-2-amine (**5**). The reaction was carried out according to the general procedure A. Column chromatography: silica, EtOAc/*n*-hexane, 1:2; Yellow oil: 96 % yield; TLC: (silica gel, EtOAc/*n*-hexane, 2:1), R_f = 0.8. ^{1}H NMR (300 MHz, $CDCl_3$) δ 7.56 (q, *J* = 8.0 Hz, 1H), 7.25 (m, 1H), 6.97 (t, *J* = 2.2 Hz, 1H), 6.90 (ddd, *J* = 8.0, 2.1, 0.8 Hz, 1H), 6.73 (dd, *J* = 8.1, 2.3 Hz, 1H), 6.66 (ddd, *J* = 8.3, 2.4, 0.8 Hz, 1H), 6.33 (dd, *J* = 7.8, 2.2 Hz, 1H), 3.83 (s, 3H); ^{13}C NMR (75 MHz, $CDCl_3$) δ 162.87 (d, *J* = 238.2 Hz), 160.49, 154.92 (d, *J* = 16.1 Hz), 142.12 (d, *J* = 8.4 Hz), 140.82, 130.03, 113.09, 108.87, 106.67, 104.30 (d, *J* = 4.2 Hz),98.29 (d, *J* = 36.1 Hz), 55.27; ^{19}F NMR (282 MHz, $CDCl_3$) δ −69.08 (d, *J* = 8.1 Hz).

6-Fluoro-N-(3-methoxyphenyl)-N-propylpyridin-2-amine (**6**). The reaction was carried out according to the general procedure B. Column chromatography: silica, EtOAc/*n*-hexane, 1:3; Yellow oil: 95% yield; TLC: (silica gel, EtOAc/*n*-hexane, 1:3), R_f = 0.75. ^{1}H NMR (400 MHz, $CDCl_3$) δ 7.35–7.27 (m, 2H), 6.95–6.65 (m, 3H), 6.12 (td, *J* = 7.6, 2.5 Hz, 2H), 3.85 (d, *J* = 7.6 Hz, 2H), 3.81 (s, 3H), 1.66 (m, 2H), 0.92 (t, *J* = 7.4 Hz, 3H); ^{13}C NMR (101 MHz, $CDCl_3$) δ 162.85 (d, *J* = 234.7 Hz), 160.87, 157.87 (d, *J* = 16.1 Hz), 145.82, 140.72 (d, *J* = 8.3 Hz), 130.50, 120.09, 113.64, 111.95, 104.78 (d, *J* = 4.1 Hz), 95.17 (d, *J* = 37.4 Hz), 55.30, 51.76, 21.05, 11.26; ^{19}F NMR (377 MHz, $CDCl_3$) δ −69.25 (d, *J* = 8.3 Hz).

6-Fluoro-N-(3-methoxyphenyl)-N-phenylpyridin-2-amine (**7**). The reaction was carried out according to the general procedure A. For this compound, higher amounts of $Pd(OAc)_2$ (84 mg, 0.375 mmol, 0.15 eq.) and Xantphos (217 mg, 0.375 mmol, 0.15 eq.) were added stepwise (3 × 0.125 mmol) to the reaction mixture over 24 h. Column chromatography: silica, EtOAc/n-hexane, 1:3; Milky oil: 46% yield; TLC: (silica gel, EtOAc/n-hexane, 1:3), R_f = 0.85. ^{1}H NMR (400 MHz, $CDCl_3$) δ 7.48 (dt, *J* = 8.4, 7.9 Hz, 1H), 7.38–7.29 (m, 2H), 7.28–7.12 (m, 4H), 6.79 (ddd, *J* = 7.9, 2.0, 0.9 Hz, 1H), 6.77–6.69 (m, 2H), 6.50 (ddd, *J* = 8.1, 2.2, 0.5 Hz, 1H), 6.34 (ddd, *J* = 7.8, 2.9, 0.5 Hz, 1H), 3.75 (s, 3H); ^{13}C NMR (101 MHz, $CDCl_3$) δ 162.43 (d, *J* = 237.8 Hz), 160.49, 157.50 (d, *J* = 15.1 Hz), 146.32, 145.06, 141.55 (d, *J* = 8.1 Hz), 130.02, 129.39, 126.62, 125.23, 119.07, 112.63, 110.74, 109.10 (d, *J* = 4.5 Hz), 99.41 (d, *J* = 37.0 Hz), 55.29; ^{19}F NMR (377 MHz, $CDCl_3$) δ −67.46 (d, *J* = 7.3 Hz).

4-((6-Fluoropyridin-2-yl)(propyl)amino)-2-methoxybenzaldehyde (**8**). The reaction was carried out according to the general procedure C. Column chromatography: silica, EtOAc/petroleum ether (PE), 1:2; Yellow oil: 57% yield; TLC: (silica gel, EtOAc/PE, 1:2), R_f = 0.55. ^{1}H NMR (300 MHz, $CDCl_3$) δ 10.35 (s, 1H), 7.82 (d, *J* = 8.4 Hz, 1H), 7.46 (dt, *J* = 8.5, 7.9 Hz, 1H), 6.88 (ddd, *J* = 8.4, 2.0, 0.7 Hz, 1H), 6.82 (d, *J* = 1.9 Hz, 1H), 6.55 (ddd, *J* = 8.1, 2.4, 0.5 Hz, 1H), 6.30 (ddd, *J* = 7.8, 2.9, 0.5 Hz, 1H), 3.98–3.89 (m, 2H), 3.88 (s, 3H), 1.69 (dq, *J* = 14.8, 7.4 Hz, 2H), 0.94 (t, *J* = 7.4 Hz, 3H); ^{13}C NMR (75 MHz, $CDCl_3$) δ 189.19, 163.05 (d, *J* = 244.3 Hz), 161.72, 159.68 (d, *J* = 15.1 Hz), 149.95, 140.12 (d, *J* = 8.1 Hz), 130.33, 118.77, 111.37 (d, *J* = 4.5 Hz), 106.62, 100.47 (d, *J* = 37.0 Hz), 101.76, 55.99, 49.89, 20.95, 11.38; ^{19}F NMR (282 MHz, $CDCl_3$) δ −68.09 (d, *J* = 8.6 Hz).

4-((6-Fluoropyridin-2-yl)(phenyl)amino)-2-methoxybenzaldehyde (**9**). The reaction was carried out according to the general procedure C. Column chromatography: silica, EtOAc/*n*-hexane, 1:3; Yellow oil: 68% yield; TLC: (silica gel, EtOAc/*n*-hexane, 1:3), R_f = 0.60. ^{1}H NMR (300 MHz, $CDCl_3$) δ 10.32 (s, 1H), 7.73

(d, J = 8.5 Hz, 1H), 7.59 (q, J = 8.0 Hz, 1H), 7.46–7.37 (m, 2H), 7.33–7.25 (m, 1H), 7.24–7.16 (m, 2H), 6.78 (d, J = 2.0 Hz, 1H), 6.69 (ddd, J = 8.5, 2.0, 0.8 Hz, 1H), 6.60 (dd, J = 8.0, 1.7 Hz, 1H), 6.54–6.46 (m, 1H), 3.77 (s, 3H); ^{13}C NMR (75 MHz, $CDCl_3$) δ 188.37, 162.91 (d, J = 235.1 Hz), 162.63,156.61 (d, J = 14.9 Hz), 152.14, 144.37, 142.13 (d, J = 8.1 Hz), 130.06, 129.50, 127.66, 126.70, 120.65, 116.19, 111.59 (d, J = 4.6 Hz), 106.62, 101.86 (d, J = 36.6 Hz), 55.60; ^{19}F NMR (282 MHz, $CDCl_3$) δ −66.92 (d, J = 8.5 Hz).

*(E)-2-Cyano-3-(4-((6-fluoropyridin-2-yl)(propyl)amino)-2-methoxyphenyl)acrylic Acid (**1**).* The reaction was carried out according to the general procedure C. Yellow solid: 95% yield; TLC: (silica gel, $CHCl_3$/MeOH/acetic acid (AcOH), 95:5:0.1), R_f = 0.60. ^{1}H NMR (400 MHz, $CDCl_3/CD_3OD$) δ 8.63 (s, 1H), 8.30 (d, J = 8.7 Hz, 1H), 7.46 (q, J = 8.2 Hz, 1H), 6.86 (dd, J = 8.7, 2.1 Hz, 1H), 6.74 (d, J = 2.1 Hz, 1H), 6.59 (dd, J = 8.1, 2.2 Hz, 1H), 6.31 (dd, J = 7.8, 2.8 Hz, 1H), 3.93–3.86 (m, 2H), 3.80 (s, 3H), 1.65 (h, J = 7.4 Hz, 2H), 0.90 (t, J = 7.4 Hz, 3H); ^{13}C NMR (101 MHz, $CDCl_3/CD_3OD$) δ 164.86, 162.72 (d, J = 237.5 Hz), 160.52, 156.27 (d, J = 15.2 Hz), 151.55, 148.32, 141.46 (d, J = 8.3 Hz), 133.13, 130.43, 116.63, 116.39, 108.28 (d, J = 4.3 Hz), 106.26, 100.01, 99.02 (d, J = 36.9 Hz), 55.72, 51.83, 21.14, 11.14; ^{19}F NMR (376 MHz, $CDCl_3/CD_3OD$) δ -68.23 (dt, J = 8.3, 2.2 Hz).HR-MS (ESI) m/z:calcd. for $[C_{18}H_{17}FN_3O]^+$ = 310.1350; found = 310.1332 $[M–CO_2H]^+$.

*(E)-2-Cyano-3-(4-((6-fluoropyridin-2-yl)(phenyl)amino)-2-methoxyphenyl)acrylic Acid (**2**).* The reaction was carried out according to the general procedure C. Orange solid: 98% yield; TLC: (silica gel, $CHCl_3$/MeOH/AcOH), 95:5:0.1), R_f = 0.75.^{1}H NMR (400 MHz, $CDCl_3$) δ 8.75 (s, 1H), 8.37 (d, J = 8.8 Hz, 1H), 7.65 (q, J = 8.0 Hz, 1H), 7.47 (t, J = 7.7 Hz, 2H), 7.41–7.17 (m, 3H), 6.80 (d, J = 1.9 Hz, 1H), 6.73 (dd, J = 8.8, 1.9 Hz, 1H), 6.69–6.61 (m, 1H), 6.58 (dd, J = 7.9, 2.7 Hz, 1H), 3.79 (s, 3H); ^{13}C NMR (101 MHz, $CDCl_3$) δ 167.91, 162.31 (d, J = 240.5 Hz), 160.76, 156.25 (d, J = 14.6 Hz), 152.17, 149.60, 143.99, 142.34 (d, J = 8.2 Hz), 130.35, 130.24, 127.87, 127.16, 116.26, 115.94, 115.58, 112.29 (d, J = 4.5 Hz), 105.47, 102.54 (d, J = 36.5 Hz), 97.31, 55.82; ^{19}F NMR (377 MHz, $CDCl_3$) δ -66.88 (d, J = 8.2 Hz).HR-MS (ESI) m/z: calcd. for $[C_{21}H_{15}FN_3O]^{+\cdot}$ = 344.1194; found = 344.1180 $[M–CO_2H]^+$.

*N-(3-Methoxyphenyl)-6-nitropyridin-2-amine (**12**).* The reaction was carried out according to the general procedure A. Column chromatography: silica, EtOAc/n-hexane, 1:1; Yellow solid: 80 % yield; TLC: (silica gel, EtOAc/n-hexane, 1:1), R_f = 0.65. ^{1}H NMR (400 MHz, $CDCl_3$) δ 7.78–7.70 (m, 1H), 7.63 (dd, J = 7.6, 0.6 Hz, 1H), 7.31–7.24 (m, 1H), 7.23–7.19 (m, 1H), 7.14 (dd, J = 8.2, 0.6 Hz, 1H), 6.88 (ddd, J = 7.9, 2.0, 0.8 Hz, 1H), 6.71 (ddd, J = 8.3, 2.5, 0.8 Hz, 1H), 3.86 (s, 3H); ^{13}C NMR (101 MHz, $CDCl_3$) δ 160.29, 155.31, 155.06, 140.46, 139.94, 129.79, 114.77, 112.21, 109.24, 107.35, 105.65, 55.16.

*N-(3-Methoxyphenyl)-6-nitro-N-propylpyridin-2-amine (**13**).* The reaction was carried out according to the general procedure B. Column chromatography: silica, EtOAc/n-hexane, 1:3; Yellow oil: 93% yield; TLC: (silica gel, EtOAc/n-hexane, 1:3), R_f = 0.70. ^{1}H NMR (400 MHz, $CDCl_3$) δ 7.53–7.29 (m, 3H), 6.88 (dd, J = 8.3, 2.3 Hz, 1H), 6.82 (d, J = 7.9 Hz, 1H), 6.79–6.68 (m, 1H), 6.59 (d, J = 8.2 Hz, 1H), 3.95 (t, J = 7.4 Hz, 2H), 3.82 (s, 3H), 1.69 (h, J = 7.4 Hz, 2H), 0.95 (t, J = 7.4 Hz, 3H); ^{13}C NMR (101 MHz, $CDCl_3$) δ 161.44, 157.92, 156.25, 145.36, 139.22, 131.23, 120.24, 114.28, 113.93, 112.86, 105.78, 55.72, 52.38, 21.21, 11.68.

*2-Methoxy-4-((6-nitropyridin-2-yl)(propyl)amino)benzaldehyde (**14**).* The reaction was carried out according to the general procedure C. Column chromatography: silica, EtOAc/PE, 1:2; Yellow oil: 92% yield; TLC: (silica gel, EtOAc/PE, 1:2), R_f = 0.60. ^{1}H NMR (400 MHz, $CDCl_3$) δ 10.40 (s, 1H), 7.89 (d, J = 8.3 Hz, 1H), 7.63–7.53 (m, 2H), 6.94–6.89 (m, 2H), 6.88 (d, J = 1.9 Hz, 1H), 4.03 (t, J = 7.4 Hz, 2H), 3.91 (s, 3H), 1.74 (h, J = 7.4 Hz, 2H), 0.97 (t, J = 7.4 Hz, 3H); ^{13}C NMR (101 MHz, $CDCl_3$) δ 188.37, 163.12, 156.66, 155.98, 151.33, 139.56, 130.32, 122.69, 118.05, 115.38, 108.86, 107.32, 55.84, 52.30, 21.08, 11.38.

*(E)-2-Cyano-3-(2-methoxy-4-((6-nitropyridin-2-yl)(propyl)amino)phenyl)acrylic Acid (**15**).* The reaction was carried out according to the general procedure C. Yellow solid: >98% yield; TLC: (silica gel, $CHCl_3$/MeOH/AcOH), 95:5:0.1), R_f = 0.70. ^{1}H NMR (400 MHz, $CDCl_3/CD_3OD$) δ 8.62 (s, 1H), 8.30 (d, J = 8.5 Hz, 1H),7.58 (t, J = 7.9 Hz, 1H), 7.51 (d, J = 7.6 Hz, 1H), 6.92 (d, J = 8.3 Hz, 1H), 6.89 (dd, J = 8.6, 1.7 Hz, 1H), 6.80 (d, J = 1.5 Hz, 1H), 3.98 (t, J = 7.4 Hz, 2H), 3.82 (s, 3H), 1.68 (h, J = 7.4 Hz, 2H), 0.91

(t, $J = 7.3$ Hz, 3H); ^{13}C NMR (101 MHz, $CDCl_3/CD_3OD$) δ 164.39, 160.51, 156.43, 155.70, 150.30, 148.24, 139.62, 130.62, 118.14, 117.66, 116.35, 115.78, 107.90, 107.54, 101.63, 55.82, 52.13, 20.95, 11.16. HR-MS (ESI) m/z calcd. for $[C_{18}H_{17}N_4O_3]^{+\cdot}$= 337.1295; found = 337.1283 $[M–CO_2H]^{+\cdot}$.

3.2. Assessment of the MCT1 Inhibition by [^{14}C]lactate Uptake Assay

Inhibition of the MCT1-mediated lactate transport was determined using the rat brain endothelial cell line (RBE4, a gift from F. Roux research group [40]) as previously described [26]. PCR analysis and Western Blot demonstrated that only the MCT1 isoform is expressed by RBE4 cells.

3.3. Radiochemistry

3.3.1. General Methods

No-carrier-added [^{18}F]fluoride was produced via the [^{18}O(p,n)^{18}F] nuclear reaction by irradiation of an [^{18}O]H_2O target (Hyox 18 enriched water, Rotem Industries Ltd., Arava, Israel) on a Cyclone 18/9 (IBA RadioPharma Solutions, Lourain-La-Neuve, Belgium) with fixed energy proton beam using Nirta [^{18}F]fluoride XL target. Radio thin layer chromatography (radio-TLC) was performed on silica gel (ALUGRAM SIL G/UV254, Machery-Nagel, Düren, Germany) pre-coated plates with a mixture of dichloromethane (DCM)/MeOH (4:1) as eluent. The plates were exposed to storage phosphor screens (BAS IP MS 2025 E, GE Healthcare Europe GmbH, Freiburg, Germany) and recorded using the Amersham Typhoon RGB Biomolecular Imager (GE Healthcare Life Sciences). Images were quantified with the ImageQuant TL8.1 software (GE Healthcare Life Sciences).

Analytical chromatographic separations were performed on a JASCO LC-2000 system, incorporating a PU-2080Plus pump, AS-2055Plus auto injector (100 μL sample loop), and a UV-2070Plus detector coupled with a gamma radioactivity HPLC flow detector (Gabi Star, raytest Isotopenmessgeräte GmbH, Straubenhardt, Germany). Data analysis was performed with the Galaxy chromatography software (version 1.10.0.5590, Agilent Technologies Deutschland GmbH, Waldbronn, Germany) using the chromatograms obtained at 254 and 370 nm. Reprosil-Pur C18-AQ column (250 × 4.6 mm; 5 μm; Dr. Maisch HPLC GmbH; Ammerbuch-Entingen, Germany) with an eluent mixture of ACN/20 mM NH_4OAc (aq., pH 6.8) and a flow of 1.0 mL/min were used (gradient: eluent A 10% ACN/20 mM NH_4OAc (aq.); eluent B 90% ACN/20 mM NH_4OAc (aq.); 0–5 min 100% A, 5–20 min up to 62% B, 20–21 min up to 100% B, 21–26 min 100% B, 26–27 min up to 100% A, 27–35 min 100% A; isocratic: 30% MeOH/20 mM NH_4OAc (aq.), flow: 0.75 mL/min, UV detection at 370 nm).

Semi-preparative HPLC separation was performed by using the HPLC system implemented in the TRACERlab FX2 N synthesizer (GE Healthcare). A Reprosil-Pur 120 CN column (250 × 20 mm, 10 μm, Dr. Maisch HPLC GmbH, Germany) was used with 45% MeOH/20 mM NH_4OAc (aq.) as eluent mixture and a flow rate of 7.0 mL/min. The ammonium acetate concentration stated as aq. 20 mM NH_4OAc, corresponds to the concentration in the aqueous component of an eluent mixture.

The molar activities were determined based on a calibration curve carried out under isocratic HPLC conditions (Reprosil-Pur C18-AQ, 250 × 4.6 mm, 30% MeOH/20 mM NH_4OAc (aq.), flow: 0.75 mL/min) using chromatograms obtained at 370 nm as an appropriate maximum of UV absorbance.

3.3.2. Radiosynthesis of [^{18}F]**1**

No carrier added [^{18}F]fluoride in 1.5 mL water was trapped on a Sep-Pak Accell Plus QMA Carbonate Plus light cartridge (Waters GmbH, Eschborn, Germany). The activity was eluted with 400 μL of an aqueous solution of potassium carbonate (K_2CO_3, 1.8 mg, 13 μmol) into a 4 mL V-shape vial prefilled with Kryptofix® 2.2.2 ($K_{2.2.2}$, 11 mg, 29 μmol) in 1 mL ACN. The aqueous [^{18}F]fluoride was azeotropically dried under vacuum and nitrogen flow within 7–10 min using a single mode microwave (75 W, at 50–60 °C, power cycling mode; Discover PETWave from CEM GmbH, Kamp-Lintfort, Germany) [60]. Two aliquots of ACN (2 × 1.0 mL) were added during the drying procedure and the final complex was obtained in a dried form. A solution of 1.0 mg of the nitro precursor **15** in 750 μL

DMSO was added, and the ^{18}F-labeling was performed at 130 °C. To determine the radiochemical yields of the labeling process, samples were taken at different time points (5, 10, 15, and 20 min) and analyzed by radio-HPLC and radio-TLC.

After cooling to < 30 °C, the reaction mixture was diluted with 2.0 mL aqueous NH_4HCO_2 (adjusted to pH 4 with formic acid) and 2.0 mL MeOH/water (1:/1) and directly applied to an isocratic semi-preparative RP-HPLC for isolation of [^{18}F]**1**. The collected radiotracer fraction was diluted with 40 mL water to perform final purification by sorption on a Sep-Pak® C18 light cartridge (Waters, GmbH, Eschborn, Germany) and successive elution with 1.3 mL of ethanol. The ethanolic solution was concentrated under a gentle argon stream at 70 °C to a final volume of 10–50 μL. Afterwards, the radiotracer was diluted in isotonic saline to obtain a final product containing 10% of EtOH (*v*/*v*).

3.3.3. Determination of In Vitro Stability and log $D_{7.4}$ of [^{18}F]**1**

In vitro stability was investigated by incubation of about 5 MBq of [^{18}F]**1** in phosphate-buffered saline (PBS, pH 7.4), *n*-octanol, saline and ethanol (500 μL) at 40 °C up to 60 min. Samples were taken at 60 min and the radio-TLC and radio-HPLC analyses were performed.

The lipophilicity of [^{18}F]**1** was experimentally determined by partitioning a small amount of the radiotracer between *n*-octanol and PBS (pH 7.4) at room temperature using the conventional shake-flask method. The radiotracer (15 μL, ~800 kBq) was added to the tubes containing a mixture of *n*-octanol and PBS (3.0 mL, n = 4). After shaking for 20 min using the mechanical shaker (HS250 basic, IKA Labortechnik GmbH & Co. KG, Staufen, Germany), the samples were centrifuged for 5 min at 5000 rpm, followed by separation of the phases. Aliquots were taken from the organic and the aqueous phases (1 mL of each) and activity was measured in a γ-counter (PerkinElmer Wallac Wizard 1480 Gamma Counter, manufactured by WALLAC, Turku, Finland). For the second extraction, another 1 mL aliquot of the organic layer was mixed with 2.0 mL *n*-octanol and 3.0 mL of PBS and was subjected to the same procedure. The distribution coefficient (D) was calculated as [activity (cpm/mL) in *n*-octanol]/[activity (cpm/mL) in PBS, pH 7.4] stated as the decade logarithm (log $D_{7.4}$).

3.4. *Animal Studies*

3.4.1. General Information

All experimental work including animals has been conducted in accordance with the national legislation on the use of animals for research (Tierschutzgesetz (TierSchG), Tierschutz-Versuchstierverordnung (TierSchVersV)) and has been approved by the responsible research ethics committee (TVV 18/18, DD24.1-5131/446/19, Landesdirektion Sachsen, 20 June, 2018). Female CD-1 mice, 10–12 weeks, were obtained from the Medizinisch-ExperimentellesZentrum at Universität Leipzig. For the time of the experiments, the animals were kept in a dedicated climatic chamber with free access to water and food under a 12:12 h dark:light cycle at a constant temperature of 24 °C.

3.4.2. In Vitro Autoradiographic Analysis of Binding Sites of [^{18}F]**1** in Mouse Kidney

The kidneys was isolated after cervical dislocation from one CD-1 mouse, frozen rapidly in isopentane at −25 °C for 5 min, and stored at −25 °C until the sectioning. Cryosections (transversal, 10 μm) were obtained using a microtome (MICROM HM560, Thermo Scientific Microm, Fisher Scientific GmbH, Schwerte, Germany), mounted on microscopy slides (SuperFrost, Thermo Scientific Menzel, Fisher Scientific GmbH, Schwerte, Germany), dried for ~2 h at room temperature, and stored at −25 °C until the autoradiography study. For the experiment, the slides were taken out from the freezer, the cryosections dried under a stream of cold air, and pre-incubated with PBS for 15 min at room temperature. The incubation solution was decanted, the slices dried again under a stream of cold air, and covered afterwards with the incubation solution ([^{18}F]**1**, 198 kBq/mL PBS or 1.19 nM at the time of incubation, without (total binding) or with co-incubation with 10^{-5}, 10^{-7}, and 10^{-9} M α-CHC-Na). Incubation at room temperature was terminated after 60 min, the slides were washed twice in 50 mM

TRIS-HCl, pH 7.4 at 4 °C, on ice for two minutes each followed by dipping in ice-cold demineralized water for 5 s and rapid drying under a stream of cold air. Afterwards, the slides were exposed to a phosphor imager plate (BAS-IP TR 2025, FujiFilm Corporation, Tokyo, Japan) along with standards obtained by pipetting and drying 1 μL of each concentration of a serial dilution of the radiotracer solution on to a microscopic slide.

3.4.3. Analysis of Radiometabolites of [^{18}F]**1** in Mouse

The radiotracer [^{18}F]**1** (32.84 MBq in 200 μL isotonic saline) was injected in an awake female CD-1 mouse (12 weeks old, 31 g) via the tail vein. After 30 min, the animal was slightly anesthetized with isoflurane, and blood was collected from retro-orbital bleeding followed by cervical dislocation. Blood plasma was separated by centrifugation of the blood sample at 10,000 rpm for 2 min. Brain was also isolated, cleaned by pouring PBS and homogenized in demineralized water (~2 mL/g tissue) in a borosilicate glass with a PTFE plunger by 10 strokes at 1000 rpm (POTTER S, Homogenizer, B. Braun Biotech, Sartorius AG, Göttingen, Germany). Blood plasma and brain homogenate were provided for preparation of samples for radio-HPLC analyses as described in the following.

RP-HPLC: Protein precipitation was performed by addition of an ice-cold ACN/H_2O mixture (9:1) to the plasma and brain samples in a ratio of 4:1 (*v*/*v*: solvent/tissue sample, n = 2). The samples were vortexed for 2 min, incubated on ice for 3 min, and the suspensions were centrifuged at 10,000 rpm at 4 °C for 5 min. For the second extraction, the precipitates were re-dissolved in 100 μL of the solvent mixture, vortexed for 3 min, incubated on ice for 5 min and subjected to the same centrifuging procedure. The combined supernatants (total volume between 1–2 mL) were concentrated at 70 °C under argon flow to a final volume of approximately 100 μL and were analyzed by analytical radio-HPLC. A Reprosil-Pur C18-AQ column (250 mm × 4.6 mm; 5 μm) was used as stationary phase and elution was done using the gradient mode as described in Section 3.3.1. To determine the percentage of radioactivity in the supernatants compared to total activity, aliquots of each step as well as the precipitates were quantified by gamma counting.

MLC: Preparation of the plasma and brain samples was performed as already described [47,48]. A Reprosil-Pur C18-AQ column (250 × 4.6 mm, particle size: 10 μm) coupled with a pre-column of 10 mm length was used. Separations were performed by using an isocratic mode with an aqueous eluent containing 50 mM sodium dodecyl sulfate and 10 mM Na_2HPO_4 at a flow rate of 1.0 mL/min.

3.4.4. Small Animal Micro-PET/MR Studies

The dynamic biodistribution of the radiotracers was assessed by small animal PET (nanoscan, Mediso, Hungary) over 60 min PET with a subsequently T1 weighted MR. Anaesthetized (2% isofluran, carrier gas mixture of 40% air and 60% O_2) female CD-1 mice (bodyweight = 30.3 ± 1.1 g) were kept during imaging on a heated animal bed to sustain body temperature and were pretreated with vehicle (0.9% saline) and α-CHC-Na (25 mg/kg bodyweight) prior to tracer application ([^{18}F]**1**: 5.8 ± 0.2 MBq, 1.1 fmol/g bodyweight and [^{18}F]FACH: 5.9 ± 0.5 MBq, 3.7 ± 1.8 fmol/g), whereby all injections were administered intravenously. The acquisitions were performed in normal mode and a coincidence Mode 1–5. For subsequent dynamic reconstructions, list mode data were sorted into sinograms (12 × 10 s, 6 × 30 s, 5 × 60 s, and 10 × 300 s). The frames were reconstructed by Ordered Subset Expectation Maximization applied to 3D sinograms (OSEM3D) with an attenuation correction with 4 iterations, 6 subsets and a voxel size of 0.4 mm^3 (Nucline v2.01, Mediso, Hungary). Analyses of reconstructed studies were performed with PMOD software (v4.005, PMOD Technologies LLC, Zurich, Switzerland) and results are expressed in Standardized Uptake Value (SUV).

4. Conclusions

In summary, two new analogs of FACH, **1** and **2**, were synthesized and the former, with moderate MCT1 inhibition, was regarded to be a good PET candidate and therefore chosen for labeling with fluorine-18. Although the partition coefficient log $D_{7.4}$ of [^{18}F]**1** was 2-fold higher than the one of [^{18}F]FACH, the brain accumulation of both radiotracers was in a similar moderate range. This demonstrates that log $D_{7.4}$ alone does not govern passive diffusion into the brain, which is also reflected by comparing log $D_{7.4}$ with calculated log K_{BB} (brain-blood partition coefficient). Nevertheless, the high uptake of [^{18}F]**1** in kidney and other peripheral MCT-expressing organs together with the strong inhibition by specific drugs provide evidence that this radiotracer is suitable for future investigation of MCT imaging with PET. Moreover, these results suggest that further structural modifications towards improving MCT-mediated transport might result in higher brain uptake in vivo.

5. Patents

The nitro- or bromo- precursor for the radiosynthesis of the structurally modified analogs of FACH is subject of a patent application by Helmholtz-Zentrum Dresden-Rossendorf (DMPA registration No. 10 2019 112 040.3) with following contributing inventors: Rareş-Petru Moldovan, Masoud Sadeghzadeh, Barbara Wenzel, Mathias Kranz, Steffen Fischer, Rodrigo Teodoro, Friedrich-Alexander Ludwig, Magali Toussaint and Peter Brust.

Author Contributions: Conceptualization, M.S., B.W., W.D.-C., R.-P.M., L.R.D. and P.B.; Data curation, D.G., M.T., F.-A.L., and G.S.; Formal analysis, D.G., W.D.-C., F.L., S.J., and S.K.J.; Funding acquisition, M.S., L.R.D., and P.B.; Investigation, M.S., B.W., D.G., W.D.-C., M.T., S.J., S.K.J., G.S., and V.R.M.; Methodology, M.S., B.W., S.F., R.T., G.S., and V.R.M.; Project administration, M.S. and P.B.; Resources, W.D.-C., R.T., S.F., and V.R.M.; Software, D.G. and G.S.; Supervision, L.R.D. and P.B.; Validation, B.W., D.G., W.D.-C, R.-P.M., F.-A.L., R.T., S.K.J., V.R.M., L.R.D., and P.B.; Visualization, M.S.; Writing—original draft, M.S., B.W., G.S., and D.G.; Writing—review & editing, M.S., B.W., D.G., W.D.-C., M.T., R.-P.M., S.F., F.-A.L., R.T., S.J., S.K.J., G.S., V.R.M., L.R.D., and P.B. All authors have read and agreed to the published version of the manuscript.

Acknowledgments: The Alexander von Humboldt Foundation and the University of Minnesota Duluth are acknowledged for financial supports. We are thankful to K. Franke and A. Mansel for providing [^{18}F]fluoride as well as Matthias Scheunemann and Susann Schröder for their scientific supports. We also thank the staff of the Institute of Analytical Chemistry, Department of Chemistry and Mineralogy of the University of Leipzig, for recording and processing the NMR and HR-MS spectra.

References

1. Halestrap, A.P.; Meredith, D. The SLC16 gene family—From monocarboxylate transporters (MCTs) to aromatic amino acid transporters and beyond. *Pflüger, Archiv für die Gesammte Physiologie des Menschen und der Thiere* **2004**, *447*, 619–628. [CrossRef] [PubMed]
2. Jones, R.S.; Morris, A.M.E. Monocarboxylate Transporters: Therapeutic Targets and Prognostic Factors in Disease. *Clin. Pharmacol. Ther.* **2016**, *100*, 454–463. [CrossRef] [PubMed]
3. Halestrap, A.P.; Wilson, M.C. The monocarboxylate transporter family—Role and regulation. *IUBMB Life* **2011**, *64*, 109–119. [CrossRef]
4. Hong, C.S.; Graham, N.A.; Gu, W.; Camacho, C.E.; Mah, V.; Maresh, E.L.; Alavi, M.; Bagryanova, L.; Krotee, P.A.L.; Gardner, B.K.; et al. MCT1 Modulates Cancer Cell Pyruvate Export and Growth of Tumors that Co-express MCT1 and MCT4. *Cell Rep.* **2016**, *14*, 1590–1601. [CrossRef] [PubMed]
5. Park, S.J.; Smith, C.P.; Wilbur, R.R.; Cain, C.P.; Kallu, S.R.; Valasapalli, S.; Sahoo, A.; Guda, M.R.; Tsung, A.J.; Velpula, K.K. An overview of MCT1 and MCT4 in GMB: Small molecule transporters with large implications. *Am. J. Cancer Res.* **2018**, *8*, 1967–1976. [PubMed]
6. Cao, Y.-W.; Liu, Y.; Dong, Z.; Guo, L.; Kang, E.-H.; Wang, Y.-H.; Zhang, W.; Niu, H.-T. Monocarboxylate transporters MCT1 and MCT4 are independent prognostic biomarkers for the survival of patients with clear cell renal cell carcinoma and those receiving therapy targeting angiogenesis. *Urol. Oncol. Semin. Orig. Investig.* **2018**, *36*, 311.e15–311.e25. [CrossRef]
7. Marchiq, I.; Pouysségur, J. Hypoxia, cancer metabolism and the therapeutic benefit of targeting lactate/H(+) symporters. *J. Mol. Med.* **2015**, *94*, 155–171. [CrossRef]

8. Roy, D.; Sheng, G.Y.; Herve, S.; Carvalho, E.; Mahanty, A.; Yuan, S.; Sun, L. Interplay between cancer cell cycle and metabolism: Challenges, targets and therapeutic opportunities. *Biomed. Pharm.* **2017**, *89*, 288–296. [CrossRef]
9. Zhu, A.; Lee, D.; Shim, H. Metabolic positron emission tomography imaging in cancer detection and therapy response. *Semin. Oncol.* **2011**, *38*, 55–69. [CrossRef]
10. O'Neill, H.; Malik, V.; Johnston, C.; Reynolds, J.V.; O'Sullivan, J. Can the Efficacy of [^{18}F]FDG-PET/CT in Clinical Oncology Be Enhanced by Screening Biomolecular Profiles? *Pharmaceuticals* **2019**, *12*, 16. [CrossRef]
11. Endo, K.; Oriuchi, N.; Higuchi, T.; Iida, Y.; Hanaoka, H.; Miyakubo, M.; Ishikita, T.; Koyama, K. PET and PET/CT using ^{18}F-FDG in the diagnosis and management of cancer patients. *Int. J. Clin. Oncol.* **2006**, *11*, 286–296. [CrossRef] [PubMed]
12. Ganapathy-Kanniappan, S.; Geschwind, J.-F. Tumor glycolysis as a target for cancer therapy: Progress and prospects. *Mol. Cancer* **2013**, *12*, 152. [CrossRef] [PubMed]
13. Draoui, N.; Feron, O. Lactate shuttles at a glance: From physiological paradigms to anti-cancer treatments. *Dis. Model. Mech.* **2011**, *4*, 727–732. [CrossRef] [PubMed]
14. Ocaña, M.C.; Poveda, B.M.; Quesada, A.R.; Medina, M. Ángel Metabolism within the tumor microenvironment and its implication on cancer progression: An ongoing therapeutic target. *Med. Res. Rev.* **2018**, *39*, 70–113. [CrossRef] [PubMed]
15. Beinat, C.; Patel, C.; Haywood, T.; Murty, S.; Alam, I.; Xie, Y.; Gandhi, H.; Holley, D.; Gambhir, S. Evaluation of [^{18}F]DASA-23 for non-invasive measurement of aberrantly expressed pyruvate kinase M2 in glioblastoma: Preclinical and first in human studies. *J. Nucl. Med.* **2019**, *60*, 52.
16. Fu, Y.; Liu, S.; Yin, S.; Niu, W.; Xiong, W.; Tan, M.; Li, G.; Zhou, M. The reverse Warburg effect is likely to be an Achilles' heel of cancer that can be exploited for cancer therapy. *Oncotarget* **2017**, *8*, 57813–57825. [CrossRef]
17. Herrero, P.; Dence, C.S.; Coggan, A.R.; Kisrieva-Ware, Z.; Eisenbeis, P.; Gropler, R.J. L-3-^{11}C-Lactate as a PET Tracer of Myocardial Lactate Metabolism: A Feasibility Study. *J. Nucl. Med.* **2007**, *48*, 2046–2055. [CrossRef]
18. Yokoi, F.; Hara, T.; Iio, M.; Nonaka, I.; Satoyoshi, E. 1-[^{11}C]pyruvate turnover in brain and muscle of patients with mitochondrial encephalomyopathy. A study with positron emission tomography (PET). *J. Neurol. Sci.* **1990**, *99*, 339–348. [CrossRef]
19. Graham, K.; Müller, A.; Lehmann, L.; Koglin, N.; Dinkelborg, L.; Siebeneicher, H. [^{18}F]Fluoropyruvate: Radiosynthesis and initial biological evaluation. *J. Label. Compd. Radiopharm.* **2014**, *57*, 164–171. [CrossRef]
20. Van Hée, V.F.; Labar, D.; Dehon, G.; Grasso, D.; Grégoire, V.; Muccioli, G.G.; Frédérick, R.; Sonveaux, P. Radiosynthesis and validation of (±)-[^{18}F]-3-fluoro-2-hydroxypropionate ([18F]-FLac) as a PET tracer of lactate to monitor MCT1-dependent lactate uptake in tumors. *Oncotarget* **2017**, *8*, 24415. [CrossRef]
21. Tateishi, H.; Tsuji, A.B.; Kato, K.; Sudo, H.; Sugyo, A.; Hanakawa, T.; Zhang, M.-R.; Saga, T.; Arano, Y.; Higashi, T. Synthesis and evaluation of ^{11}C-labeled coumarin analog as an imaging probe for detecting monocarboxylate transporters expression. *Bioorganic Med. Chem. Lett.* **2017**, *27*, 4893–4897. [CrossRef] [PubMed]
22. Wang, X.; Levi, A.J.; Halestrap, A.P. Substrate and inhibitor specificities of the monocarboxylate transporters of single rat heart cells. *Am. J. Physiol. Circ. Physiol.* **1996**, *270*, H476–H484. [CrossRef] [PubMed]
23. Hildyard, J.C.W.; Halestrap, A.P. Identification of the mitochondrial pyruvate carrier in Saccharomyces cerevisiae. *Biochem. J.* **2003**, *374*, 607–611. [CrossRef] [PubMed]
24. Gurrapu, S.; Jonnalagadda, S.; Alam, M.A.; Nelson, G.L.; Sneve, M.G.; Drewes, L.R.; Mereddy, V.R. Monocarboxylate Transporter 1 Inhibitors as Potential Anticancer Agents. *ACS Med. Chem. Lett.* **2015**, *6*, 558–561. [CrossRef] [PubMed]
25. Jonnalagadda, S.; Jonnalagadda, S.K.; Ronayne, C.T.; Nelson, G.L.; Solano, L.N.; Rumbley, J.; Holy, J.; Mereddy, V.R.; Drewes, L.R. Novel N,N-dialkyl cyanocinnamic acids as monocarboxylate transporter 1 and 4 inhibitors. *Oncotarget* **2019**, *10*, 2355–2368. [CrossRef] [PubMed]
26. Sadeghzadeh, M.; Moldovan, R.-P.; Fischer, S.; Wenzel, B.; Ludwig, F.-A.; Teodoro, R.; Deuther-Conrad, W.; Jonnalagadda, S.; Jonnalagadda, S.K.; Gudelis, E.; et al. Development and radiosynthesis of the first ^{18}F-labeled inhibitor of monocarboxylate transporters (MCTs). *J. Label. Compd. Radiopharm.* **2019**, *62*, 411–424. [CrossRef]
27. Sadeghzadeh, M.; Moldovan, R.; Wenzel, B.; Kranz, M.; Deuther-Conrad, W.; Toussaint, M.; Fischer, S.; Ludwig, F.-A.; Teodoro, R.; Jonnalagadda, S.; et al. Development of the first F-18-labeled MCT1/MCT4 lactate

transport inhibitor: Radiosynthesis and preliminary in vivo evaluation in mice. In Proceedings of the 23rd International Symposium on Radiopharmaceutical Sciences, Beijing, China, 26–31 May 2019; Volume 62, pp. S59–S60.

28. Sadeghzadeh, M.; Moldovan, R.-P.; Teodoro, R.; Brust, P.; Wenzel, B. One-step radiosynthesis of the MCTs imaging agent [^{18}F]FACH by aliphatic 18F-labelling of a methylsulfonate precursor containing an unprotected carboxylic acid group. *Sci. Rep.* **2019**, *9*, 1–8. [CrossRef]
29. Colen, C.B.; Seraji-Bozorgzad, N.; Marples, B.; Galloway, M.; Sloan, A.E.; Mathupala, S.P. Metabolic Remodeling Of Malignant Gliomas For Enhanced Sensitization During Radiotherapy. *Neurosurgery* **2006**, *59*, 1313–1324. [CrossRef]
30. Mathupala, S.P.; Colen, C.B.; Parajuli, P.; Sloan, A.E. Lactate and malignant tumors: A therapeutic target at the end stage of glycolysis. *J. Bioenerg. Biomembr.* **2007**, *39*, 73–77. [CrossRef]
31. Omori, K.; Tachikawa, M.; Hirose, S.; Taii, A.; Akanuma, S.-I.; Hosoya, K.-I.; Terasaki, T. Developmental changes in transporter and receptor protein expression levels at the rat blood-brain barrier based on quantitative targeted absolute proteomics. *Drug Metab. Pharmacokinet.* **2020**, *35*, 117–123. [CrossRef]
32. Colen, C.B.; Shen, Y.; Ghoddoussi, F.; Yu, P.; Francis, T.B.; Koch, B.J.; Monterey, M.D.; Galloway, M.; Sloan, A.E.; Mathupala, S.P. Metabolic Targeting of Lactate Efflux by Malignant Glioma Inhibits Invasiveness and Induces Necrosis: An In Vivo Study. *Neoplasia* **2011**, *13*, 620–632. [CrossRef] [PubMed]
33. Miranda-Gonçalves, V.; Honavar, I.; Pinheiro, C.; Martinho, O.; Pires, M.; Pinheiro, C.; Cordeiro, M.; Bebiano, G.; Costa, P.; Palmeirim, I.; et al. Monocarboxylate transporters (MCTs) in gliomas: Expression and exploitation as therapeutic targets. *Neuro Oncol.* **2012**, *15*, 172–188. [CrossRef] [PubMed]
34. Serafimova, I.M.; Pufall, M.A.; Krishnan, S.; Duda, K.; Cohen, M.S.; Maglathlin, R.L.; McFarland, J.M.; Miller, R.M.; Frödin, M.; Taunton, J. Reversible targeting of noncatalytic cysteines with chemically tuned electrophiles. *Nat. Methods* **2012**, *8*, 471–476. [CrossRef] [PubMed]
35. Halestrap, A.P. The mechanism of the inhibition of the mitochondrial pyruvate transportater by α-cyanocinnamate derivatives. *Biochem. J.* **1976**, *156*, 181–183. [CrossRef] [PubMed]
36. Koley, M.; Wimmer, L.; Schnürch, M.; Mihovilovic, M.D. Regioselective Syntheses of 2,3-Substituted Pyridines by Orthogonal Cross-Coupling Strategies. *Eur. J. Org. Chem.* **2011**, *2011*, 1972–1979. [CrossRef]
37. Begouin, A.; Hesse, S.; Queiroz, M.J.R.P.; Kirsch, G. Palladium-Catalyzed Buchwald–Hartwig Coupling of Deactivated Aminothiophenes with Substituted Halopyridines. *Eur. J. Org. Chem.* **2007**, *2007*, 1678–1682. [CrossRef]
38. Schumacher, R.A.; Hopper, A.T.; Tehim, A.; Hess, H.-E.; Unterbeck, A.; Kuester, E.; Brubaker, W.F.; Dunn, R.F. Phosphodiesterase 4 Inhibitors, including N-Substituted Aniline and Diphenylamine Analogs. U.S. Patents 7,405,230 B2, 29 July 2008.
39. Vilsmeier, A.; Haack, A. Über die einwirkung von halogenphosphor auf alkyl-formanilide. Eine neue methode zur darstellung sekundärer und tertiärer P-alkylamino-benzaldehyde. *Eur. J. Inorg. Chem.* **1927**, *60*, 4. [CrossRef]
40. Roux, F.; Couraud, P.-O. Rat brain endothelial cell lines for the study of blood-brain barrier permeability and transport functions. *Cell. Mol. Neurobiol.* **2005**, *25*, 41–57. [CrossRef]
41. Pike, V.W. PET radiotracers: Crossing the blood–brain barrier and surviving metabolism. *Trends Pharmacol. Sci.* **2009**, *30*, 431–440. [CrossRef]
42. US EPA. *Estimation Programs Interface Suite™ for Microsoft® Windows*; Version 4.1; EPA: Washington, DC, USA, 2012.
43. *ACD/Percepta*, Version 2726; ACD/Labs 2015 Release (Build 2726 27 November 2014); ACD/Labs: Toronto, ON, Canada. Available online: www.acdlabs.com (accessed on 4 May 2020).
44. Schüürmann, G. Ecotoxic Modes of Action of Chemical Substances. In *Ecotoxicology: Ecological Fundamentals, Chemical Exposure and Biological Effects*; Schüürmann, G., Markert, B., Eds.; John Wiley; Spektrum Akademischer Verlag: New York, NY, USA, 1998; pp. 665–749.
45. Wang, Q.; Lu, Y.; Yuan, M.; Darling, I.M.; Repasky, E.A.; Morris, A.M.E. Characterization of Monocarboxylate Transport in Human Kidney HK-2 Cells. *Mol. Pharm.* **2006**, *3*, 675–685. [CrossRef]
46. Becker, H.M.; Mohebbi, N.; Perna, A.; Ganapathy, V.; Capasso, G.; Wagner, C.A. Localization of members of MCT monocarboxylate transporter family *Slc16* in the kidney and regulation during metabolic acidosis. *Am. J. Physiol. Physiol.* **2010**, *299*, F141–F154. [CrossRef] [PubMed]
47. Lindemann, M.; Hinz, S.; Deuther-Conrad, W.; Namasivayam, V.; Dukic-Stefanovic, S.; Teodoro, R.; Toussaint, M.; Kranz, M.; Juhl, C.; Steinbach, J.; et al. Radiosynthesis and in vivo evaluation of a fluorine-18

labeled pyrazine based radioligand for PET imaging of the adenosine A 2B receptor. *Bioorganic Med. Chem.* **2018**, *26*, 4650–4663. [CrossRef] [PubMed]
48. Nakao, R.; Amini, N.; Halldin, C. Simultaneous Determination of Protein-Free and Total Positron Emission Tomography Radioligand Concentrations in Plasma Using High-Performance Frontal Analysis Followed by Mixed Micellar Liquid Chromatography: Application to [^{11}C]PBR28 in Human Plasma. *Anal. Chem.* **2013**, *85*, 8728–8734. [CrossRef] [PubMed]
49. Pierre, K.; Pellerin, L. Monocarboxylate transporters in the central nervous system: Distribution, regulation and function. *J. Neurochem.* **2005**, *94*, 1–14. [CrossRef] [PubMed]
50. Vijay, N.; Morris, A.M.E. Role of monocarboxylate transporters in drug delivery to the brain. *Curr. Pharm. Des.* **2014**, *20*, 1487–1498. [CrossRef] [PubMed]
51. Spector, R. Micronutrient Homeostasis in Mammalian Brain and Cerebrospinal Fluid. *J. Neurochem.* **1989**, *53*, 1667–1674. [CrossRef]
52. Friedland, R.P.; Mathis, C.A.; Budinger, T.F.; Moyer, B.R.; Rosen, M. Labeled choline and phosphorylcholine: Body distribution and brain autoradiography: Concise communication. *J. Nucl. Med.* **1983**, *24*, 812–815.
53. Rosen, M.A.; Jones, R.M.; Yano, Y.; Budinger, T.F. Carbon-11 choline: Synthesis, purification, and brain uptake inhibition by 2-dimethylaminoethanol. *J. Nucl. Med.* **1985**, *26*, 1424–1428.
54. Hara, T.; Kosaka, N.; Shinoura, N.; Kondo, T. PET imaging of brain tumor with [methyl-^{11}C]choline. *J. Nucl. Med.* **1997**, *38*, 842–847.
55. Dardel, N.T.; Gómez-Río, M.; Triviño-Ibáñez, E.; Llamas-Elvira, J.M. Clinical applications of PET using C-11/F-18-choline in brain tumours: A systematic review. *Clin. Transl. Imaging* **2017**, *5*, 101–119. [CrossRef]
56. Evangelista, L.; Briganti, A.; Fanti, S.; Joniau, S.; Reske, S.; Schiavina, R.; Stief, C.; Thalmann, G.N.; Picchio, M. New Clinical Indications for ^{18}F/^{11}C-choline, New Tracers for Positron Emission Tomography and a Promising Hybrid Device for Prostate Cancer Staging: A Systematic Review of the Literature. *Eur. Urol.* **2016**, *70*, 161–175. [CrossRef] [PubMed]
57. Bergersen, L.H. Is lactate food for neurons? Comparison of monocarboxylate transporter subtypes in brain and muscle. *Neuroscience* **2007**, *145*, 11–19. [CrossRef]
58. Perez-Escuredo, J.; Van Hée, V.; Sboarina, M.; Falces, J.; Payen, V.L.; Pellerin, L.; Sonveaux, P. Monocarboxylate transporters in the brain and in cancer. *Biochim. Biophys. Acta (BBA) Bioenerg.* **2016**, *1863*, 2481–2497. [CrossRef] [PubMed]
59. Miranda-Gonçalves, V.; Bezerra, F.; Costa-Almeida, R.; Freitas-Cunha, M.; Soares, R.; Martinho, O.; Reis, R.M.; Pinheiro, C.; Baltazar, F. Monocarboxylate transporter 1 is a key player in glioma-endothelial cell crosstalk. *Mol. Carcinog.* **2017**, *56*, 2630–2642. [CrossRef]
60. Teodoro, R.; Wenzel, B.; Oh-Nishi, A.; Fischer, S.; Peters, D.; Suhara, T.; Deuther-Conrad, W.; Brust, P. A high-yield automated radiosynthesis of the alpha 7 nicotinic receptor radioligand [^{18}F]NS10743. *Appl. Radiat. Isot.* **2015**, *95*, 76–84. [CrossRef] [PubMed]

6

Current Landscape and Emerging Fields of PET Imaging in Patients with Brain Tumors

Jan-Michael Werner [1], Philipp Lohmann [2], Gereon R. Fink [1,2], Karl-Josef Langen [2,3] and Norbert Galldiks [1,2,*,†]

1 Department of Neurology, Faculty of Medicine and University Hospital Cologne, University of Cologne, Kerpener St. 62, 50937 Cologne, Germany; jan-michael.werner@uk-koeln.de (J.-M.W.); gereon.fink@uk-koeln.de (G.R.F.)
2 Institute of Neuroscience and Medicine (INM-3, -4), Research Center Juelich, Leo-Brandt-St., 52425 Juelich, Germany; p.lohmann@fz-juelich.de (P.L.); k.j.langen@fz-juelich.de (K.-J.L.)
3 Department of Nuclear Medicine, University Hospital Aachen, 52074 Aachen, Germany
* Correspondence: n.galldiks@fz-juelich.de or norbert.galldiks@uk-koeln.de

† Center of Integrated Oncology (CIO), Universities of Aachen, Bonn, Cologne, and Duesseldorf, Germany.

Academic Editor: Peter Brust

Abstract: The number of positron-emission tomography (PET) tracers used to evaluate patients with brain tumors has increased substantially over the last years. For the management of patients with brain tumors, the most important indications are the delineation of tumor extent (e.g., for planning of resection or radiotherapy), the assessment of treatment response to systemic treatment options such as alkylating chemotherapy, and the differentiation of treatment-related changes (e.g., pseudoprogression or radiation necrosis) from tumor progression. Furthermore, newer PET imaging approaches aim to address the need for noninvasive assessment of tumoral immune cell infiltration and response to immunotherapies (e.g., T-cell imaging). This review summarizes the clinical value of the landscape of tracers that have been used in recent years for the above-mentioned indications and also provides an overview of promising newer tracers for this group of patients.

Keywords: amino acid; FET; FACBC; FDOPA; immunoPET; molecular imaging; glioma; brain metastases

---

1. Introduction

For the management of patients with brain tumors, clinicians frequently need to rely on imaging information obtained from anatomical magnetic resonance imaging (MRI) before, during, and after the treatment. While contrast-enhanced MRI is of paramount value in neuro-oncology, its specificity for neoplastic tissue is low, and changes of the blood-brain barrier permeability as indicated by contrast enhancement are not limited to tumor tissue [1–7]. Nevertheless, precise delineation of tumor extent, including non-enhancing tumor subregions, is decisive for several diagnostic and therapeutic steps (e.g., planning of biopsy, surgery, or radiotherapy) [7,8]. Following radio- and/or chemotherapy, neurooncologists often encounter treatment-related changes. Some of these, e.g., pseudoprogression, are difficult to differentiate from actual tumor progression with conventional MRI alone [6–12]. Pseudoprogression describes a phenomenon characterized by an increase of contrast enhancement without clinical deterioration, and which disappears again over time without any treatment change [3,9,13–16]. Such treatment-related changes may occur early (in the case of pseudoprogression typically within the first 12 weeks after chemoradiation completion) or late (several months or even years after radiotherapy in the case 31 of radiation necrosis) [7,8,17].

Furthermore, surrogates of treatment response or progression obtained from MRI (e.g., a decrease of contrast enhancement or the fluid-attenuated inversion recovery (FLAIR) signal hyperintensity) may be unspecific. They can be influenced by inflammation, infarction, and reactive changes after surgery [2,6,12,18]. If treatment-related changes remain unidentified, an effective treatment may be erroneously terminated prematurely. The latter may also harm survival and mislead study results evaluating novel treatment approaches for tumor relapse [19].

To overcome these diagnostic challenges, imaging techniques with higher diagnostic accuracy than conventional MRI offering more than just anatomical information are needed. Apart from advanced MRI techniques, positron-emission tomography (PET) imaging has been evaluated over the past decades. It has been shown that PET imaging offers additional value in neuro-oncology since it enables the non-invasive evaluation of molecular and metabolic features of brain tumors. PET, therefore, is of great value for the indications mentioned above, which are of particular clinical interest [7,8,10,20]. Consequently, the PET task force of the Response Assessment in Neuro-Oncology (RANO) working group highlighted the additional clinical value of PET imaging using amino acid tracers compared to anatomical MRI. Accordingly, its widespread clinical use was recommended in patients with glioma and brain metastases [17,21].

The continuously growing landscape of PET tracers enables the evaluation of many biochemical processes in patients with brain tumors. With the advent of newer treatment options in neuro-oncology, in particular, targeted therapy and various immunotherapy options, the needs for additional information derived from neuroimaging in terms of characterization of the tumor environment, the evaluation of tumoral drug accumulation, immune cell infiltration, and the diagnosis of treatment-related changes following these newer treatment options are steadily increasing. Some of these requirements may be met by the existing landscape of well-established PET tracers, while others can be addressed by newer ones [22,23].

This review summarizes the value of PET tracers that have been used in brain tumors in recent years for the most relevant clinical indications. Furthermore, more unique but promising PET tracers are summarized and discussed.

2. Methods

A PubMed search using the terms "PET", "positron", "tracer", "glioma", "brain metastases", "FDG", "amino acid", "methionine", "FET", "FDOPA", "FACBC", "AMT", "TSPO", "GE-180", "FLT", "FAZA", "EGFR", "VEGF", "immunoPET", "isocitrate dehydrogenase", "radiotherapy", "T-cell imaging", "reporter gene", "radiation necrosis", "pseudoprogression", "tumor extent", "response assessment", "treatment-related changes", and combinations thereof was performed until January 2020. The PET tracers were evaluated regarding their clinical value for the delineation of tumor extent, diagnosis of treatment-related changes, the assessment of treatment response (Table 1), and according to the information provided by newer PET probes (Table 2).

Table 1. Frequently used PET tracers for the delineation of tumor extent, diagnosis of treatment-related changes, and the assessment of treatment response in brain tumor imaging.

Imaging Target and Corresponding Tracers	Delineation of Tumor Extent	Diagnosis of Treatment-Related Changes	Assessment of Treatment Response
Glucose metabolism			
$[^{18}F]$FDG	-	+	-
Amino acid transport			
$[^{18}F]$FET	++	++ [1]	++ [2]
$[^{11}C]$MET	++	+	++
$[^{18}F]$FDOPA	++	++	++
$[^{11}C]$AMT	(++)	(++)	n.a.
$[^{18}F]$FACBC	(++)	n.a.	n.a.
Mitochondrial translocator protein (TSPO)			
$[^{18}F]$GE-180	unclear	n.a.	n.a.
Cellular proliferation			
$[^{18}F]$FLT	-	+	++ [3]
Hypoxia			
$[^{18}F]$FMISO	n.a.	n.a.	(++) [3]
$[^{18}F]$FAZA	n.a.	n.a.	(++) [3]
Perfusion			
$[^{15}O]H_2O$	n.a.	n.a.	n.a.
Angiogenesis			
$[^{89}Zr]$bevacizumab	n.a.	n.a.	n.a.

++ = high diagnostic accuracy; (++) = high diagnostic accuracy, but limited data available; + = limited diagnostic accuracy; - = not helpful; [1] = increased accuracy when using dynamic $[^{18}F]$FET PET; [2] = in enhancing and non-enhancing tumors; [3] = in patients undergoing antiangiogenic treatment with bevacizumab; $[^{11}C]$AMT = α-$[^{11}C]$-methyl-L-tryptophan; $[^{18}F]$FACB = anti-1-amino-3-$[^{18}F]$fluorocyclobutane-1-carboxylic acid; $[^{18}F]$FAZA = $[^{18}F]$flouroazomycin arabinoside; $[^{18}F]$FDG = $[^{18}F]$-2-fluoro-2-deoxy-D-glucose; $[^{18}F]$FDOPA = 3,4-dihydroxy-6-$[^{18}F]$fluoro-L-phenylalanine; $[^{18}F]$FET = O-(2-$[^{18}F]$fluoroethyl)-L-tyrosine; $[^{18}F]$FLT = 3′-deoxy-3′-$[^{18}F]$flurothymidine; $[^{18}F]$FMISO = $[^{18}F]$fluoromisonidazole; $[^{15}O]H_2O$ = radiolabeled water; $[^{11}C]$MET = $[^{11}C]$methyl-L-methionine; n.a. = only preliminary or no data available.

Table 2. Promising PET tracers for the evaluation of newer treatment options.

Tracer	Target	Mechanism
Imaging of the EGFR family		
[^{11}C]erlotinib	EGFR	TKI-mediated imaging
[^{89}Zr]Zr-DFO-nimotuzumab	EGFR	Antibody-mediated imaging
[^{11}C]PD153035	EGFR	TKI-mediated imaging
[^{89}Zr]pertuzumab	HER2	Antibody-mediated imaging
[^{64}Cu]-DOTA-trastuzumab	HER2	Antibody-mediated imaging
Immuno-Imaging		
[^{89}Zr]nivolumab	PD-1	Antibody-mediated imaging
[^{89}Zr]atezolizumab	PD-L1	Antibody-mediated imaging
[^{18}F]BMS-986192	PD-L1	PET imaging using an engineered target-binding protein (adnectin)
[^{89}Zr]IAB22M2C	CD8+ T-cells	Antibody fragment-mediated imaging
[^{18}F]CFA	DCK	Targeting of the deoxy-cytidine kinase
[^{18}F]FHBG	HSV1-tk	Imaging of reporter gene expression
Imaging of IDH mutations		
[^{18}F]AGI-5198	IDH-mutant cells	Imaging of the mutant IDH enzyme using a radiolabeled IDH1 inhibitor
[^{18}F]-labeled triazinediamine analogue	IDH-mutant cells	Imaging of the mutant IDH enzyme
Radiolabeled butyl-phenyl sulfonamide	IDH-mutant cells	Imaging of the mutant IDH enzyme
[^{11}C]acetate	IDH-mutant cells	Metabolic trapping of the tracer in IDH-mutant cells

[^{18}F]CFA = 2-chloro-2′-deoxy-2′-[^{18}F]fluoro-9-b-D-arabinofuranosyl-adenine; DCK = deoxy-cytidine kinase EGFR = epidermal growth factor receptor; [^{18}F]FHBG = 9-[4-[^{18}F]fluoro-3-(hydroxymethyl)butyl]guanine; HER2 = human epidermal growth factor receptor 2; HSV1-tk = herpes simplex virus type 1 thymidine kinase; IDH = isocitrate dehydrogenase-1 or -2; PD-1 = programmed cell death receptor-1; PD-L1 = programmed cell death protein ligand 1; TKI = tyrosine kinase inhibitor.

3. Current Landscape of PET Imaging

PET allows targeting metabolic and molecular processes in patients with brain tumors relevant to diagnosis, treatment, and prognosis that cannot be assessed with anatomic computed tomography (CT) or MR imaging. A variety of PET tracers have been evaluated predominantly in glioma patients or patients with brain metastases with the main focus on glucose metabolism, amino acid transport, proliferation, hypoxia, blood flow, or angiogenesis. This section will provide an overview of PET tracers for brain tumors that have been evaluated in human subjects in the last years, especially for those above mentioned highly relevant indications in clinical routine. An overview is presented in Table 1.

3.1. *PET Imaging of Glucose Metabolism*

[^{18}F]-2-Fluoro-2-deoxy-D-glucose ([^{18}F]FDG) is the most widespread PET tracer in nuclear medicine. In neoplastic tissue, the uptake of [^{18}F]FDG reflects the increased expression of glucose transporters and hexokinase. The latter enzyme phosphorylates glucose and [^{18}F]FDG. In the central nervous system, the physiologically high and varying uptake of [^{18}F]FDG in healthy brain parenchyma hampers the accurate delineation of the brain tumor. This limits the diagnostic accuracy for the correct identification of treatment-related changes and assessment of treatment response in gliomas and brain metastases [17,21]. It has repeatedly been shown that the diagnostic accuracy of [^{18}F]FDG regarding the differentiation of radiation-induced changes from glioma and brain metastases recurrence is inferior to other imaging modalities, including advanced MRI and amino acid PET [17,24–26]. However, [^{18}F]FDG PET seems to be of value for the delineation of tumor extent and assessment of treatment response in patients with primary central nervous system (CNS) lymphoma [27–30].

3.2. *PET Using Amino Acid PET Tracers*

Radiolabeled amino acid tracers (Figure 1) are of great interest in brain tumor imaging because of the high tumor-to-brain contrast based on the relatively high specificity for neoplastic tissue and the low uptake in healthy brain tissue [7,8,21,31–33].

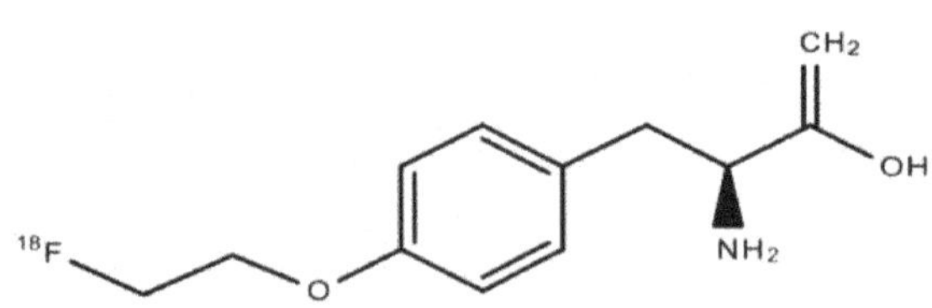

1. [^{18}F]FET

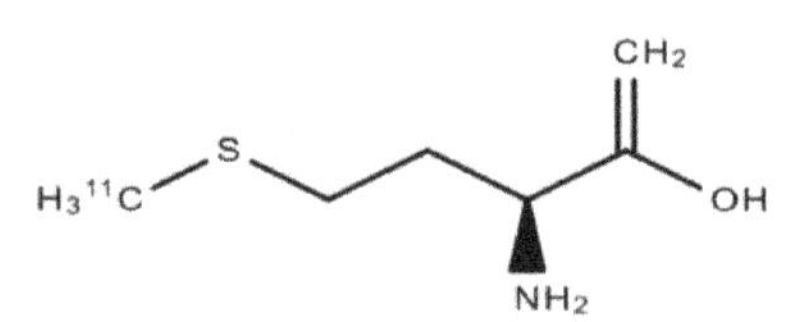

2. [^{11}C]MET

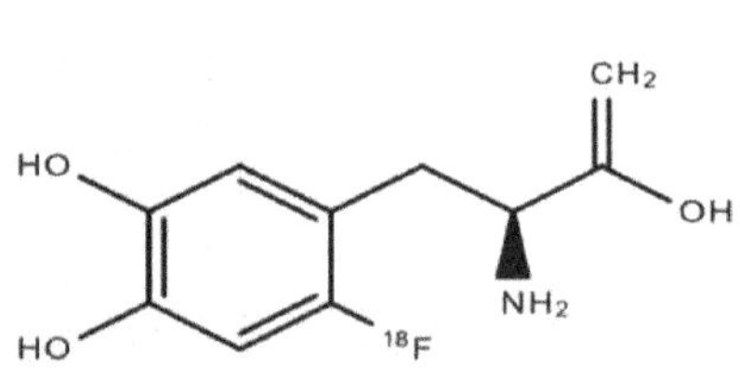

3. [^{18}F]FDOPA

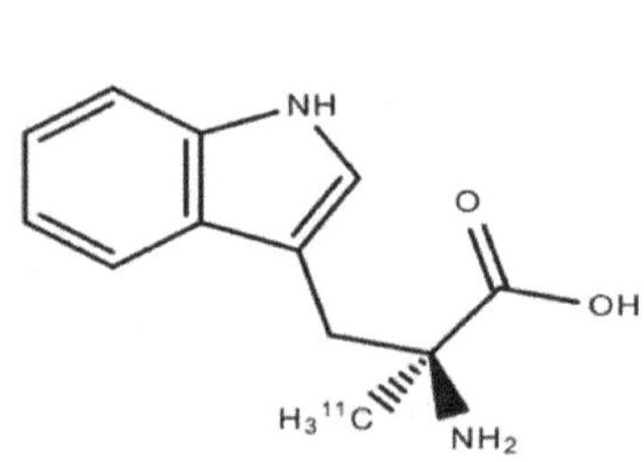

4. [^{11}C]AMT

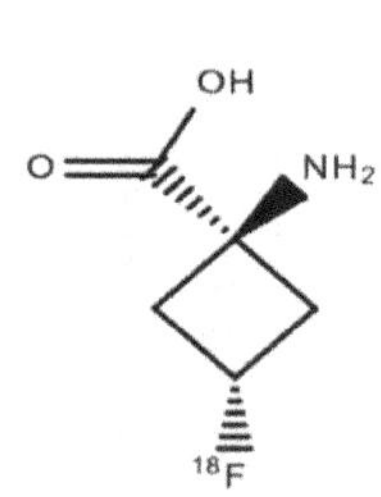

5. [^{18}F]FACBC

Figure 1. Chemical structure of radiolabeled amino acids.

3.2.1. Uptake Mechanisms of Amino Acid PET Tracers

The uptake of the amino acid tracers O-(2-[^{18}F]fluoroethyl)-L-tyrosine ([^{18}F]FET), [^{11}C]methyl-L-methionine ([^{11}C]MET), and 3,4-dihydroxy-6-[^{18}F]fluoro-L-phenylalanine ([^{18}F]FDOPA) is mainly based on the increased expression of large neutral amino acid transporters of the L-type (LAT) in gliomas and brain metastases (i.e., subtypes LAT1 and LAT2) [7,34–37]. Moreover, LAT1 overexpression correlates with malignant phenotypes and proliferation of gliomas. It is associated with glioma angiogenesis [38,39]. A critical consideration for the practical application of [^{11}C]MET compared to [^{18}F]FET or [^{18}F]FDOPA is the half-life of the [^{11}C]-isotope ([^{18}F] 110 vs. [^{11}C] 20 min) [40,41], which allows the transport of [^{18}F]FET and [^{18}F]FDOPA to PET facilities. In contrast, the use of [^{11}C]MET necessitates an on-site cyclotron. In many European centers, this logistical disadvantage has led to the replacement of [^{11}C]MET predominantly by [^{18}F]FET [7]. When using [^{18}F]FDOPA, the physiological uptake in the striatum may hamper the evaluation of tumor extent [7,42].

The L-tryptophan analogue α-[^{11}C]-methyl-L-tryptophan ([^{11}C]AMT) is another radiolabeled amino acid with uptake via the LAT system. Additionally, [^{11}C]AMT uptake is mediated via the kynurenine pathway and has a rate-limiting enzyme indoleamine 2,3-dioxygenase [43]. Indoleamine 2,3-dioxygenase is upregulated in various cancers including gliomas [44], which prompted the use of [^{11}C]AMT PET in patients with brain tumors [45].

Other tracers such as the synthetic amino acid analog anti-1-amino-3-[^{18}F]fluorocyclobutane-1-carboxylic acid ([^{18}F]FACBC or [^{18}F]fluciclovine) are also LAT-mediated but use additionally the alanine, serine, and cysteine transporter 2, which is upregulated in many human cancers [46–49].

3.2.2. Value of Amino Acid PET Tracers for Brain Tumor Patients

For the planning of diagnostic and therapeutic procedures, the precise delineation of tumor spread is essential. For example, the tumor extent as assessed by amino acid PET provides valuable information for planning stereotactic biopsies, resection, and radiotherapy [1,50–52]. For [^{11}C]MET and [^{18}F]FET, it has been shown that the delineation of tumor extent, particularly in non-enhancing gliomas, can be assessed with high accuracy using amino acid PET [51,53]. Preliminary data suggest that newer tracers such as [^{18}F]FACBC PET are also helpful in identifying metabolically active and non-contrast enhancing tumor regions in glioma patients [54–56]. Moreover, it has been shown that in the majority of cases, the metabolically active tumor burden as assessed by amino acid PET extends considerably beyond the volume of MRI contrast enhancement, which is of significant relevance for subsequent treatment planning [1,7,53,57]. Regarding the comparability of PET tracers for this indication, [^{11}C]MET, [^{18}F]FET, and [^{18}F]FDOPA seem to be equally informative [58–61]. Nevertheless, it has to be pointed out that 20–30% of grade II gliomas, according to the World Health Organization (WHO) classification of tumors of the central nervous system [62,63], show no amino acid uptake [64–66]. A negative amino acid PET, therefore, does not exclude glioma [8].

For the differentiation of treatment-related changes from tumor relapse, amino acid PET also provides valuable diagnostic information. Using [^{18}F]FET or [^{18}F]FDOPA, especially the differentiation of radiation injury from tumor relapse in glioma patients, as well as in patients with brain metastases, can be obtained with a relatively high diagnostic accuracy between 80–90% (Figure 2) [11,26,67–80]. Importantly, in glioma patients, parameters derived from dynamic [^{18}F]FET PET acquisition may further increase the diagnostic accuracy [67,74–76,78]. This has also been demonstrated in patients with brain metastases who underwent radiosurgery for brain metastases treatment [80,81]. The diagnostic accuracy of [^{11}C]MET PET regarding this clinical question is slightly lower (approximately 75%) [8,82,83], which is most probably related to the higher affinity of [^{11}C]MET for inflammation [84]. First PET studies using [^{11}C]AMT or [^{18}F]FACBC suggest that these tracers may also be of value for the differentiation of radiation injury from glioma progression [85,86].

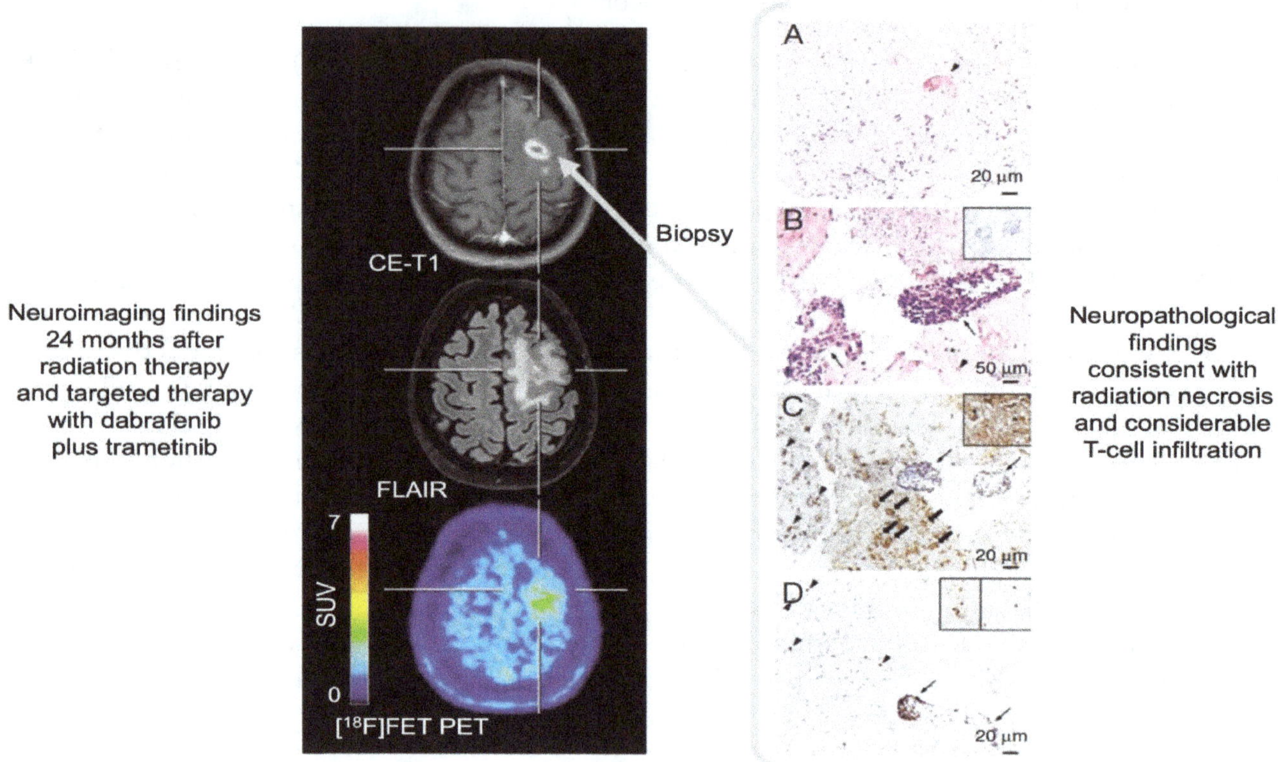

Figure 2. Radiation necrosis and chronic inflammation in a patient with brain metastases of a B-Raf proto-oncogene (BRAF)-mutated malignant melanoma who had been treated with whole-brain radiation therapy combined with concurrent dabrafenib plus trametinib. Twenty-four months later, the contrast-enhanced magnetic resonance imaging (MRI) indicates a recurrence of the brain metastases (left panel), whereas the O-(2-[^{18}F]fluoroethyl)-L-tyrosine ([^{18}F]FET) positron-emission tomography (PET) shows only insignificant metabolic activity and is consistent with the findings of treatment-related MRI changes. Neuropathological findings (right panel) after stereotactic biopsy show signs of radiation necrosis as well as considerable T-cell infiltration. (**A**) Hyaline, eosinophilic necrosis with evidence of a necrotic vessel wall (arrowhead). (**B**) Vital brain parenchyma besides necrosis with activated microglia cells (arrowhead), and blood vessels with lymphocyte infiltrates (arrows) without evidence of tumor cells (inserted box). (**C**) Adjacent to inflamed blood vessels (arrows), a resorption of necroses by macrophages (block arrows) as well as activated microglia cells (arrowheads) and astrocytes in the brain parenchyma (inserted box). (**D**) The main population of intra- and perivascular T-cell infiltrates are CD3$^+$ (arrow), but also CD4$^+$ (inserted box left) and CD8$^+$ (inserted box right) T-cells contribute to the infiltrates (modified from Galldiks et al. [10], with permission from Oxford University Press).

The advent of immunotherapy using immune checkpoint inhibitors and targeted therapy has improved the survival of cancer patients, particularly in melanoma and lung cancer. Recent trials suggest that patients with brain metastases from these tumor entities may also benefit from these agents alone or in combination [87]. Regarding patients with brain metastases treated with checkpoint inhibitors or targeted therapy (frequently combined with radiotherapy), initial data indicate that amino acid PET may provide valuable information for differentiating relapse from equivocal MRI findings related to immunotherapy-induced inflammation [10,88].

Recently, a variety of experimental treatment options has been introduced for treating patients with high-grade glioma. [^{18}F]FET PET was shown to differentiate benign MRI findings related to these experimental therapies, e.g., immunotherapy with dendritic cell vaccination or targeted therapy with regorafenib, from tumor relapse [89,90]. However, the number of patients treated with these therapies and monitored with [^{18}F]FET PET is still small, and the results should be interpreted with caution.

The assessment of the response to a particular neurooncological treatment is of clinical relevance since treatment decisions can be negatively affected by treatment-related changes. The accurate assessment of response helps both to discontinue an ineffective treatment option as early as possible and to prevent an effective treatment from being erroneously terminated prematurely with a potentially harmful influence on survival. Furthermore, the evaluation of response also helps to avoid possible treatment side effects, e.g., bone marrow depression or fatigue, and, therefore, to maintain or even improve life-quality. It has been shown in glioma patients that the assessment of response to alkylating chemotherapy (i.e., temozolomide or lomustine) using [^{11}C]MET or [^{18}F]FET PET provides valuable additional information compared to contrast-enhanced MRI. Importantly, metabolic PET responders (i.e., patients with a decrease of tumor-to-brain ratios or metabolically active tumor volumes at follow-up relative to baseline imaging) had a significantly longer survival than metabolic non-responders [91–98].

Following antiangiogenic therapy using bevacizumab, the use of reduced contrast enhancement as a surrogate marker for treatment response is not optimal due to a phenomenon called pseudoresponse [9]. Pseudoresponse describes a decrease of contrast enhancement related to a rapid restoration of the blood-brain barrier by antiangiogenic drugs [9]. However, a clinical benefit is not infrequently lacking in patients with an impressive radiological response (pseudoresponse). [^{18}F]FET and [^{18}F]FDOPA PET may provide valuable information regarding the identification of pseudoresponse [99–102]. Moreover, [^{18}F]FDOPA and [^{18}F]FET PET were also able to predict a favorable clinical outcome in bevacizumab responders [101–104].

After chemoradiation completion, newly diagnosed glioblastoma patients can be treated with tumor-treating fields therapy in addition to adjuvant temozolomide chemotherapy [105]. Initial studies suggest that amino acid PET might identify responding patients undergoing tumor-treating fields therapy, but it has to be considered that the response can also be related to the concurrently applied chemotherapy or delayed chemoradiation effects [106,107].

3.3. PET Imaging of the Mitochondrial Translocator Protein

PET ligands targeting the 18 kDa mitochondrial translocator protein (TSPO), located at the outer mitochondrial membrane and formerly known as the peripheral benzodiazepine receptor, are also of interest in neuro-oncology [108,109]. TSPO is associated with neuroinflammation due to its expression in activated microglia, endothelial cells, and infiltrating macrophages [109]. The PET ligand [^{11}C]PK11195 was one of the first ligands evaluated for TSPO expression in glioma patients [110–112].

The recently introduced TSPO ligand GE-180 labeled with [^{18}F] offers an increased binding specificity and was tested in patients with gliomas [113] and neuroinflammatory diseases such as multiple sclerosis [114–116]. Regarding the delineation of glioma extent, it has been demonstrated that the [^{18}F]GE-180 uptake volume is significantly larger than the volume of contrast enhancement [113,117]. However, when comparing [^{18}F]FET with [^{18}F]GE-180 uptake volumes intraindividually in terms of spatial distribution, the overlap is only moderate (Dice similarity coefficient, 0.55) despite comparable tumor volumes [117]. These differences might help to characterize glioma heterogeneity and warrant further studies with spatial correlation of imaging findings of [^{18}F]FET uptake to [^{18}F]GE-180 uptake with neuropathology.

3.4. PET Imaging of Cellular Proliferation

The radiolabeled nucleoside 3′-deoxy-3′-[^{18}F]fluorothymidine ([^{18}F]FLT) is a pyrimidine analogue. It is used to evaluate cellular proliferation because of its rapid incorporation into newly synthesized DNA [118]. [^{18}F]FLT is trapped intracellularly after phosphorylation by the thymidine kinase-1, a cytoplasmatic enzyme expressed during cell proliferation [46,119]. However, the requirement of a disrupted blood-brain barrier for [^{18}F]FLT uptake may limit its diagnostic use [2,120]. For example, in terms of tumor detection and delineation, [^{18}F]FLT PET was less sensitive than [^{11}C]MET PET to detect WHO grade II gliomas, which usually show no contrast enhancement [121]. Furthermore, a meta-analysis evaluating the value of [^{18}F]FLT PET for the diagnosis of glioma recurrence based on approximately 800 patients showed no superiority of [^{18}F]FLT (pooled sensitivity, 82%; pooled specificity, 76%) compared to [^{18}F]FDG (pooled sensitivity, 78%; pooled specificity, 77%) [122].

On the other hand, [^{18}F]FLT PET seems to be useful for the assessment of response to antiangiogenic therapy with bevacizumab in patients with recurrent malignant glioma. [^{18}F]FLT PET was able to identify a reduction of proliferative activity in responding patients with favorable outcome as an indicator for response compared to metabolic non-responders [123–125]. Furthermore, [^{18}F]FLT PET was used in patients with malignant melanoma brain metastases treated with targeted therapy or immunotherapy using checkpoint inhibitors [126]. In that study, responding patients showed a clearer reduction of proliferative activity as assessed by [^{18}F]FLT PET than the decrease of contrast enhancement on standard MRI.

3.5. PET Imaging of Tumor Hypoxia

Hypoxia is a key factor in treatment outcome in various cancers, including glioma. It has been shown that hypoxia is associated with tumor persistence and resistance to cancer treatment [127]. To further evaluate this phenomenon using PET, the tracer [^{18}F]fluoromisonidazole ([^{18}F]FMISO) has been developed, which is trapped in hypoxic but viable cells [46,128,129]. It has been demonstrated in glioblastoma patients that [^{18}F]FMISO PET delineates additional hypoxic tumor subregions which exceed the contrast-enhancing tumor parts, indicating that hypoxia may induce peripheral tumor growth [130]. A subsequent study showed that the metabolically active tumor volume in [^{11}C]MET PET strongly correlated with the hypoxic volume defined by [^{18}F]FMISO [131]. Importantly, the tumor area on [^{11}C]MET PET exceeded the area of the contrast enhancement on MRI in the range of 20–30%.

More recently, [^{18}F]FMISO PET has been used for monitoring the effects of antiangiogenic therapy with bevacizumab in patients with recurrent malignant glioma [132,133]. It was shown that patients who had a response in both contrast-enhanced MRI and [^{18}F]FMISO PET had significantly longer survival than patients who responded on MRI only [133].

[^{18}F]-labeled flouroazomycin arabinoside ([^{18}F]FAZA) may be a promising alternative to [^{18}F]FMISO offering an improved tumor-to-background ratio due to faster blood clearance [134,135]. Preliminary data in glioblastoma patients suggest that [^{18}F]FAZA PET might be of value for radiotherapy response assessment [136].

3.6. PET Imaging of Tumor Perfusion

The evaluation of regional cerebral blood flow (rCBF) allows identifying brain tumors with high vascularization. rCBF can be measured by PET using [^{15}O]-labeled water. However, [^{15}O]H_2O requires an on-site cyclotron because of its very short half-life (2 min) [137]. The development and easy accessibility of perfusion-weighted CT and MRI has led to various studies evaluating brain tumors outnumbering [^{15}O]H_2O PET studies by far. In direct comparisons, it has been shown that rCBF values differ considerably between CT- and MRI-based perfusion measurements and [^{15}O]H_2O PET [138,139].

In patients with malignant gliomas undergoing chemoradiation with nitrosoureas, a reduction of rCBF was evaluated using [^{15}O]H_2O PET, but data on subsequent survival as an indicator for treatment response are lacking [140,141].

3.7. PET Imaging of Angiogenesis

The vascular endothelial growth factor (VEGF) is overexpressed by most tumors, including brain tumors, and an important trigger for neovascularization [142]. Bevacizumab is a recombinant humanized monoclonal antibody against VEGF and appears to prolong progression-free survival and decrease steroid usage in patients with malignant glioma [142,143]. Based on these properties, [^{89}Zr]-labeled bevacizumab PET imaging has been evaluated for tumoral drug accumulation in pediatric patients with diffuse intrinsic pontine glioma [144]. That study demonstrated intertumoral heterogeneity of drug accumulation and may aid in selecting those patients with the greatest chance of benefit from bevacizumab [144,145]. Other studies have used [^{64}Cu]-labeled conjugates of VEGF with DOTA (1,4,7,10-tetra-azacylododecane *N,N′,N′′,N′′′*-tetraacetic acid) for PET imaging in animal models [146–148]. Similarly, these approaches suggest the clinical value for the identification of patients who will benefit from anti-VEGF therapy.

In adult glioblastoma patients, it has been demonstrated that accumulation of [^{123}I]VEGF in the tumor region of glioblastomas can be assessed using single photon emission computed tomography (SPECT) imaging [149]. Importantly, high uptake of [^{123}I]VEGF was able to identify glioblastoma patients with a poor clinical outcome.

4. Emerging Fields of PET Imaging

Currently, blockade of immune checkpoints and other immunotherapy options (i.e., vaccination strategies, oncolytic virus approaches, cell-based immunotherapy such as chimeric antigen receptor T-cells (CAR-T cells) are under evaluation in patients with brain cancer including glioma and brain metastases. Furthermore, recent study results suggest that newer-generation targeted therapies are a promising treatment option, especially in a subset of patients with brain metastases [150]. As a new treatment option, mutations of the isocitrate dehydrogenase (*IDH*) gene, which frequently occur in WHO grade II and III gliomas, have also gained interest as a potential treatment target [151,152]. All these promising treatment options impose new demands on brain imaging (e.g., imaging of immune reactions in the brain). The current body of literature suggests that PET has the potential to adapt to these needs. An overview is presented in Table 2.

4.1. PET Imaging of the Epidermal Growth Factor Receptor Family

Both the epidermal growth factor receptor (EGFR) and the human epidermal growth factor receptor 2 (HER2) are transmembrane protein receptors and belong to the EGFR family. These receptors are targets for various growth factors that mediate various cellular processes such as differentiation or proliferation. In clinical oncology, various gene mutations may lead to overexpression of these proteins and are associated with the development of a variety of cancers. Importantly, these mutations also play a significant role in various treatment options, including tyrosine kinase inhibitors and monoclonal antibodies targeting EGFR, HER2, or both [153], as well as for imaging. Especially the evaluation of a response to these targeted therapy options in patients with brain metastases (from melanoma, lung, or breast cancer) as well as in glioma patients is the indication with the highest clinical potential for EGFR- and HER2-targeted PET [154,155]. In recent years, radiolabeled EGFR and HER2 antibodies, as well as tyrosine kinase inhibitors, have been used as PET imaging agents.

For identifying EGFR overexpression, PET ligands such as [^{11}C]erlotinib, [^{11}C]PD153035, and [^{89}Zr]Zr-DFO-nimotuzumab have been used [156–158]. The most relevant PET tracers for imaging of HER2 overexpression are [^{64}Cu]DOTA-trastuzumab and [^{89}Zr]pertuzumab (Figure 3) [159,160].

4.2. Immuno-Imaging: Immuno-PET and Imaging of T-Cells

In recent years, immunotherapy with antibodies directed against immune checkpoints such as the cytotoxic T-lymphocyte antigen-4 (CTLA-4; e.g., ipilimumab), the programmed cell death receptor-1 (PD-1; e.g., pembrolizumab, nivolumab), or the programmed cell death protein ligand 1 (PD-L1; e.g., atezolizumab) have gained paramount importance in clinical oncology and neuro-oncology. However, the efficacy and responsiveness of these agents may vary considerably among different cancer types and across individuals. Biomarkers obtained from tumor tissue, such as PD-1 and PD-L1 expression, can help to select patients. However, these tissue biomarkers are limited, and some patients show no response even if the target is present [161]. Therefore, the significance of PET for predicting response to immunotherapy and patient selection increases. Among other methods, immuno-PET combines antibodies or antibody fragments with a radionuclide and takes advantage of the specificity and affinity of antibodies and the sensitivity of PET [162]. Generally, targets for immuno-PET can be T-cell markers (e.g., $CD4^+$, $CD8^+$), immune checkpoints (e.g., CTLA-4, PD-1, PD-L1), or biomarkers of the immune response (e.g., interferon-γ, interleukin-2) [23].

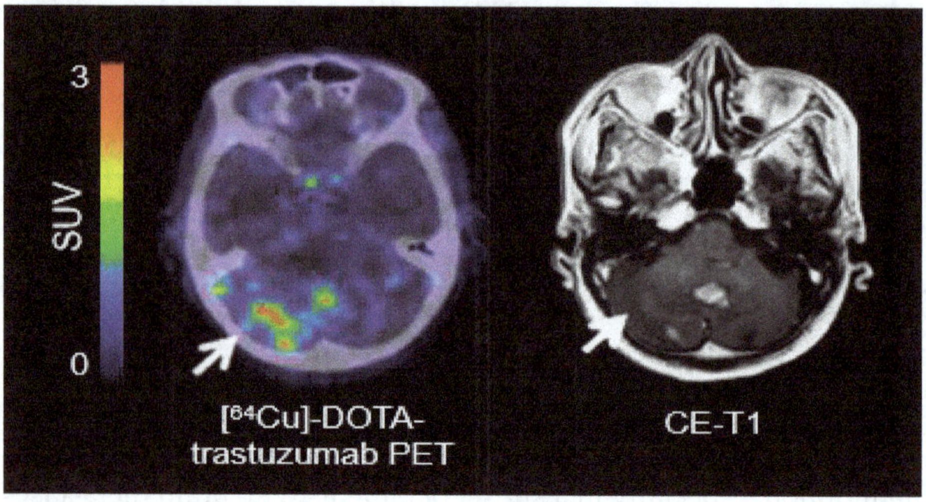

Figure 3. [^{64}Cu]-DOTA-trastuzumab positron-emission tomography (PET) and contrast-enhanced magnetic resonance imaging (MRI) performed one day after initiation of treatment with trastuzumab in a patient with a human epidermal growth factor receptor 2 (HER2)-positive breast cancer with brain metastases. In single brain metastases, [^{64}Cu]-DOTA-trastuzumab PET helps to improve lesion detection (arrow) (modified from Tamura et al. [160], with permission from the Society of Nuclear Medicine and Molecular Imaging).

First-in-human studies suggest that targeting PD-1 with [^{89}Zr]nivolumab [163] or PD-L1 with [^{89}Zr]atezolizumab [164] is useful as imaging biomarkers to non-invasively evaluate the expression of these immune checkpoints in patients with extra- and intracranial cancer [164,165]. Engineered target-binding proteins (adnectins) for PD-L1 ligands such as [^{18}F]BMS-986192 are currently under evaluation [166].

Tumor-infiltrating T-cells (such as CD8$^+$) play an essential role in the activation of immune cells in response to checkpoint inhibition [167]. Recently, it has been shown that a radiolabeled [^{89}Zr]IAB22M2C has the potential to visualize CD8$^+$ T-cell-enriched tumor tissue [168]. The assessment of immune cells infiltrating tumors has also been investigated with PET using radiolabeled clofarabine (2-chloro-2′-deoxy-2′-[^{18}F]fluoro-9-b-D-arabinofuranosyl-adenine; [^{18}F]CFA) [169]. [^{18}F]CFA is a substrate for the enzyme deoxy-cytidine kinase, which is overexpressed in immune cells such as CD8$^+$ T-cells [169]. Importantly, [^{18}F]CFA PET has shown a great clinical potential to localize and quantify immune responses in glioblastoma patients undergoing dendritic cell vaccination treatment combined with immune checkpoint blockade (Figure 4) [169].

Another interesting approach is the transfection of immune cells with a reporter gene that encodes a protein that can be specifically targeted by a radiolabeled reporter probe [170]. Imaging of reporter gene expression of cells transfected with the herpes simplex virus type 1 thymidine kinase reporter gene has been demonstrated using 9-[4-[^{18}F]fluoro-3-(hydroxymethyl)butyl]guanine ([^{18}F]FHBG) [171]. Moreover, this technique has the potential to image recently introduced cell-based therapies with CAR-T cells [23]. Accordingly, a study with recurrent high-grade glioma patients suggested that [^{18}F]FHBG PET can detect reporter gene expression in CAR-engineered cytotoxic T-lymphocytes [172].

4.3. PET Imaging of Isocitrate Dehydrogenase Mutations

In patients with malignant glioma, the modest outcome improvement following both standard therapy (i.e., chemoradiation with temozolomide) and newer treatment options (e.g., tumor-treating fields) has prompted various efforts to identify molecules that are fundamental to regulate tumor progression and provide additional options for personalized therapy in this group of patients.

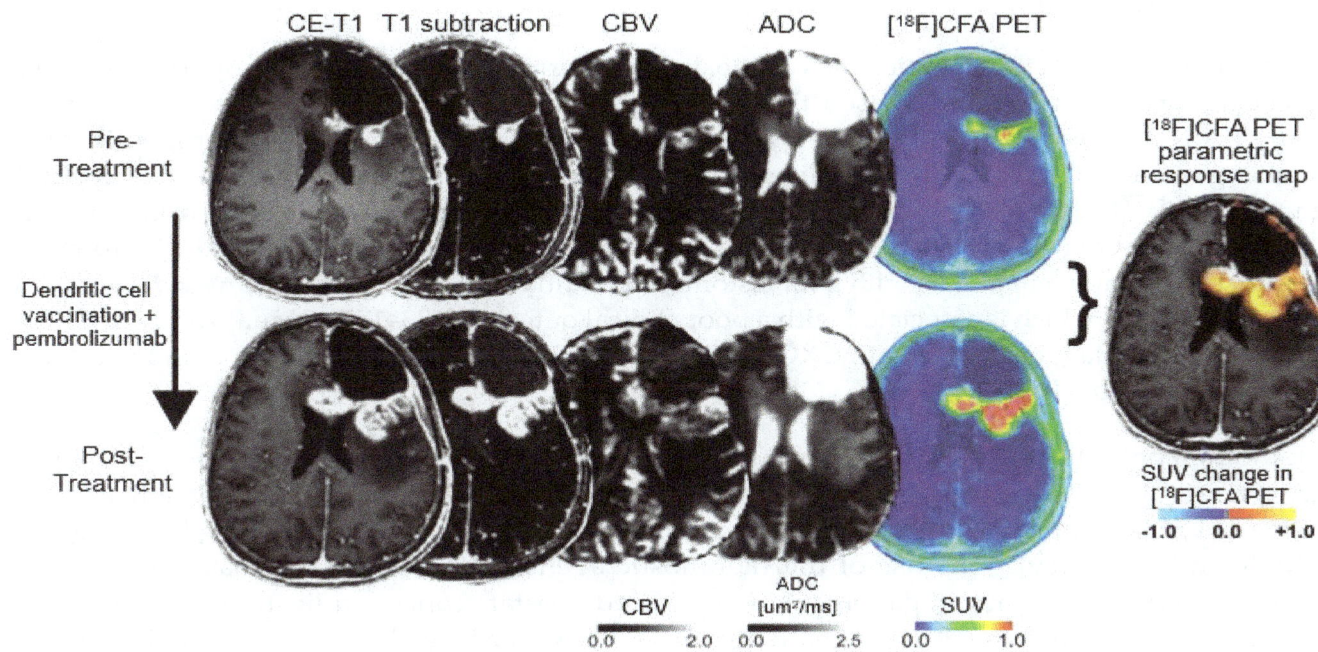

Figure 4. Detection of immune response in a patient with recurrent glioblastoma using 2-chloro-2′-deoxy-2′-[^{18}F]fluoro-9-b-D-arabinofuranosyl-adenine ([^{18}F]CFA) positron-emission tomography (PET) and advanced magnetic resonance imaging (MRI) before (upper panel) and after treatment with dendritic cell vaccination and programmed cell death receptor-1 (PD-1) blockade using pembrolizumab (lower panel). Following treatment, [^{18}F]CFA uptake is considerably increased, indicating an immune-cell infiltration, and helps distinguishing tumor progression from inflammation (modified from Antonios et al. [169], with permission from the National Academy of Sciences).

Accordingly, the enzyme isocitrate dehydrogenase (IDH) has gained interest as a potential target. IDH is an enzyme of the Krebs cycle, catalyzing the oxidative decarboxylation of isocitrate to alpha-ketoglutarate. Mutations in the *IDH1* and *IDH2* gene, frequently occurring in WHO grade II or III astrocytomas and oligodendrogliomas, result in a significant increase of the oncometabolite 2-hydroxyglutarate (2-HG) [173,174]. In cells with IDH mutant enzymes, the accumulation of 2-HG alters several downstream cellular activities, causing epigenetic dysregulation and, consequently, a block in cellular differentiation, leading to oncogenesis [175].

Therefore, mutant IDH proteins are highly attractive targets for inhibitory drugs. In glioma patients, selective oral IDH inhibitors of IDH1 (i.e., ivosidenib, BAY-1436032), pan-IDH1/2 (i.e., AG-881), and vaccination strategies targeting the IDH1R132H mutation are currently under clinical evaluation. Initial results predominantly from phase-1 studies are promising and suggest that these inhibitors are safe and have antitumoral activity [151,152,176]. Although immunohistochemistry and genomic sequencing are the methods of choice for the detection of an IDH mutation, these techniques are invasive and are not appropriate for treatment monitoring, which requires continual assessment. Furthermore, the use of magnetic resonance spectroscopy (MRS) to non-invasively evaluate 2-HG is technically challenging, and may be false-positive in 20% of cases [177,178].

Newer PET probes for imaging mutant IDH expression in gliomas may be an alternative imaging method. Recent radiochemical developments suggest that triazinediamine or butyl-phenyl sulfonamide analogs labeled with [^{18}F] are promising candidate radiotracers for noninvasive PET imaging of IDH mutations in gliomas [179,180]. Furthermore, a [^{18}F]-labeled IDH1 inhibitor (AGI-5198) has also been investigated [181]. Interestingly, Koyaso and colleagues demonstrated that [^{11}C]acetate uptake in IDH mutant cells is significantly higher than in IDH wild-type cells because of metabolic trapping [182]. Taken together, further efforts to translate these promising approaches for IDH imaging into clinical use are warranted.

4.4. PET-Based Theranostics

The combination of therapeutics and diagnostics, also termed as theranostics, supports the concept of precision oncology. One PET-based theranostic approach is the peptide receptor radionuclide therapy (PRRT), in which overexpressed tumor-specific receptors are used as a therapeutic target. By exchanging the radionuclide used for diagnostic PET such as [^{68}Ga] with a radiation source, typically β-emitters like [^{177}Lu] or [^{90}Y], the same PET tracer can be used for therapy. Although there are currently no theranostic approaches clinically established for gliomas or brain metastases, there are promising concepts. For example in patients with glioblastoma, a potential target is the overexpressed chemokine receptor-4 (CXCR4) which is associated with a poor clinical outcome [183–185]. Visualization of CXCR4 expression using diagnostic PET with CXCR4-directed [^{68}Ga]Pentixafor® has been demonstrated in glioblastoma patients [186].

Another potential target is the prostate-specific membrane antigen (PSMA) which may be overexpressed in prostate cancer and also in predominantly malignant gliomas. Diagnostic PET imaging of PSMA expression in patients with malignant glioma can be obtained using [^{68}Ga]-labeled PSMA ligands [187–189]. The use of the theranostic agent [^{177}Lu]-PSMA-617 has demonstrated favorable safety and efficacy in patients with advanced prostate cancer, indicating the potential to be also of value for patients with malignant glioma [190]. Nevertheless, the potential of theranostics needs to be further evaluated in patients with malignant gliomas.

5. Discussion

Anatomical MRI is currently the method of choice for neuroimaging of brain tumors, but PET complements this technique and provides important biological information that cannot be obtained from anatomical MRI alone. Currently, best-established PET tracers in neuro-oncology are radiolabeled amino acids targeting L-system transporters. However, a considerable number of other PET tracers have been developed for brain tumor patients and allow the evaluation of a wide range of biochemical processes. A variety of PET biomarkers offers the potential to play a clinically significant role for the monitoring of newer treatment options such as targeted therapy and immunotherapy, e.g., by providing an early assessment of response to these options, and for a more accurate differentiation of viable tumor from treatment-related changes. A major current shortcoming is the lack of large, prospective clinical trials in patients with both glioma and brain metastases for many of these PET tracers. Despite encouraging early study results in the field, it has to be further demonstrated that these tracers improve considerably patient management and outcome.

Author Contributions: Study design, writing of manuscript drafts: J.W. and N.G. Revising manuscript, approving final content of the manuscript: All. All authors have read and agreed to the published version of the manuscript.

References

1. Lohmann, P.; Stavrinou, P.; Lipke, K.; Bauer, E.K.; Ceccon, G.; Werner, J.M.; Neumaier, B.; Fink, G.R.; Shah, N.J.; Langen, K.J.; et al. FET PET reveals considerable spatial differences in tumour burden compared to conventional MRI in newly diagnosed glioblastoma. *Eur. J. Nucl. Med. Mol. Imaging* **2019**, *46*, 591–602. [CrossRef]
2. Dhermain, F.G.; Hau, P.; Lanfermann, H.; Jacobs, A.H.; van den Bent, M.J. Advanced MRI and PET imaging for assessment of treatment response in patients with gliomas. *Lancet Neurol.* **2010**, *9*, 906–920. [CrossRef]
3. Brandsma, D.; Stalpers, L.; Taal, W.; Sminia, P.; van den Bent, M.J. Clinical features, mechanisms, and management of pseudoprogression in malignant gliomas. *Lancet Oncol.* **2008**, *9*, 453–461. [CrossRef]

4. Hygino da Cruz, L.C., Jr.; Rodriguez, I.; Domingues, R.C.; Gasparetto, E.L.; Sorensen, A.G. Pseudoprogression and pseudoresponse: Imaging challenges in the assessment of posttreatment glioma. *AJNR Am. J. Neuroradiol.* **2011**, *32*, 1978–1985. [CrossRef]
5. Yang, I.; Aghi, M.K. New advances that enable identification of glioblastoma recurrence. *Nat. Rev. Clin. Oncol.* **2009**, *6*, 648–657. [CrossRef]
6. Kumar, A.J.; Leeds, N.E.; Fuller, G.N.; Van Tassel, P.; Maor, M.H.; Sawaya, R.E.; Levin, V.A. Malignant gliomas: MR imaging spectrum of radiation therapy- and chemotherapy-induced necrosis of the brain after treatment. *Radiology* **2000**, *217*, 377–384. [CrossRef] [PubMed]
7. Langen, K.J.; Galldiks, N.; Hattingen, E.; Shah, N.J. Advances in neuro-oncology imaging. *Nat. Rev. Neurol.* **2017**, *13*, 279–289. [CrossRef]
8. Galldiks, N.; Lohmann, P.; Albert, N.L.; Tonn, J.C.; Langen, K.-J. Current status of PET imaging in neuro-oncology. *Neurooncol. Adv.* **2019**, *1*. [CrossRef]
9. Brandsma, D.; van den Bent, M.J. Pseudoprogression and pseudoresponse in the treatment of gliomas. *Curr. Opin. Neurol.* **2009**, *22*, 633–638. [CrossRef]
10. Galldiks, N.; Kocher, M.; Ceccon, G.; Werner, J.M.; Brunn, A.; Deckert, M.; Pope, W.B.; Soffietti, R.; Le Rhun, E.; Weller, M.; et al. Imaging challenges of immunotherapy and targeted therapy in patients with brain metastases: Response, progression, and pseudoprogression. *Neuro Oncol.* **2020**, *22*, 17–30. [CrossRef]
11. Galldiks, N.; Dunkl, V.; Stoffels, G.; Hutterer, M.; Rapp, M.; Sabel, M.; Reifenberger, G.; Kebir, S.; Dorn, F.; Blau, T.; et al. Diagnosis of pseudoprogression in patients with glioblastoma using O-(2-[18F]fluoroethyl)-L-tyrosine PET. *Eur. J. Nucl. Med. Mol. Imaging* **2015**, *42*, 685–695. [CrossRef] [PubMed]
12. Ahluwalia, M.S.; Wen, P.Y. Antiangiogenic therapy for patients with glioblastoma: Current challenges in imaging and future directions. *Expert Rev. Anticancer Ther.* **2011**, *11*, 653–656. [CrossRef]
13. Taal, W.; Brandsma, D.; de Bruin, H.G.; Bromberg, J.E.; Swaak-Kragten, A.T.; Smitt, P.A.; van Es, C.A.; van den Bent, M.J. Incidence of early pseudo-progression in a cohort of malignant glioma patients treated with chemoirradiation with temozolomide. *Cancer* **2008**, *113*, 405–410. [CrossRef]
14. Radbruch, A.; Fladt, J.; Kickingereder, P.; Wiestler, B.; Nowosielski, M.; Baumer, P.; Schlemmer, H.P.; Wick, A.; Heiland, S.; Wick, W.; et al. Pseudoprogression in patients with glioblastoma: Clinical relevance despite low incidence. *Neuro Oncol.* **2015**, *17*, 151–159. [CrossRef]
15. Galldiks, N.; Kocher, M.; Langen, K.J. Pseudoprogression after glioma therapy: An update. *Expert Rev. Neurother.* **2017**, *17*, 1109–1115. [CrossRef] [PubMed]
16. Young, R.J.; Gupta, A.; Shah, A.D.; Graber, J.J.; Zhang, Z.; Shi, W.; Holodny, A.I.; Omuro, A.M. Potential utility of conventional MRI signs in diagnosing pseudoprogression in glioblastoma. *Neurology* **2011**, *76*, 1918–1924. [CrossRef] [PubMed]
17. Galldiks, N.; Langen, K.J.; Albert, N.L.; Chamberlain, M.; Soffietti, R.; Kim, M.M.; Law, I.; Le Rhun, E.; Chang, S.; Schwarting, J.; et al. PET imaging in patients with brain metastasis-report of the RANO/PET group. *Neuro Oncol.* **2019**, *21*, 585–595. [CrossRef] [PubMed]
18. Wen, P.Y.; Macdonald, D.R.; Reardon, D.A.; Cloughesy, T.F.; Sorensen, A.G.; Galanis, E.; Degroot, J.; Wick, W.; Gilbert, M.R.; Lassman, A.B.; et al. Updated response assessment criteria for high-grade gliomas: Response assessment in neuro-oncology working group. *J. Clin. Oncol.* **2010**, *28*, 1963–1972. [CrossRef]
19. Reardon, D.A.; Weller, M. Pseudoprogression: Fact or wishful thinking in neuro-oncology? *Lancet Oncol.* **2018**, *19*, 1561–1563. [CrossRef]
20. Nandu, H.; Wen, P.Y.; Huang, R.Y. Imaging in neuro-oncology. *Ther. Adv. Neurol. Disord.* **2018**, *11*. [CrossRef]
21. Albert, N.L.; Weller, M.; Suchorska, B.; Galldiks, N.; Soffietti, R.; Kim, M.M.; la Fougere, C.; Pope, W.; Law, I.; Arbizu, J.; et al. Response Assessment in Neuro-Oncology working group and European Association for Neuro-Oncology recommendations for the clinical use of PET imaging in gliomas. *Neuro Oncol.* **2016**, *18*, 1199–1208. [CrossRef] [PubMed]
22. Wei, W.; Ni, D.; Ehlerding, E.B.; Luo, Q.Y.; Cai, W. PET Imaging of Receptor Tyrosine Kinases in Cancer. *Mol. Cancer Ther.* **2018**, *17*, 1625–1636. [CrossRef] [PubMed]
23. Wei, W.; Jiang, D.; Ehlerding, E.B.; Luo, Q.; Cai, W. Noninvasive PET Imaging of T cells. *Trends Cancer* **2018**, *4*, 359–373. [CrossRef] [PubMed]

24. Chernov, M.; Hayashi, M.; Izawa, M.; Ochiai, T.; Usukura, M.; Abe, K.; Ono, Y.; Muragaki, Y.; Kubo, O.; Hori, T.; et al. Differentiation of the radiation-induced necrosis and tumor recurrence after gamma knife radiosurgery for brain metastases: Importance of multi-voxel proton MRS. *Min-Minim. Invasive Neurosurg.* **2005**, *48*, 228–234. [CrossRef]
25. Hatzoglou, V.; Yang, T.J.; Omuro, A.; Gavrilovic, I.; Ulaner, G.; Rubel, J.; Schneider, T.; Woo, K.M.; Zhang, Z.; Peck, K.K.; et al. A prospective trial of dynamic contrast-enhanced MRI perfusion and fluorine-18 FDG PET-CT in differentiating brain tumor progression from radiation injury after cranial irradiation. *Neuro Oncol.* **2016**, *18*, 873–880. [CrossRef]
26. Tomura, N.; Kokubun, M.; Saginoya, T.; Mizuno, Y.; Kikuchi, Y. Differentiation between Treatment-Induced Necrosis and Recurrent Tumors in Patients with Metastatic Brain Tumors: Comparison among (11)C-Methionine-PET, FDG-PET, MR Permeability Imaging, and MRI-ADC-Preliminary Results. *AJNR Am. J. Neuroradiol.* **2017**, *38*, 1520–1527. [CrossRef]
27. Palmedo, H.; Urbach, H.; Bender, H.; Schlegel, U.; Schmidt-Wolf, I.G.; Matthies, A.; Linnebank, M.; Joe, A.; Bucerius, J.; Biersack, H.J.; et al. FDG-PET in immunocompetent patients with primary central nervous system lymphoma: Correlation with MRI and clinical follow-up. *Eur. J. Nucl. Med. Mol. Imaging* **2006**, *33*, 164–168. [CrossRef]
28. Birsen, R.; Blanc, E.; Willems, L.; Burroni, B.; Legoff, M.; Le Ray, E.; Pilorge, S.; Salah, S.; Quentin, A.; Deau, B.; et al. Prognostic value of early 18F-FDG PET scanning evaluation in immunocompetent primary CNS lymphoma patients. *Oncotarget* **2018**, *9*, 16822–16831. [CrossRef]
29. Chiavazza, C.; Pellerino, A.; Ferrio, F.; Cistaro, A.; Soffietti, R.; Ruda, R. Primary CNS Lymphomas: Challenges in Diagnosis and Monitoring. *Biomed. Res. Int.* **2018**, *2018*, 3606970. [CrossRef]
30. Herholz, K.; Langen, K.J.; Schiepers, C.; Mountz, J.M. Brain tumors. *Semin. Nucl. Med.* **2012**, *42*, 356–370. [CrossRef]
31. Langen, K.J.; Watts, C. Neuro-oncology: Amino acid PET for brain tumours—Ready for the clinic? *Nat. Rev. Neurol.* **2016**, *12*, 375–376. [CrossRef] [PubMed]
32. Law, I.; Albert, N.L.; Arbizu, J.; Boellaard, R.; Drzezga, A.; Galldiks, N.; la Fougere, C.; Langen, K.J.; Lopci, E.; Lowe, V.; et al. Joint EANM/EANO/RANO practice guidelines/SNMMI procedure standards for imaging of gliomas using PET with radiolabelled amino acids and [(18)F]FDG: Version 1.0. *Eur. J. Nucl. Med. Mol. Imaging* **2019**, *46*, 540–557. [CrossRef] [PubMed]
33. Drake, L.R.; Hillmer, A.T.; Cai, Z. Approaches to PET Imaging of Glioblastoma. *Molecules* **2020**, *25*, 568. [CrossRef]
34. Youland, R.S.; Kitange, G.J.; Peterson, T.E.; Pafundi, D.H.; Ramiscal, J.A.; Pokorny, J.L.; Giannini, C.; Laack, N.N.; Parney, I.F.; Lowe, V.J.; et al. The role of LAT1 in (18)F-DOPA uptake in malignant gliomas. *J. Neurooncol.* **2013**, *111*, 11–18. [CrossRef] [PubMed]
35. Papin-Michault, C.; Bonnetaud, C.; Dufour, M.; Almairac, F.; Coutts, M.; Patouraux, S.; Virolle, T.; Darcourt, J.; Burel-Vandenbos, F. Study of LAT1 Expression in Brain Metastases: Towards a Better Understanding of the Results of Positron Emission Tomography Using Amino Acid Tracers. *PLoS ONE* **2016**, *11*, e0157139. [CrossRef] [PubMed]
36. Wiriyasermkul, P.; Nagamori, S.; Tominaga, H.; Oriuchi, N.; Kaira, K.; Nakao, H.; Kitashoji, T.; Ohgaki, R.; Tanaka, H.; Endou, H.; et al. Transport of 3-fluoro-L-alpha-methyl-tyrosine by tumor-upregulated L-type amino acid transporter 1: A cause of the tumor uptake in PET. *J. Nucl. Med.* **2012**, *53*, 1253–1261. [CrossRef]
37. Okubo, S.; Zhen, H.N.; Kawai, N.; Nishiyama, Y.; Haba, R.; Tamiya, T. Correlation of L-methyl-11C-methionine (MET) uptake with L-type amino acid transporter 1 in human gliomas. *J. Neurooncol.* **2010**, *99*, 217–225. [CrossRef] [PubMed]
38. Haining, Z.; Kawai, N.; Miyake, K.; Okada, M.; Okubo, S.; Zhang, X.; Fei, Z.; Tamiya, T. Relation of LAT1/4F2hc expression with pathological grade, proliferation and angiogenesis in human gliomas. *BMC Clin. Pathol.* **2012**, *12*, 4. [CrossRef]
39. Kracht, L.W.; Friese, M.; Herholz, K.; Schroeder, R.; Bauer, B.; Jacobs, A.; Heiss, W.D. Methyl-[11C]-l-methionine uptake as measured by positron emission tomography correlates to microvessel density in patients with glioma. *Eur. J. Nucl. Med. Mol. Imaging* **2003**, *30*, 868–873. [CrossRef]
40. Langen, K.J.; Hamacher, K.; Weckesser, M.; Floeth, F.; Stoffels, G.; Bauer, D.; Coenen, H.H.; Pauleit, D. O-(2-[18F]fluoroethyl)-L-tyrosine: Uptake mechanisms and clinical applications. *Nucl. Med. Biol.* **2006**, *33*, 287–294. [CrossRef]

41. Galldiks, N.; Law, I.; Pope, W.B.; Arbizu, J.; Langen, K.J. The use of amino acid PET and conventional MRI for monitoring of brain tumor therapy. *Neuroimage Clin.* **2017**, *13*, 386–394. [CrossRef] [PubMed]
42. Cicone, F.; Filss, C.P.; Minniti, G.; Rossi-Espagnet, C.; Papa, A.; Scaringi, C.; Galldiks, N.; Bozzao, A.; Shah, N.J.; Scopinaro, F.; et al. Volumetric assessment of recurrent or progressive gliomas: Comparison between F-DOPA PET and perfusion-weighted MRI. *Eur. J. Nucl. Med. Mol. Imaging* **2015**, *42*, 905–915. [CrossRef]
43. Juhasz, C.; Dwivedi, S.; Kamson, D.O.; Michelhaugh, S.K.; Mittal, S. Comparison of amino acid positron emission tomographic radiotracers for molecular imaging of primary and metastatic brain tumors. *Mol. Imaging* **2014**, *13*. [CrossRef]
44. Uyttenhove, C.; Pilotte, L.; Theate, I.; Stroobant, V.; Colau, D.; Parmentier, N.; Boon, T.; Van den Eynde, B.J. Evidence for a tumoral immune resistance mechanism based on tryptophan degradation by indoleamine 2,3-dioxygenase. *Nat. Med.* **2003**, *9*, 1269–1274. [CrossRef] [PubMed]
45. Batista, C.E.; Juhasz, C.; Muzik, O.; Kupsky, W.J.; Barger, G.; Chugani, H.T.; Mittal, S.; Sood, S.; Chakraborty, P.K.; Chugani, D.C. Imaging correlates of differential expression of indoleamine 2,3-dioxygenase in human brain tumors. *Mol. Imaging Biol.* **2009**, *11*, 460–466. [CrossRef] [PubMed]
46. Choudhary, G.; Langen, K.J.; Galldiks, N.; McConathy, J. Investigational PET tracers for high-grade gliomas. *Q. J. Nucl. Med. Mol. Imaging* **2018**, *62*, 281–294. [CrossRef] [PubMed]
47. Fuchs, B.C.; Bode, B.P. Amino acid transporters ASCT2 and LAT1 in cancer: Partners in crime? *Semin. Cancer Biol.* **2005**, *15*, 254–266. [CrossRef] [PubMed]
48. Scalise, M.; Pochini, L.; Console, L.; Losso, M.A.; Indiveri, C. The Human SLC1A5 (ASCT2) Amino Acid Transporter: From Function to Structure and Role in Cell Biology. *Front. Cell Dev. Biol.* **2018**, *6*, 96. [CrossRef]
49. Schuster, D.M.; Nanni, C.; Fanti, S.; Oka, S.; Okudaira, H.; Inoue, Y.; Sorensen, J.; Owenius, R.; Choyke, P.; Turkbey, B.; et al. Anti-1-amino-3-18F-fluorocyclobutane-1-carboxylic acid: Physiologic uptake patterns, incidental findings, and variants that may simulate disease. *J. Nucl. Med.* **2014**, *55*, 1986–1992. [CrossRef]
50. Hayes, A.R.; Jayamanne, D.; Hsiao, E.; Schembri, G.P.; Bailey, D.L.; Roach, P.J.; Khasraw, M.; Newey, A.; Wheeler, H.R.; Back, M. Utilizing 18F-fluoroethyltyrosine (FET) positron emission tomography (PET) to define suspected nonenhancing tumor for radiation therapy planning of glioblastoma. *Pract. Radiat. Oncol.* **2018**, *8*, 230–238. [CrossRef]
51. Kracht, L.W.; Miletic, H.; Busch, S.; Jacobs, A.H.; Voges, J.; Hoevels, M.; Klein, J.C.; Herholz, K.; Heiss, W.D. Delineation of brain tumor extent with [11C]L-methionine positron emission tomography: Local comparison with stereotactic histopathology. *Clin. Cancer Res.* **2004**, *10*, 7163–7170. [CrossRef] [PubMed]
52. Lopez, W.O.; Cordeiro, J.G.; Albicker, U.; Doostkam, S.; Nikkhah, G.; Kirch, R.D.; Trippel, M.; Reithmeier, T. Correlation of (18)F-fluoroethyl tyrosine positron-emission tomography uptake values and histomorphological findings by stereotactic serial biopsy in newly diagnosed brain tumors using a refined software tool. *Onco Targets Ther.* **2015**, *8*, 3803–3815. [CrossRef] [PubMed]
53. Pauleit, D.; Floeth, F.; Hamacher, K.; Riemenschneider, M.J.; Reifenberger, G.; Muller, H.W.; Zilles, K.; Coenen, H.H.; Langen, K.J. O-(2-[18F]fluoroethyl)-L-tyrosine PET combined with MRI improves the diagnostic assessment of cerebral gliomas. *Brain* **2005**, *128*, 678–687. [CrossRef] [PubMed]
54. Bogsrud, T.V.; Londalen, A.; Brandal, P.; Leske, H.; Panagopoulos, I.; Borghammer, P.; Bach-Gansmo, T. 18F-Fluciclovine PET/CT in Suspected Residual or Recurrent High-Grade Glioma. *Clin. Nucl. Med.* **2019**. [CrossRef] [PubMed]
55. Michaud, L.; Beattie, B.J.; Akhurst, T.; Dunphy, M.; Zanzonico, P.; Finn, R.; Mauguen, A.; Schoder, H.; Weber, W.A.; Lassman, A.B.; et al. (18)F-Fluciclovine ((18)F-FACBC) PET imaging of recurrent brain tumors. *Eur. J. Nucl. Med. Mol. Imaging* **2019**. [CrossRef] [PubMed]
56. Tsuyuguchi, N.; Terakawa, Y.; Uda, T.; Nakajo, K.; Kanemura, Y. Diagnosis of Brain Tumors Using Amino Acid Transport PET Imaging with (18)F-fluciclovine: A Comparative Study with L-methyl-(11)C-methionine PET Imaging. *Asia Ocean. J. Nucl. Med. Biol.* **2017**, *5*, 85–94. [CrossRef] [PubMed]
57. Galldiks, N.; Ullrich, R.; Schroeter, M.; Fink, G.R.; Jacobs, A.H.; Kracht, L.W. Volumetry of [(11)C]-methionine PET uptake and MRI contrast enhancement in patients with recurrent glioblastoma multiforme. *Eur. J. Nucl. Med. Mol. Imaging* **2010**, *37*, 84–92. [CrossRef]

58. Grosu, A.L.; Astner, S.T.; Riedel, E.; Nieder, C.; Wiedenmann, N.; Heinemann, F.; Schwaiger, M.; Molls, M.; Wester, H.J.; Weber, W.A. An interindividual comparison of O-(2-[18F]fluoroethyl)-L-tyrosine (FET)- and L-[methyl-11C]methionine (MET)-PET in patients with brain gliomas and metastases. *Int. J. Radiat. Oncol. Biol. Phys.* **2011**, *81*, 1049–1058. [CrossRef]
59. Becherer, A.; Karanikas, G.; Szabo, M.; Zettinig, G.; Asenbaum, S.; Marosi, C.; Henk, C.; Wunderbaldinger, P.; Czech, T.; Wadsak, W.; et al. Brain tumour imaging with PET: A comparison between [18F]fluorodopa and [11C]methionine. *Eur. J. Nucl. Med. Mol. Imaging* **2003**, *30*, 1561–1567. [CrossRef]
60. Kratochwil, C.; Combs, S.E.; Leotta, K.; Afshar-Oromieh, A.; Rieken, S.; Debus, J.; Haberkorn, U.; Giesel, F.L. Intra-individual comparison of (1)(8)F-FET and (1)(8)F-DOPA in PET imaging of recurrent brain tumors. *Neuro Oncol.* **2014**, *16*, 434–440. [CrossRef]
61. Lapa, C.; Linsenmann, T.; Monoranu, C.M.; Samnick, S.; Buck, A.K.; Bluemel, C.; Czernin, J.; Kessler, A.F.; Homola, G.A.; Ernestus, R.I.; et al. Comparison of the amino acid tracers 18F-FET and 18F-DOPA in high-grade glioma patients. *J. Nucl. Med.* **2014**, *55*, 1611–1616. [CrossRef] [PubMed]
62. Louis, D.N.; Perry, A.; Reifenberger, G.; von Deimling, A.; Figarella-Branger, D.; Cavenee, W.K.; Ohgaki, H.; Wiestler, O.D.; Kleihues, P.; Ellison, D.W. The 2016 World Health Organization Classification of Tumors of the Central Nervous System: A summary. *Acta Neuropathol.* **2016**, *131*, 803–820. [CrossRef] [PubMed]
63. Louis, D.N.; Ohgaki, H.; Wiestler, O.D.; Cavenee, W.K.; Burger, P.C.; Jouvet, A.; Scheithauer, B.W.; Kleihues, P. The 2007 WHO classification of tumours of the central nervous system. *Acta Neuropathol.* **2007**, *114*, 97–109. [CrossRef] [PubMed]
64. Pichler, R.; Dunzinger, A.; Wurm, G.; Pichler, J.; Weis, S.; Nussbaumer, K.; Topakian, R.; Aigner, R.M. Is there a place for FET PET in the initial evaluation of brain lesions with unknown significance? *Eur. J. Nucl. Med. Mol. Imaging* **2010**, *37*, 1521–1528. [CrossRef] [PubMed]
65. Hutterer, M.; Nowosielski, M.; Putzer, D.; Jansen, N.L.; Seiz, M.; Schocke, M.; McCoy, M.; Gobel, G.; la Fougere, C.; Virgolini, I.J.; et al. [18F]-fluoro-ethyl-L-tyrosine PET: A valuable diagnostic tool in neuro-oncology, but not all that glitters is glioma. *Neuro Oncol.* **2013**, *15*, 341–351. [CrossRef]
66. Jansen, N.L.; Graute, V.; Armbruster, L.; Suchorska, B.; Lutz, J.; Eigenbrod, S.; Cumming, P.; Bartenstein, P.; Tonn, J.C.; Kreth, F.W.; et al. MRI-suspected low-grade glioma: Is there a need to perform dynamic FET PET? *Eur. J. Nucl. Med. Mol. Imaging* **2012**, *39*, 1021–1029. [CrossRef]
67. Werner, J.M.; Stoffels, G.; Lichtenstein, T.; Borggrefe, J.; Lohmann, P.; Ceccon, G.; Shah, N.J.; Fink, G.R.; Langen, K.J.; Kabbasch, C.; et al. Differentiation of treatment-related changes from tumour progression: A direct comparison between dynamic FET PET and ADC values obtained from DWI MRI. *Eur. J. Nucl. Med. Mol. Imaging* **2019**, *46*, 1889–1901. [CrossRef]
68. Kebir, S.; Fimmers, R.; Galldiks, N.; Schafer, N.; Mack, F.; Schaub, C.; Stuplich, M.; Niessen, M.; Tzaridis, T.; Simon, M.; et al. Late Pseudoprogression in Glioblastoma: Diagnostic Value of Dynamic O-(2-[18F]fluoroethyl)-L-Tyrosine PET. *Clin. Cancer Res.* **2016**, *22*, 2190–2196. [CrossRef]
69. Popperl, G.; Gotz, C.; Rachinger, W.; Gildehaus, F.J.; Tonn, J.C.; Tatsch, K. Value of O-(2-[18F]fluoroethyl)-L-tyrosine PET for the diagnosis of recurrent glioma. *Eur. J. Nucl. Med. Mol. Imaging* **2004**, *31*, 1464–1470. [CrossRef]
70. Rachinger, W.; Goetz, C.; Popperl, G.; Gildehaus, F.J.; Kreth, F.W.; Holtmannspotter, M.; Herms, J.; Koch, W.; Tatsch, K.; Tonn, J.C. Positron emission tomography with O-(2-[18F]fluoroethyl)-l-tyrosine versus magnetic resonance imaging in the diagnosis of recurrent gliomas. *Neurosurgery* **2005**, *57*, 505–511. [CrossRef]
71. Mihovilovic, M.I.; Kertels, O.; Hanscheid, H.; Lohr, M.; Monoranu, C.M.; Kleinlein, I.; Samnick, S.; Kessler, A.F.; Linsenmann, T.; Ernestus, R.I.; et al. O-(2-((18)F)fluoroethyl)-L-tyrosine PET for the differentiation of tumour recurrence from late pseudoprogression in glioblastoma. *J. Neurol. Neurosurg. Psychiatry* **2019**, *90*, 238–239. [CrossRef] [PubMed]
72. Mehrkens, J.H.; Popperl, G.; Rachinger, W.; Herms, J.; Seelos, K.; Tatsch, K.; Tonn, J.C.; Kreth, F.W. The positive predictive value of O-(2-[18F]fluoroethyl)-L-tyrosine (FET) PET in the diagnosis of a glioma recurrence after multimodal treatment. *J. Neurooncol.* **2008**, *88*, 27–35. [CrossRef] [PubMed]
73. Jena, A.; Taneja, S.; Gambhir, A.; Mishra, A.K.; D'Souza, M.M.; Verma, S.M.; Hazari, P.P.; Negi, P.; Jhadav, G.K.; Sogani, S.K. Glioma Recurrence Versus Radiation Necrosis: Single-Session Multiparametric Approach Using Simultaneous O-(2-18F-Fluoroethyl)-L-Tyrosine PET/MRI. *Clin. Nucl. Med.* **2016**, *41*, e228–e236. [CrossRef] [PubMed]

74. Pyka, T.; Hiob, D.; Preibisch, C.; Gempt, J.; Wiestler, B.; Schlegel, J.; Straube, C.; Zimmer, C. Diagnosis of glioma recurrence using multiparametric dynamic 18F-fluoroethyl-tyrosine PET-MRI. *Eur. J. Radiol.* **2018**, *103*, 32–37. [CrossRef]
75. Galldiks, N.; Stoffels, G.; Filss, C.; Rapp, M.; Blau, T.; Tscherpel, C.; Ceccon, G.; Dunkl, V.; Weinzierl, M.; Stoffel, M.; et al. The use of dynamic O-(2-18F-fluoroethyl)-l-tyrosine PET in the diagnosis of patients with progressive and recurrent glioma. *Neuro Oncol.* **2015**, *17*, 1293–1300. [CrossRef]
76. Ceccon, G.; Lohmann, P.; Stoffels, G.; Judov, N.; Filss, C.P.; Rapp, M.; Bauer, E.; Hamisch, C.; Ruge, M.I.; Kocher, M.; et al. Dynamic O-(2-18F-fluoroethyl)-L-tyrosine positron emission tomography differentiates brain metastasis recurrence from radiation injury after radiotherapy. *Neuro Oncol.* **2017**, *19*, 281–288. [CrossRef]
77. Tsuyuguchi, N.; Sunada, I.; Iwai, Y.; Yamanaka, K.; Tanaka, K.; Takami, T.; Otsuka, Y.; Sakamoto, S.; Ohata, K.; Goto, T.; et al. Methionine positron emission tomography of recurrent metastatic brain tumor and radiation necrosis after stereotactic radiosurgery: Is a differential diagnosis possible? *J. Neurosurg.* **2003**, *98*, 1056–1064. [CrossRef]
78. Galldiks, N.; Stoffels, G.; Filss, C.P.; Piroth, M.D.; Sabel, M.; Ruge, M.I.; Herzog, H.; Shah, N.J.; Fink, G.R.; Coenen, H.H.; et al. Role of O-(2-(18)F-fluoroethyl)-L-tyrosine PET for differentiation of local recurrent brain metastasis from radiation necrosis. *J. Nucl. Med.* **2012**, *53*, 1367–1374. [CrossRef]
79. Lizarraga, K.J.; Allen-Auerbach, M.; Czernin, J.; DeSalles, A.A.; Yong, W.H.; Phelps, M.E.; Chen, W. (18)F-FDOPA PET for differentiating recurrent or progressive brain metastatic tumors from late or delayed radiation injury after radiation treatment. *J. Nucl. Med.* **2014**, *55*, 30–36. [CrossRef]
80. Cicone, F.; Minniti, G.; Romano, A.; Papa, A.; Scaringi, C.; Tavanti, F.; Bozzao, A.; Maurizi Enrici, R.; Scopinaro, F. Accuracy of F-DOPA PET and perfusion-MRI for differentiating radionecrotic from progressive brain metastases after radiosurgery. *Eur. J. Nucl. Med. Mol. Imaging* **2015**, *42*, 103–111. [CrossRef]
81. Terakawa, Y.; Tsuyuguchi, N.; Iwai, Y.; Yamanaka, K.; Higashiyama, S.; Takami, T.; Ohata, K. Diagnostic accuracy of 11C-methionine PET for differentiation of recurrent brain tumors from radiation necrosis after radiotherapy. *J. Nucl. Med.* **2008**, *49*, 694–699. [CrossRef] [PubMed]
82. Nihashi, T.; Dahabreh, I.J.; Terasawa, T. Diagnostic accuracy of PET for recurrent glioma diagnosis: A meta-analysis. *AJNR Am. J. Neuroradiol.* **2013**, *34*, 944–950. [CrossRef] [PubMed]
83. Minamimoto, R.; Saginoya, T.; Kondo, C.; Tomura, N.; Ito, K.; Matsuo, Y.; Matsunaga, S.; Shuto, T.; Akabane, A.; Miyata, Y.; et al. Differentiation of Brain Tumor Recurrence from Post-Radiotherapy Necrosis with 11C-Methionine PET: Visual Assessment versus Quantitative Assessment. *PLoS ONE* **2015**, *10*, e0132515. [CrossRef]
84. Salber, D.; Stoffels, G.; Pauleit, D.; Oros-Peusquens, A.M.; Shah, N.J.; Klauth, P.; Hamacher, K.; Coenen, H.H.; Langen, K.J. Differential uptake of O-(2-18F-fluoroethyl)-L-tyrosine, L-3H-methionine, and 3H-deoxyglucose in brain abscesses. *J. Nucl. Med.* **2007**, *48*, 2056–2062. [CrossRef] [PubMed]
85. Alkonyi, B.; Barger, G.R.; Mittal, S.; Muzik, O.; Chugani, D.C.; Bahl, G.; Robinette, N.L.; Kupsky, W.J.; Chakraborty, P.K.; Juhasz, C. Accurate differentiation of recurrent gliomas from radiation injury by kinetic analysis of alpha-11C-methyl-L-tryptophan PET. *J. Nucl. Med.* **2012**, *53*, 1058–1064. [CrossRef] [PubMed]
86. Henderson, F.; Brem, S.; O'Rourke, D.M.; Nasrallah, M.; Buch, V.P.; Young, A.J.; Doot, R.K.; Pantel, A.; Desai, A.; Bagley, S.J.; et al. 18F-Fluciclovine PET to distinguish treatment-related effects from disease progression in recurrent glioblastoma: PET fusion with MRI guides neurosurgical sampling. *Neurooncol. Pract.* **2019**. [CrossRef]
87. Long, G.V.; Atkinson, V.; Lo, S.; Sandhu, S.; Guminski, A.D.; Brown, M.P.; Wilmott, J.S.; Edwards, J.; Gonzalez, M.; Scolyer, R.A.; et al. Combination nivolumab and ipilimumab or nivolumab alone in melanoma brain metastases: A multicentre randomised phase 2 study. *Lancet Oncol.* **2018**, *19*, 672–681. [CrossRef]
88. Galldiks, N.; Abdulla, D.S.Y.; Scheffler, M.; Schweinsberg, V.; Schlaak, M.; Kreuzberg, N.; Landsberg, J.; Lohmann, P.; Ceccon, G.; Werner, J.M.; et al. Treatment monitoring of immunotherapy and targeted therapy using FET PET in patients with melanoma and lung cancer brain metastases: Initial experiences. *J. Clin. Oncol.* **2019**, *37*, e13525. [CrossRef]
89. Kristin Schmitz, A.; Sorg, R.V.; Stoffels, G.; Grauer, O.M.; Galldiks, N.; Steiger, H.J.; Kamp, M.A.; Langen, K.J.; Sabel, M.; Rapp, M. Diagnostic impact of additional O-(2-[18F]fluoroethyl)-L-tyrosine ((18)F-FET) PET following immunotherapy with dendritic cell vaccination in glioblastoma patients. *Br. J. Neurosurg.* **2019**. [CrossRef]

90. Galldiks, N.; Werner, J.M.; Tscherpel, C.; Fink, G.R.; Langen, K.J. Imaging findings following regorafenib in malignant gliomas: FET PET adds valuable information to anatomical MRI. *Neurooncol. Adv.* **2019**, *1*. [CrossRef]
91. Galldiks, N.; Kracht, L.W.; Burghaus, L.; Ullrich, R.T.; Backes, H.; Brunn, A.; Heiss, W.D.; Jacobs, A.H. Patient-tailored, imaging-guided, long-term temozolomide chemotherapy in patients with glioblastoma. *Mol. Imaging* **2010**, *9*, 40–46. [CrossRef] [PubMed]
92. Galldiks, N.; Kracht, L.W.; Burghaus, L.; Thomas, A.; Jacobs, A.H.; Heiss, W.D.; Herholz, K. Use of 11C-methionine PET to monitor the effects of temozolomide chemotherapy in malignant gliomas. *Eur. J. Nucl. Med. Mol. Imaging* **2006**, *33*, 516–524. [CrossRef] [PubMed]
93. Herholz, K.; Kracht, L.W.; Heiss, W.D. Monitoring the effect of chemotherapy in a mixed glioma by C-11-methionine PET. *J. Neuroimaging* **2003**, *13*, 269–271. [CrossRef] [PubMed]
94. Galldiks, N.; Langen, K.J.; Holy, R.; Pinkawa, M.; Stoffels, G.; Nolte, K.W.; Kaiser, H.J.; Filss, C.P.; Fink, G.R.; Coenen, H.H.; et al. Assessment of treatment response in patients with glioblastoma using O-(2-18F-fluoroethyl)-L-tyrosine PET in comparison to MRI. *J. Nucl. Med.* **2012**, *53*, 1048–1057. [CrossRef] [PubMed]
95. Piroth, M.D.; Pinkawa, M.; Holy, R.; Klotz, J.; Nussen, S.; Stoffels, G.; Coenen, H.H.; Kaiser, H.J.; Langen, K.J.; Eble, M.J. Prognostic value of early [18F]fluoroethyltyrosine positron emission tomography after radiochemotherapy in glioblastoma multiforme. *Int. J. Radiat. Oncol. Biol. Phys.* **2011**, *80*, 176–184. [CrossRef] [PubMed]
96. Wyss, M.; Hofer, S.; Bruehlmeier, M.; Hefti, M.; Uhlmann, C.; Bartschi, E.; Buettner, U.W.; Roelcke, U. Early metabolic responses in temozolomide treated low-grade glioma patients. *J. Neurooncol.* **2009**, *95*, 87–93. [CrossRef]
97. Roelcke, U.; Wyss, M.T.; Nowosielski, M.; Ruda, R.; Roth, P.; Hofer, S.; Galldiks, N.; Crippa, F.; Weller, M.; Soffietti, R. Amino acid positron emission tomography to monitor chemotherapy response and predict seizure control and progression-free survival in WHO grade II gliomas. *Neuro Oncol.* **2016**, *18*, 744–751. [CrossRef]
98. Suchorska, B.; Unterrainer, M.; Biczok, A.; Sosnova, M.; Forbrig, R.; Bartenstein, P.; Tonn, J.C.; Albert, N.L.; Kreth, F.W. (18)F-FET-PET as a biomarker for therapy response in non-contrast enhancing glioma following chemotherapy. *J. Neurooncol.* **2018**, *139*, 721–730. [CrossRef]
99. Galldiks, N.; Rapp, M.; Stoffels, G.; Dunkl, V.; Sabel, M.; Langen, K.J. Earlier diagnosis of progressive disease during bevacizumab treatment using O-(2-18F-fluorethyl)-L-tyrosine positron emission tomography in comparison with magnetic resonance imaging. *Mol. Imaging* **2013**, *12*, 273–276. [CrossRef]
100. Morana, G.; Piccardo, A.; Garre, M.L.; Nozza, P.; Consales, A.; Rossi, A. Multimodal magnetic resonance imaging and 18F-L-dihydroxyphenylalanine positron emission tomography in early characterization of pseudoresponse and nonenhancing tumor progression in a pediatric patient with malignant transformation of ganglioglioma treated with bevacizumab. *J. Clin. Oncol.* **2013**, *31*, e1. [CrossRef]
101. Hutterer, M.; Nowosielski, M.; Putzer, D.; Waitz, D.; Tinkhauser, G.; Kostron, H.; Muigg, A.; Virgolini, I.J.; Staffen, W.; Trinka, E.; et al. O-(2-18F-fluoroethyl)-L-tyrosine PET predicts failure of antiangiogenic treatment in patients with recurrent high-grade glioma. *J. Nucl. Med.* **2011**, *52*, 856–864. [CrossRef] [PubMed]
102. Galldiks, N.; Rapp, M.; Stoffels, G.; Fink, G.R.; Shah, N.J.; Coenen, H.H.; Sabel, M.; Langen, K.-J. Response assessment of bevacizumab in patients with recurrent malignant glioma using [18F]Fluoroethyl-l-tyrosine PET in comparison to MRI. *Eur. J. Nucl. Med. Mol. Imaging* **2012**, *40*, 22–33. [CrossRef] [PubMed]
103. Galldiks, N.; Dunkl, V.; Ceccon, G.; Tscherpel, C.; Stoffels, G.; Law, I.; Henriksen, O.M.; Muhic, A.; Poulsen, H.S.; Steger, J.; et al. Early treatment response evaluation using FET PET compared to MRI in glioblastoma patients at first progression treated with bevacizumab plus lomustine. *Eur. J. Nucl. Med. Mol. Imaging* **2018**, *45*, 2377–2386. [CrossRef] [PubMed]
104. Schwarzenberg, J.; Czernin, J.; Cloughesy, T.F.; Ellingson, B.M.; Pope, W.B.; Grogan, T.; Elashoff, D.; Geist, C.; Silverman, D.H.; Phelps, M.E.; et al. Treatment response evaluation using 18F-FDOPA PET in patients with recurrent malignant glioma on bevacizumab therapy. *Clin. Cancer Res.* **2014**, *20*, 3550–3559. [CrossRef]
105. Stupp, R.; Taillibert, S.; Kanner, A.; Read, W.; Steinberg, D.; Lhermitte, B.; Toms, S.; Idbaih, A.; Ahluwalia, M.S.; Fink, K.; et al. Effect of Tumor-Treating Fields Plus Maintenance Temozolomide vs Maintenance Temozolomide Alone on Survival in Patients With Glioblastoma: A Randomized Clinical Trial. *JAMA* **2017**, *318*, 2306–2316. [CrossRef]

106. Bosnyak, E.; Barger, G.R.; Michelhaugh, S.K.; Robinette, N.L.; Amit-Yousif, A.; Mittal, S.; Juhasz, C. Amino Acid PET Imaging of the Early Metabolic Response During Tumor-Treating Fields (TTFields) Therapy in Recurrent Glioblastoma. *Clin. Nucl. Med.* **2018**, *43*, 176–179. [CrossRef]
107. Ceccon, G.; Lazaridis, L.; Stoffels, G.; Rapp, M.; Weber, M.; Blau, T.; Lohmann, P.; Kebir, S.; Herrmann, K.; Fink, G.R.; et al. Use of FET PET in glioblastoma patients undergoing neurooncological treatment including tumour-treating fields: Initial experience. *Eur. J. Nucl. Med. Mol. Imaging* **2018**, *45*, 1626–1635. [CrossRef]
108. Chen, M.K.; Baidoo, K.; Verina, T.; Guilarte, T.R. Peripheral benzodiazepine receptor imaging in CNS demyelination: Functional implications of anatomical and cellular localization. *Brain* **2004**, *127*, 1379–1392. [CrossRef]
109. Papadopoulos, V.; Baraldi, M.; Guilarte, T.R.; Knudsen, T.B.; Lacapere, J.J.; Lindemann, P.; Norenberg, M.D.; Nutt, D.; Weizman, A.; Zhang, M.R.; et al. Translocator protein (18kDa): New nomenclature for the peripheral-type benzodiazepine receptor based on its structure and molecular function. *Trends Pharmacol. Sci.* **2006**, *27*, 402–409. [CrossRef]
110. Schweitzer, P.J.; Fallon, B.A.; Mann, J.J.; Kumar, J.S. PET tracers for the peripheral benzodiazepine receptor and uses thereof. *Drug Discov. Today* **2010**, *15*, 933–942. [CrossRef]
111. Su, Z.; Roncaroli, F.; Durrenberger, P.F.; Coope, D.J.; Karabatsou, K.; Hinz, R.; Thompson, G.; Turkheimer, F.E.; Janczar, K.; Du Plessis, D.; et al. The 18-kDa mitochondrial translocator protein in human gliomas: An 11C-(R)PK11195 PET imaging and neuropathology study. *J. Nucl. Med.* **2015**, *56*, 512–517. [CrossRef] [PubMed]
112. Su, Z.; Herholz, K.; Gerhard, A.; Roncaroli, F.; Du Plessis, D.; Jackson, A.; Turkheimer, F.; Hinz, R. [(1)(1)C]-(R)PK11195 tracer kinetics in the brain of glioma patients and a comparison of two referencing approaches. *Eur. J. Nucl. Med. Mol. Imaging* **2013**, *40*, 1406–1419. [CrossRef] [PubMed]
113. Albert, N.L.; Unterrainer, M.; Fleischmann, D.F.; Lindner, S.; Vettermann, F.; Brunegraf, A.; Vomacka, L.; Brendel, M.; Wenter, V.; Wetzel, C.; et al. TSPO PET for glioma imaging using the novel ligand (18)F-GE-180: First results in patients with glioblastoma. *Eur. J. Nucl. Med. Mol. Imaging* **2017**, *44*, 2230–2238. [CrossRef] [PubMed]
114. Vomacka, L.; Albert, N.L.; Lindner, S.; Unterrainer, M.; Mahler, C.; Brendel, M.; Ermoschkin, L.; Gosewisch, A.; Brunegraf, A.; Buckley, C.; et al. TSPO imaging using the novel PET ligand [(18)F]GE-180: Quantification approaches in patients with multiple sclerosis. *EJNMMI Res.* **2017**, *7*, 89. [CrossRef] [PubMed]
115. Unterrainer, M.; Mahler, C.; Vomacka, L.; Lindner, S.; Havla, J.; Brendel, M.; Boning, G.; Ertl-Wagner, B.; Kumpfel, T.; Milenkovic, V.M.; et al. TSPO PET with [(18)F]GE-180 sensitively detects focal neuroinflammation in patients with relapsing-remitting multiple sclerosis. *Eur. J. Nucl. Med. Mol. Imaging* **2018**, *45*, 1423–1431. [CrossRef] [PubMed]
116. Sridharan, S.; Raffel, J.; Nandoskar, A.; Record, C.; Brooks, D.J.; Owen, D.; Sharp, D.; Muraro, P.A.; Gunn, R.; Nicholas, R. Confirmation of Specific Binding of the 18-kDa Translocator Protein (TSPO) Radioligand [(18)F]GE-180: A Blocking Study Using XBD173 in Multiple Sclerosis Normal Appearing White and Grey Matter. *Mol. Imaging Biol.* **2019**, *21*, 935–944. [CrossRef]
117. Unterrainer, M.; Fleischmann, D.F.; Diekmann, C.; Vomacka, L.; Lindner, S.; Vettermann, F.; Brendel, M.; Wenter, V.; Ertl-Wagner, B.; Herms, J.; et al. Comparison of (18)F-GE-180 and dynamic (18)F-FET PET in high grade glioma: A double-tracer pilot study. *Eur. J. Nucl. Med. Mol. Imaging* **2019**, *46*, 580–590. [CrossRef]
118. Shields, A.F.; Grierson, J.R.; Dohmen, B.M.; Machulla, H.J.; Stayanoff, J.C.; Lawhorn-Crews, J.M.; Obradovich, J.E.; Muzik, O.; Mangner, T.J. Imaging proliferation in vivo with [F-18]FLT and positron emission tomography. *Nat. Med.* **1998**, *4*, 1334–1336. [CrossRef]
119. van Waarde, A.; Elsinga, P.H. Proliferation markers for the differential diagnosis of tumor and inflammation. *Curr. Pharm. Des.* **2008**, *14*, 3326–3339. [CrossRef]
120. Saga, T.; Kawashima, H.; Araki, N.; Takahashi, J.A.; Nakashima, Y.; Higashi, T.; Oya, N.; Mukai, T.; Hojo, M.; Hashimoto, N.; et al. Evaluation of primary brain tumors with FLT-PET: Usefulness and limitations. *Clin. Nucl. Med.* **2006**, *31*, 774–780. [CrossRef]
121. Jacobs, A.H.; Thomas, A.; Kracht, L.W.; Li, H.; Dittmar, C.; Garlip, G.; Galldiks, N.; Klein, J.C.; Sobesky, J.; Hilker, R.; et al. 18F-fluoro-L-thymidine and 11C-methylmethionine as markers of increased transport and proliferation in brain tumors. *J. Nucl. Med.* **2005**, *46*, 1948–1958. [PubMed]

122. Li, Z.; Yu, Y.; Zhang, H.; Xu, G.; Chen, L. A meta-analysis comparing 18F-FLT PET with 18F-FDG PET for assessment of brain tumor recurrence. *Nucl. Med. Commun.* **2015**, *36*, 695–701. [CrossRef] [PubMed]
123. Chen, W.; Delaloye, S.; Silverman, D.H.; Geist, C.; Czernin, J.; Sayre, J.; Satyamurthy, N.; Pope, W.; Lai, A.; Phelps, M.E.; et al. Predicting treatment response of malignant gliomas to bevacizumab and irinotecan by imaging proliferation with [18F] fluorothymidine positron emission tomography: A pilot study. *J. Clin. Oncol.* **2007**, *25*, 4714–4721. [CrossRef] [PubMed]
124. Schwarzenberg, J.; Czernin, J.; Cloughesy, T.F.; Ellingson, B.M.; Pope, W.B.; Geist, C.; Dahlbom, M.; Silverman, D.H.; Satyamurthy, N.; Phelps, M.E.; et al. 3′-deoxy-3′-18F-fluorothymidine PET and MRI for early survival predictions in patients with recurrent malignant glioma treated with bevacizumab. *J. Nucl. Med.* **2012**, *53*, 29–36. [CrossRef] [PubMed]
125. Harris, R.J.; Cloughesy, T.F.; Pope, W.B.; Nghiemphu, P.L.; Lai, A.; Zaw, T.; Czernin, J.; Phelps, M.E.; Chen, W.; Ellingson, B.M. 18F-FDOPA and 18F-FLT positron emission tomography parametric response maps predict response in recurrent malignant gliomas treated with bevacizumab. *Neuro Oncol.* **2012**, *14*, 1079–1089. [CrossRef]
126. Nguyen, N.C.; Yee, M.K.; Tuchayi, A.M.; Kirkwood, J.M.; Tawbi, H.; Mountz, J.M. Targeted Therapy and Immunotherapy Response Assessment with F-18 Fluorothymidine Positron-Emission Tomography/Magnetic Resonance Imaging in Melanoma Brain Metastasis: A Pilot Study. *Front. Oncol.* **2018**, *8*, 18. [CrossRef]
127. Bell, C.; Dowson, N.; Fay, M.; Thomas, P.; Puttick, S.; Gal, Y.; Rose, S. Hypoxia imaging in gliomas with 18F-fluoromisonidazole PET: Toward clinical translation. *Semin. Nucl. Med.* **2015**, *45*, 136–150. [CrossRef]
128. Rasey, J.S.; Koh, W.J.; Evans, M.L.; Peterson, L.M.; Lewellen, T.K.; Graham, M.M.; Krohn, K.A. Quantifying regional hypoxia in human tumors with positron emission tomography of [18F]fluoromisonidazole: A pretherapy study of 37 patients. *Int. J. Radiat. Oncol. Biol. Phys.* **1996**, *36*, 417–428. [CrossRef]
129. Rajendran, J.G.; Krohn, K.A. F-18 fluoromisonidazole for imaging tumor hypoxia: Imaging the microenvironment for personalized cancer therapy. *Semin. Nucl. Med.* **2015**, *45*, 151–162. [CrossRef]
130. Swanson, K.R.; Chakraborty, G.; Wang, C.H.; Rockne, R.; Harpold, H.L.; Muzi, M.; Adamsen, T.C.; Krohn, K.A.; Spence, A.M. Complementary but distinct roles for MRI and 18F-fluoromisonidazole PET in the assessment of human glioblastomas. *J. Nucl. Med.* **2009**, *50*, 36–44. [CrossRef]
131. Kawai, N.; Maeda, Y.; Kudomi, N.; Miyake, K.; Okada, M.; Yamamoto, Y.; Nishiyama, Y.; Tamiya, T. Correlation of biological aggressiveness assessed by 11C-methionine PET and hypoxic burden assessed by 18F-fluoromisonidazole PET in newly diagnosed glioblastoma. *Eur. J. Nucl. Med. Mol. Imaging* **2011**, *38*, 441–450. [CrossRef] [PubMed]
132. Barajas, R.F.; Krohn, K.A.; Link, J.M.; Hawkins, R.A.; Clarke, J.L.; Pampaloni, M.H.; Cha, S. Glioma FMISO PET/MR Imaging Concurrent with Antiangiogenic Therapy: Molecular Imaging as a Clinical Tool in the Burgeoning Era of Personalized Medicine. *Biomedicines* **2016**, *4*, 24. [CrossRef] [PubMed]
133. Yamaguchi, S.; Hirata, K.; Toyonaga, T.; Kobayashi, K.; Ishi, Y.; Motegi, H.; Kobayashi, H.; Shiga, T.; Tamaki, N.; Terasaka, S.; et al. Change in 18F-Fluoromisonidazole PET Is an Early Predictor of the Prognosis in the Patients with Recurrent High-Grade Glioma Receiving Bevacizumab Treatment. *PLoS ONE* **2016**, *11*, e0167917. [CrossRef] [PubMed]
134. Piert, M.; Machulla, H.J.; Picchio, M.; Reischl, G.; Ziegler, S.; Kumar, P.; Wester, H.J.; Beck, R.; McEwan, A.J.; Wiebe, L.I.; et al. Hypoxia-specific tumor imaging with 18F-fluoroazomycin arabinoside. *J. Nucl. Med.* **2005**, *46*, 106–113.
135. Postema, E.J.; McEwan, A.J.; Riauka, T.A.; Kumar, P.; Richmond, D.A.; Abrams, D.N.; Wiebe, L.I. Initial results of hypoxia imaging using 1-alpha-D: -(5-deoxy-5-[18F]-fluoroarabinofuranosyl)-2-nitroimidazole (18F-FAZA). *Eur. J. Nucl. Med. Mol. Imaging* **2009**, *36*, 1565–1573. [CrossRef]
136. Mapelli, P.; Zerbetto, F.; Incerti, E.; Conte, G.M.; Bettinardi, V.; Fallanca, F.; Anzalone, N.; Di Muzio, N.; Gianolli, L.; Picchio, M. 18F-FAZA PET/CT Hypoxia Imaging of High-Grade Glioma Before and After Radiotherapy. *Clin. Nucl. Med.* **2017**, *42*, e525–e526. [CrossRef]
137. Ter-Pogossian, M.M.; Eichling, J.O.; Davis, D.O.; Welch, M.J. The measure in vivo of regional cerebral oxygen utilization by means of oxyhemoglobin labeled with radioactive oxygen-15. *J. Clin. Investig.* **1970**, *49*, 381–391. [CrossRef]

138. Ludemann, L.; Warmuth, C.; Plotkin, M.; Forschler, A.; Gutberlet, M.; Wust, P.; Amthauer, H. Brain tumor perfusion: Comparison of dynamic contrast enhanced magnetic resonance imaging using T1, T2, and T2* contrast, pulsed arterial spin labeling, and H2(15)O positron emission tomography. *Eur. J. Radiol.* **2009**, *70*, 465–474. [CrossRef]
139. Gruner, J.M.; Paamand, R.; Kosteljanetz, M.; Broholm, H.; Hojgaard, L.; Law, I. Brain perfusion CT compared with (1)(5)O-H(2)O PET in patients with primary brain tumours. *Eur. J. Nucl. Med. Mol. Imaging* **2012**, *39*, 1691–1701. [CrossRef]
140. Ogawa, T.; Uemura, K.; Shishido, F.; Yamaguchi, T.; Murakami, M.; Inugami, A.; Kanno, I.; Sasaki, H.; Kato, T.; Hirata, K.; et al. Changes of cerebral blood flow, and oxygen and glucose metabolism following radiochemotherapy of gliomas: A PET study. *J. Comput. Assist. Tomogr.* **1988**, *12*, 290–297. [CrossRef]
141. Mineura, K.; Yasuda, T.; Kowada, M.; Ogawa, T.; Shishido, F.; Uemura, K. Positron emission tomographic evaluation of radiochemotherapeutic effect on regional cerebral hemocirculation and metabolism in patients with gliomas. *J. Neurooncol.* **1987**, *5*, 277–285. [CrossRef]
142. Jain, R.K.; di Tomaso, E.; Duda, D.G.; Loeffler, J.S.; Sorensen, A.G.; Batchelor, T.T. Angiogenesis in brain tumours. *Nat. Rev. Neurosci.* **2007**, *8*, 610–622. [CrossRef] [PubMed]
143. Levin, V.A.; Bidaut, L.; Hou, P.; Kumar, A.J.; Wefel, J.S.; Bekele, B.N.; Grewal, J.; Prabhu, S.; Loghin, M.; Gilbert, M.R.; et al. Randomized double-blind placebo-controlled trial of bevacizumab therapy for radiation necrosis of the central nervous system. *Int. J. Radiat. Oncol. Biol. Phys.* **2011**, *79*, 1487–1495. [CrossRef] [PubMed]
144. Jansen, M.H.; Veldhuijzen van Zanten, S.E.M.; van Vuurden, D.G.; Huisman, M.C.; Vugts, D.J.; Hoekstra, O.S.; van Dongen, G.A.; Kaspers, G.L. Molecular Drug Imaging: (89)Zr-Bevacizumab PET in Children with Diffuse Intrinsic Pontine Glioma. *J. Nucl. Med.* **2017**, *58*, 711–716. [CrossRef] [PubMed]
145. Veldhuijzen van Zanten, S.E.M.; Sewing, A.C.P.; van Lingen, A.; Hoekstra, O.S.; Wesseling, P.; Meel, M.H.; van Vuurden, D.G.; Kaspers, G.J.L.; Hulleman, E.; Bugiani, M. Multiregional Tumor Drug-Uptake Imaging by PET and Microvascular Morphology in End-Stage Diffuse Intrinsic Pontine Glioma. *J. Nucl. Med.* **2018**, *59*, 612–615. [CrossRef]
146. Hsu, A.R.; Cai, W.; Veeravagu, A.; Mohamedali, K.A.; Chen, K.; Kim, S.; Vogel, H.; Hou, L.C.; Tse, V.; Rosenblum, M.G.; et al. Multimodality molecular imaging of glioblastoma growth inhibition with vasculature-targeting fusion toxin VEGF121/rGel. *J. Nucl. Med.* **2007**, *48*, 445–454.
147. Chen, K.; Cai, W.; Li, Z.B.; Wang, H.; Chen, X. Quantitative PET imaging of VEGF receptor expression. *Mol. Imaging Biol.* **2009**, *11*, 15–22. [CrossRef]
148. Cai, W.; Chen, K.; Mohamedali, K.A.; Cao, Q.; Gambhir, S.S.; Rosenblum, M.G.; Chen, X. PET of vascular endothelial growth factor receptor expression. *J. Nucl. Med.* **2006**, *47*, 2048–2056.
149. Rainer, E.; Wang, H.; Traub-Weidinger, T.; Widhalm, G.; Fueger, B.; Chang, J.; Zhu, Z.; Marosi, C.; Haug, A.; Hacker, M.; et al. The prognostic value of [(123)I]-vascular endothelial growth factor ([(123)I]-VEGF) in glioma. *Eur. J. Nucl. Med. Mol. Imaging* **2018**, *45*, 2396–2403. [CrossRef]
150. Wu, Y.L.; Ahn, M.J.; Garassino, M.C.; Han, J.Y.; Katakami, N.; Kim, H.R.; Hodge, R.; Kaur, P.; Brown, A.P.; Ghiorghiu, D.; et al. CNS Efficacy of Osimertinib in Patients With T790M-Positive Advanced Non-Small-Cell Lung Cancer: Data From a Randomized Phase III Trial (AURA3). *J. Clin. Oncol.* **2018**, *36*, 2702–2709. [CrossRef]
151. Pusch, S.; Krausert, S.; Fischer, V.; Balss, J.; Ott, M.; Schrimpf, D.; Capper, D.; Sahm, F.; Eisel, J.; Beck, A.C.; et al. Pan-mutant IDH1 inhibitor BAY 1436032 for effective treatment of IDH1 mutant astrocytoma in vivo. *Acta Neuropathol.* **2017**, *133*, 629–644. [CrossRef] [PubMed]
152. Mellinghoff, I.K.; Penas-Prado, M.; Peters, K.B.; Cloughesy, T.F.; Burris, H.A.; Maher, E.A.; Janku, F.; Cote, G.M.; Fuente, M.I.D.L.; Clarke, J.; et al. Phase 1 study of AG-881, an inhibitor of mutant IDH1/IDH2, in patients with advanced IDH-mutant solid tumors, including glioma. *J. Clin. Oncol.* **2018**, *36*, 2002. [CrossRef]
153. Bublil, E.M.; Yarden, Y. The EGF receptor family: Spearheading a merger of signaling and therapeutics. *Curr. Opin. Cell Biol.* **2007**, *19*, 124–134. [CrossRef] [PubMed]
154. Hatanpaa, K.J.; Burma, S.; Zhao, D.; Habib, A.A. Epidermal growth factor receptor in glioma: Signal transduction, neuropathology, imaging, and radioresistance. *Neoplasia* **2010**, *12*, 675–684. [CrossRef]

155. Kelly, W.J.; Shah, N.J.; Subramaniam, D.S. Management of Brain Metastases in Epidermal Growth Factor Receptor Mutant Non-Small-Cell Lung Cancer. *Front. Oncol.* **2018**, *8*, 208. [CrossRef]
156. Weber, B.; Winterdahl, M.; Memon, A.; Sorensen, B.S.; Keiding, S.; Sorensen, L.; Nexo, E.; Meldgaard, P. Erlotinib accumulation in brain metastases from non-small cell lung cancer: Visualization by positron emission tomography in a patient harboring a mutation in the epidermal growth factor receptor. *J. Thorac. Oncol.* **2011**, *6*, 1287–1289. [CrossRef]
157. Tang, Y.; Hu, Y.; Liu, W.; Chen, L.; Zhao, Y.; Ma, H.; Yang, J.; Yang, Y.; Liao, J.; Cai, J.; et al. A radiopharmaceutical [(89)Zr]Zr-DFO-nimotuzumab for immunoPET with epidermal growth factor receptor expression in vivo. *Nucl. Med. Biol.* **2019**, *70*, 23–31. [CrossRef]
158. Sun, J.; Cai, L.; Zhang, K.; Zhang, A.; Pu, P.; Yang, W.; Gao, S. A pilot study on EGFR-targeted molecular imaging of PET/CT With 11C-PD153035 in human gliomas. *Clin. Nucl. Med.* **2014**, *39*, e20–e26. [CrossRef]
159. Ulaner, G.A.; Lyashchenko, S.K.; Riedl, C.; Ruan, S.; Zanzonico, P.B.; Lake, D.; Jhaveri, K.; Zeglis, B.; Lewis, J.S.; O'Donoghue, J.A. First-in-Human Human Epidermal Growth Factor Receptor 2-Targeted Imaging Using (89)Zr-Pertuzumab PET/CT: Dosimetry and Clinical Application in Patients with Breast Cancer. *J. Nucl. Med.* **2018**, *59*, 900–906. [CrossRef]
160. Tamura, K.; Kurihara, H.; Yonemori, K.; Tsuda, H.; Suzuki, J.; Kono, Y.; Honda, N.; Kodaira, M.; Yamamoto, H.; Yunokawa, M.; et al. 64Cu-DOTA-trastuzumab PET imaging in patients with HER2-positive breast cancer. *J. Nucl. Med.* **2013**, *54*, 1869–1875. [CrossRef]
161. van der Veen, E.L.; Bensch, F.; Glaudemans, A.; Lub-de Hooge, M.N.; de Vries, E.G.E. Molecular imaging to enlighten cancer immunotherapies and underlying involved processes. *Cancer Treat. Rev.* **2018**, *70*, 232–244. [CrossRef] [PubMed]
162. Decazes, P.; Bohn, P. Immunotherapy by Immune Checkpoint Inhibitors and Nuclear Medicine Imaging: Current and Future Applications. *Cancers* **2020**, *12*, 371. [CrossRef] [PubMed]
163. Cole, E.L.; Kim, J.; Donnelly, D.J.; Smith, R.A.; Cohen, D.; Lafont, V.; Morin, P.E.; Huang, R.Y.; Chow, P.L.; Hayes, W.; et al. Radiosynthesis and preclinical PET evaluation of (89)Zr-nivolumab (BMS-936558) in healthy non-human primates. *Bioorg. Med. Chem.* **2017**, *25*, 5407–5414. [CrossRef]
164. Bensch, F.; van der Veen, E.L.; Lub-de Hooge, M.N.; Jorritsma-Smit, A.; Boellaard, R.; Kok, I.C.; Oosting, S.F.; Schroder, C.P.; Hiltermann, T.J.N.; van der Wekken, A.J.; et al. (89)Zr-atezolizumab imaging as a non-invasive approach to assess clinical response to PD-L1 blockade in cancer. *Nat. Med.* **2018**, *24*, 1852–1858. [CrossRef] [PubMed]
165. Niemeijer, A.N.; Leung, D.; Huisman, M.C.; Bahce, I.; Hoekstra, O.S.; van Dongen, G.; Boellaard, R.; Du, S.; Hayes, W.; Smith, R.; et al. Whole body PD-1 and PD-L1 positron emission tomography in patients with non-small-cell lung cancer. *Nat. Commun.* **2018**, *9*, 4664. [CrossRef] [PubMed]
166. Donnelly, D.J.; Smith, R.A.; Morin, P.; Lipovsek, D.; Gokemeijer, J.; Cohen, D.; Lafont, V.; Tran, T.; Cole, E.L.; Wright, M.; et al. Synthesis and Biologic Evaluation of a Novel (18)F-Labeled Adnectin as a PET Radioligand for Imaging PD-L1 Expression. *J. Nucl. Med.* **2018**, *59*, 529–535. [CrossRef]
167. Tumeh, P.C.; Harview, C.L.; Yearley, J.H.; Shintaku, I.P.; Taylor, E.J.; Robert, L.; Chmielowski, B.; Spasic, M.; Henry, G.; Ciobanu, V.; et al. PD-1 blockade induces responses by inhibiting adaptive immune resistance. *Nature* **2014**, *515*, 568–571. [CrossRef]
168. Pandit-Taskar, N.; Postow, M.; Hellmann, M.; Harding, J.; Barker, C.; O'Donoghue, J.; Ziolkowska, M.; Ruan, S.; Lyashchenko, S.; Tsai, F.; et al. First-in-human imaging with (89)Zr-Df-IAB22M2C anti-CD8 minibody in patients with solid malignancies: Preliminary pharmacokinetics, biodistribution, and lesion targeting. *J. Nucl. Med.* **2019**. [CrossRef]
169. Antonios, J.P.; Soto, H.; Everson, R.G.; Moughon, D.L.; Wang, A.C.; Orpilla, J.; Radu, C.; Ellingson, B.M.; Lee, J.T.; Cloughesy, T.; et al. Detection of immune responses after immunotherapy in glioblastoma using PET and MRI. *Proc. Natl. Acad. Sci. USA* **2017**, *114*, 10220–10225. [CrossRef]
170. Nair-Gill, E.D.; Shu, C.J.; Radu, C.G.; Witte, O.N. Non-invasive imaging of adaptive immunity using positron emission tomography. *Immunol. Rev.* **2008**, *221*, 214–228. [CrossRef]
171. Min, J.J.; Iyer, M.; Gambhir, S.S. Comparison of [18F]FHBG and [14C]FIAU for imaging of HSV1-tk reporter gene expression: Adenoviral infection vs stable transfection. *Eur. J. Nucl. Med. Mol. Imaging* **2003**, *30*, 1547–1560. [CrossRef] [PubMed]

172. Keu, K.V.; Witney, T.H.; Yaghoubi, S.; Rosenberg, J.; Kurien, A.; Magnusson, R.; Williams, J.; Habte, F.; Wagner, J.R.; Forman, S.; et al. Reporter gene imaging of targeted T cell immunotherapy in recurrent glioma. *Sci. Transl. Med.* **2017**, *9*. [CrossRef] [PubMed]
173. Yan, H.; Parsons, D.W.; Jin, G.; McLendon, R.; Rasheed, B.A.; Yuan, W.; Kos, I.; Batinic-Haberle, I.; Jones, S.; Riggins, G.J.; et al. IDH1 and IDH2 mutations in gliomas. *N. Engl. J. Med.* **2009**, *360*, 765–773. [CrossRef] [PubMed]
174. Dang, L.; White, D.W.; Gross, S.; Bennett, B.D.; Bittinger, M.A.; Driggers, E.M.; Fantin, V.R.; Jang, H.G.; Jin, S.; Keenan, M.C.; et al. Cancer-associated IDH1 mutations produce 2-hydroxyglutarate. *Nature* **2009**, *462*, 739–744. [CrossRef]
175. Lu, C.; Ward, P.S.; Kapoor, G.S.; Rohle, D.; Turcan, S.; Abdel-Wahab, O.; Edwards, C.R.; Khanin, R.; Figueroa, M.E.; Melnick, A.; et al. IDH mutation impairs histone demethylation and results in a block to cell differentiation. *Nature* **2012**, *483*, 474–478. [CrossRef]
176. Platten, M.; Schilling, D.; Bunse, L.; Wick, A.; Bunse, T.; Riehl, D.; Karapanagiotou-Schenkel, I.; Harting, I.; Sahm, F.; Schmitt, A.; et al. A mutation-specific peptide vaccine targeting IDH1R132H in patients with newly diagnosed malignant astrocytomas: A first-in-man multicenter phase I clinical trial of the German Neurooncology Working Group (NOA-16). *J. Clin. Oncol.* **2018**, *36*, 2001. [CrossRef]
177. Suh, C.H.; Kim, H.S.; Paik, W.; Choi, C.; Ryu, K.H.; Kim, D.; Woo, D.C.; Park, J.E.; Jung, S.C.; Choi, C.G.; et al. False-Positive Measurement at 2-Hydroxyglutarate MR Spectroscopy in Isocitrate Dehydrogenase Wild-Type Glioblastoma: A Multifactorial Analysis. *Radiology* **2019**, *291*, 752–762. [CrossRef]
178. Choi, C.; Ganji, S.K.; DeBerardinis, R.J.; Hatanpaa, K.J.; Rakheja, D.; Kovacs, Z.; Yang, X.L.; Mashimo, T.; Raisanen, J.M.; Marin-Valencia, I.; et al. 2-hydroxyglutarate detection by magnetic resonance spectroscopy in IDH-mutated patients with gliomas. *Nat. Med.* **2012**, *18*, 624–629. [CrossRef]
179. Chitneni, S.K.; Reitman, Z.J.; Gooden, D.M.; Yan, H.; Zalutsky, M.R. Radiolabeled inhibitors as probes for imaging mutant IDH1 expression in gliomas: Synthesis and preliminary evaluation of labeled butyl-phenyl sulfonamide analogs. *Eur. J. Med. Chem.* **2016**, *119*, 218–230. [CrossRef]
180. Chitneni, S.K.; Yan, H.; Zalutsky, M.R. Synthesis and Evaluation of a (18)F-Labeled Triazinediamine Analogue for Imaging Mutant IDH1 Expression in Gliomas by PET. *ACS Med. Chem. Lett.* **2018**, *9*, 606–611. [CrossRef]
181. Chitneni, S.K.; Reitman, Z.J.; Spicehandler, R.; Gooden, D.M.; Yan, H.; Zalutsky, M.R. Synthesis and evaluation of radiolabeled AGI-5198 analogues as candidate radiotracers for imaging mutant IDH1 expression in tumors. *Bioorg. Med. Chem. Lett.* **2018**, *28*, 694–699. [CrossRef] [PubMed]
182. Koyasu, S.; Shimizu, Y.; Morinibu, A.; Saga, T.; Nakamoto, Y.; Togashi, K.; Harada, H. Increased (14)C-acetate accumulation in IDH-mutated human glioblastoma: Implications for detecting IDH-mutated glioblastoma with (11)C-acetate PET imaging. *J. Neurooncol.* **2019**, *145*, 441–447. [CrossRef] [PubMed]
183. Burger, J.A.; Kipps, T.J. CXCR4: A key receptor in the crosstalk between tumor cells and their microenvironment. *Blood* **2006**, *107*, 1761–1767. [CrossRef]
184. Bian, X.W.; Yang, S.X.; Chen, J.H.; Ping, Y.F.; Zhou, X.D.; Wang, Q.L.; Jiang, X.F.; Gong, W.; Xiao, H.L.; Du, L.L.; et al. Preferential expression of chemokine receptor CXCR4 by highly malignant human gliomas and its association with poor patient survival. *Neurosurgery* **2007**, *61*, 570–579. [CrossRef] [PubMed]
185. Bailly, C.; Vidal, A.; Bonnemaire, C.; Kraeber-Bodere, F.; Cherel, M.; Pallardy, A.; Rousseau, C.; Garcion, E.; Lacoeuille, F.; Hindre, F.; et al. Potential for Nuclear Medicine Therapy for Glioblastoma Treatment. *Front. Pharmacol.* **2019**, *10*, 772. [CrossRef]
186. Lapa, C.; Luckerath, K.; Kleinlein, I.; Monoranu, C.M.; Linsenmann, T.; Kessler, A.F.; Rudelius, M.; Kropf, S.; Buck, A.K.; Ernestus, R.I.; et al. (68)Ga-Pentixafor-PET/CT for Imaging of Chemokine Receptor 4 Expression in Glioblastoma. *Theranostics* **2016**, *6*, 428–434. [CrossRef]
187. Wernicke, A.G.; Edgar, M.A.; Lavi, E.; Liu, H.; Salerno, P.; Bander, N.H.; Gutin, P.H. Prostate-specific membrane antigen as a potential novel vascular target for treatment of glioblastoma multiforme. *Arch. Pathol. Lab. Med.* **2011**, *135*, 1486–1489. [CrossRef]
188. Schwenck, J.; Tabatabai, G.; Skardelly, M.; Reischl, G.; Beschorner, R.; Pichler, B.; la Fougere, C. In vivo visualization of prostate-specific membrane antigen in glioblastoma. *Eur. J. Nucl. Med. Mol. Imaging* **2015**, *42*, 170–171. [CrossRef]

189. Unterrainer, M.; Niyazi, M.; Ruf, V.; Bartenstein, P.; Albert, N.L. The endothelial prostate-specific membrane antigen is highly expressed in gliosarcoma and visualized by [68Ga]-PSMA-11 PET: A theranostic outlook for brain tumor patients? *Neuro Oncol.* **2017**, *19*, 1698–1699. [CrossRef]
190. Rahbar, K.; Ahmadzadehfar, H.; Kratochwil, C.; Haberkorn, U.; Schafers, M.; Essler, M.; Baum, R.P.; Kulkarni, H.R.; Schmidt, M.; Drzezga, A.; et al. German Multicenter Study Investigating 177Lu-PSMA-617 Radioligand Therapy in Advanced Prostate Cancer Patients. *J. Nucl. Med.* **2017**, *58*, 85–90. [CrossRef]

7

Positron Emission Tomography (PET) Radiopharmaceuticals in Multiple Myeloma

Christos Sachpekidis [1,*], Hartmut Goldschmidt [2] and Antonia Dimitrakopoulou-Strauss [1]

1 Clinical Cooperation Unit Nuclear Medicine, German Cancer Research Center, 69120 Heidelberg, Germany; a.dimitrakopoulou-strauss@dkfz.de
2 Department of Internal Medicine V, University Hospital Heidelberg and National Center for Tumor Diseases (NCT), 69120 Heidelberg, Germany; Hartmut.Goldschmidt@med.uni-heidelberg.de
* Correspondence: c.sachpekidis@dkfz-heidelberg.de or christos_saxpe@yahoo.gr

Academic Editor: Anne Roivainen

Abstract: Multiple myeloma (MM) is a plasma cell disorder, characterized by clonal proliferation of malignant plasma cells in the bone marrow. Bone disease is the most frequent feature and an end-organ defining indicator of MM. In this context, imaging plays a pivotal role in the management of the malignancy. For several decades whole-body X-ray survey (WBXR) has been applied for the diagnosis and staging of bone disease in MM. However, the serious drawbacks of WBXR have led to its gradual replacement from novel imaging modalities, such as computed tomography (CT), magnetic resonance imaging (MRI) and positron emission tomography/computed tomography (PET/CT). PET/CT, with the tracer ^{18}F-fluorodeoxyglucose (^{18}F-FDG), is now considered a powerful diagnostic tool for the detection of medullary and extramedullary disease at the time of diagnosis, a reliable predictor of survival as well as the most robust modality for treatment response evaluation in MM. On the other hand, ^{18}F-FDG carries its own limitations as a radiopharmaceutical, including a rather poor sensitivity for the detection of diffuse bone marrow infiltration, a relatively low specificity, and the lack of widely applied, established criteria for image interpretation. This has led to the development of several alternative PET tracers, some of which with promising results regarding MM detection. The aim of this review article is to outline the major applications of PET/CT with different radiopharmaceuticals in the clinical practice of MM.

Keywords: multiple myeloma; positron emission tomography/computed tomography; radiopharmaceuticals; ^{18}F-fluorodeoxyglucose

---

1. Introduction

Multiple myeloma (MM) is a neoplastic plasma cell disorder, characterized by the uncontrolled, clonal proliferation of plasma cells in the bone marrow. It is the second most common hematologic malignancy after non-Hodgkin's lymphoma accounting for approximately 1% of neoplastic diseases, and the most common primary tumor of the skeleton [1]. MM is almost always preceded from a premalignant precursor condition (monoclonal gammopathy of undetermined significance, MGUS), which then develops into asymptomatic or smoldering myeloma (SMM) and, finally, into symptomatic disease [2]. Bone involvement in the form of focal osteolytic lesions—the hallmark radiographic sign of MM—represents a marker of disease-related end-organ damage, necessitating immediate initiation of treatment [3]. Bone disease is a major cause of morbidity and mortality for patients suffering from MM. Since practically all patients develop bone involvement during the course of the disease [4], its reliable identification represents a pivotal diagnostic challenge. Historically, skeletal damage has been assessed by conventional, whole-body X-ray survey (WBXR), which was the standard imaging approach for

MM. Nevertheless, this modality carries several limitations, including a low sensitivity—requiring a more than 30% bone demineralization before an osteolytic lesion becomes evident—its failure to detect extramedullary disease (EMD), which is a significant adverse prognostic factor of MM, and its poor performance in treatment response assessment [5]. The drawbacks of planar radiography have been overcome in recent years with the development and introduction in clinical practice of myeloma of novel imaging modalities, namely whole-body computed tomography (CT), magnetic resonance imaging (MRI) and positron emission tomography/computed tomography (PET/CT). These techniques offer a higher sensitivity than WBXR, leading to its gradual substitution by them.

It is undisputable that the role of PET/CT with the radiotracer ^{18}F-fluorodeoxyglucose (^{18}F-FDG) in MM has been upgraded with an increasing amount of literature highlighting its value in diagnosis, prognosis and treatment response evaluation of the disease. According to the latest update of the International Myeloma Working group (IMWG), the detection of one or more osteolytic lesions on CT or PET/CT fulfills the criteria of bone disease and, therefore, of symptomatic MM requiring treatment [4].

This review article provides an overview of the position of PET/CT in MM management with focus on the most widely used tracer ^{18}F-FDG. In addition, the main data published on new PET tracers targeting different molecular pathways involved in MM pathogenesis are presented.

2. ^{18}F-FDG PET/CT in MM

PET/CT is a whole-body imaging technique combining the functional information of PET with the morphological assessment provided by CT. ^{18}F-FDG, the workhorse of PET imaging, is a biomarker of intracellular glucose metabolism. The tracer is actively transported into cells by the glucose transporter proteins (GLUT), which are expressed at a high degree in tumor cells due to their enhanced glucose demands. ^{18}F-FDG, as a glucose analogue, is taken up by the neoplastic cells, undergoes phosphorylation and then gets trapped intracellularly, since ^{18}F-FDG is not a substrate for further metabolic processing by either phosphohexose isomerase or glucose-6-phosphate dehydrogenase [6].

^{18}F-FDG PET/CT has become nowadays a standard imaging technique in several tumor entities. Due to its ability in providing whole-body evaluations in a single session, the modality can assess the extent of oncological disease in a satisfying manner. In MM in particular, PET/CT can detect with a high sensitivity and specificity both medullary and extramedullary lesions [7]. Another important advantage of PET is the potential of quantification of tracer uptake by means of the index standardized uptake value (SUV), which reflects the amount of tracer activity in a particular region of interest. This quantification of tracer uptake aids in objective interpretation of PET/CT scans in addition to obtaining cross-sectional imaging and assessing ^{18}F-FDG uptake visually, particularly in terms of patient follow-up. Furthermore—and most importantly—^{18}F-FDG PET/CT can assess the metabolic burden and activity of MM in different stages of the disease due to its ability in differentiating between metabolically active and inactive lesions, with significant implications in treatment response assessment [5,7].

2.1. ^{18}F-FDG PET/CT in the Diagnosis and Staging of MM

^{18}F-FDG PET/CT has been proven to be a very useful modality for the whole-body evaluation of the active burden of MM. Its reported sensitivity and specificity for assessment of medullary and extramedullary disease extent ranges from 80–100% [7–12]. The uptake pattern, SUV and different pharmacokinetic parameters of ^{18}F-FDG correlate with the percentage of bone marrow plasma cells [13] (Figure 1).

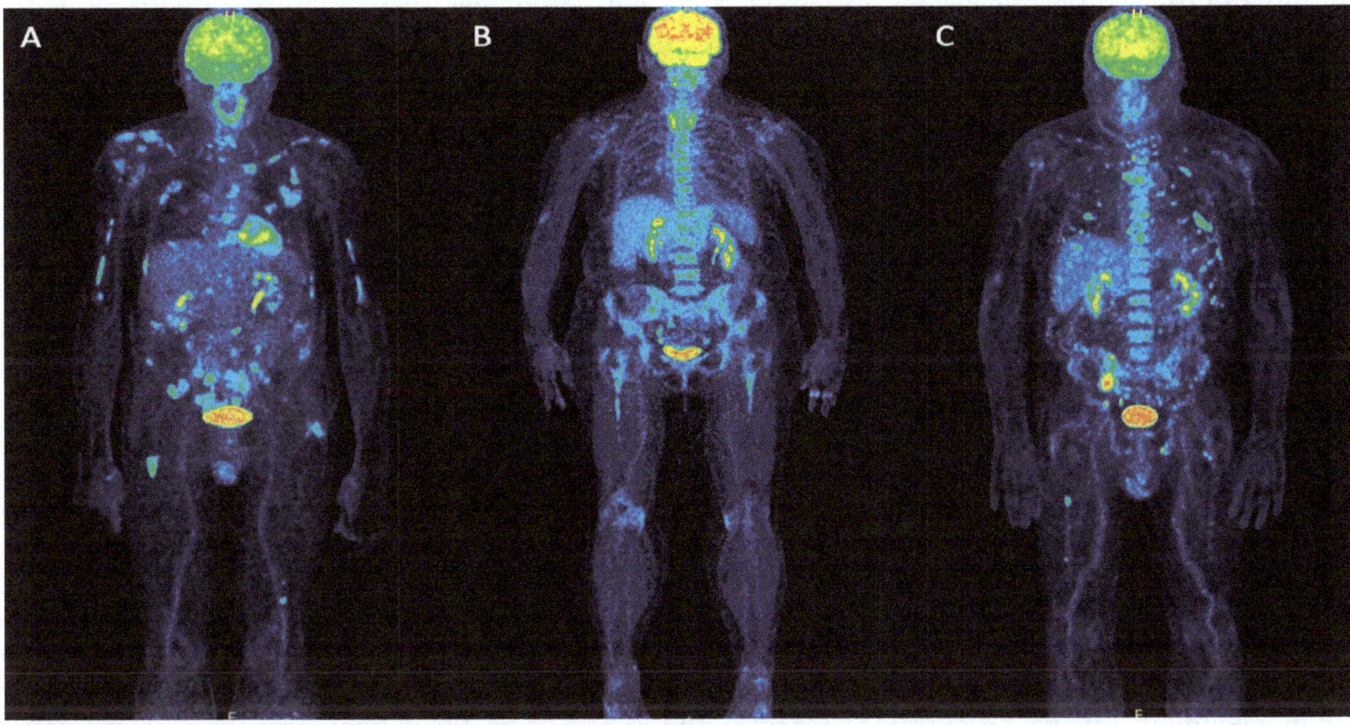

Figure 1. Maximum intensity projection (MIP) PET/CT images of newly diagnosed MM patients before treatment, representing examples of different pathologic patterns of ^{18}F-FDG uptake. (**A**) demonstrates a patient with multiple focal lesions in the skeleton. (**B**) depicts a patient with intense diffuse tracer uptake in the bone marrow of the axial skeleton and the proximal humeri and femora without clearly delineated focal lesions. (**C**) shows a patient with a mixed pattern of ^{18}F-FDG uptake with intense, diffuse uptake in the axial skeleton and multiple, focal bone marrow lesions.

PET/CT has been compared with other imaging modalities and has been shown to be superior to WBXR and comparable to MRI. In particular, a prospective study comparing ^{18}F-FDG PET/CT with WBXR and pelvic-spinal MRI highlighted the superiority of PET/CT to WBXR in 46% of cases (sensitivity 92% vs. 61%). The sensitivity of PET/CT in the spine was inferior to MRI, underestimating the disease in a third of the patients; however, ^{18}F-FDG PET/CT detected sites of active disease in areas outside the field of the MRI view [8]. Similarly, the results of a systematic review of 18 studies comparing the above-mentioned modalities showed a higher sensitivity of MRI at detecting diffuse disease of the spine, while ^{18}F-FDG PET/CT was more sensitive than WBXR with regard to detection of bone lesions [10]. In another systematic review of 17 studies no significant differences were found between ^{18}F-FDG PET/CT (sensitivity 91%, specificity 69%) and MRI (sensitivity 88%, specificity 68%) regarding detection rate of bone disease [11]. Recently, the prospective French IMAJEM study revealed no difference in the detection of bone lesions at diagnosis when comparing PET/CT and MRI with the former being positive in 95% and the latter in 91% of the patients [12].

Interestingly, there is a lack of studies regarding the comparison of ^{18}F-FDG PET/CT with whole-body CT. According to the recently published consensus statement by the IMWG, although whole-body low-dose CT is the preferred method for the detection of lytic bone lesions in MM, ^{18}F-FDG PET/CT should be considered as a valuable option, because of its ability to identify lytic lesions and extramedullary masses. Moreover, in cases of WBXR-negativity and whole-body MRI-unavailability, ^{18}F-FDG PET/CT is recommended for the differentiation between active and smoldering MM [7].

Further, the newly emerging, hybrid PET/MRI technique seems highly attractive in the diagnostic approach of MM since it combines two modalities with a high potential in myeloma evaluation in a single exam. The results of the only prospective study comparing PET/CT with PET/MRI demonstrated good image quality provided by PET/MRI and high correlation between the modalities regarding the number of detected active lesions and SUV values [14]. However, further studies are warranted to evaluate the potential role of this novel technique in the diagnostics and management of MM.

2.2. *Prognostic Value of ^{18}F-FDG PET/CT in MM*

^{18}F-FDG PET/CT is a reliable outcome predictor and is regarded as the elective technique for treatment response evaluation of MM due to its ability to distinguish active from inactive sites of disease [9,12,15]. In newly diagnosed, symptomatic MM patients, three independent PET factors have been recognized to affect both progression-free survival (PFS) and overall survival (OS) in different prospective studies. These parameters are the number of focal, ^{18}F-FDG-avid lesions, the SUV_{max} of the lesions, and the presence of EMD. Bartel et al. were the first to show in a group of 239 MM patients treated upfront with novel agents and double autologous stem-cell transplantation (ASCT) that the presence of more than three ^{18}F-FDG-avid focal lesions was related to fundamental features of myeloma biology and genomics and was the leading independent parameter associated with inferior PFS and OS [9]. A few years later, in a study by Zamagni et al., including 192 MM patients treated with thalidomide-dexamethasone induction therapy and double ASCT, it was shown that the presence at baseline of at least three focal lesions, a $SUV_{max} > 4.2$ of the hottest lesion, and the presence of EMD adversely affected 4-year estimates of PFS, while $SUV_{max} > 4.2$ and EMD were also correlated with shorter OS [15]. Further, the IMAJEM study highlighted the role of EMD as an independent, adverse prognostic factor for both PFS and OS in 134 patients receiving a combination of lenalidomide, bortezomib, and dexamethasone with or without ASCT, followed by lenalidomide maintenance [12]. The prognostic significance of the three established PET risk factors was recently confirmed in a prospective study of 48 MM patients treated with induction treatment and ASCT. In that study it was also shown that not only quantitative PET parameters from focal lesions, but also those from reference bone marrow samples, are associated with adverse PFS in the disease [16].

Apart from its predictive role in symptomatic MM, ^{18}F-FDG PET/CT has shown prognostic value in asymptomatic SMM patients. Although existing data are relatively limited, the first published results reflect the potential role of the modality in predicting the risk of progression from SMM to symptomatic disease. Siontis et al. studied a group of 122 SMM patients and found that the 2-year risk of progression to active MM was 75% in patients with a positive PET/CT (with or without lytic lesions), compared to 30% in patients with a negative PET/CT. The median time to progression (TTP) was 21 months for the PET/CT positive group, while the respective TTP for the PET/CT negative group was 60 months [17]. In another prospective, multicentric study of 120 SMM patients and a median follow-up of 2.2 years, patients with a positive PET study without underlying osteolysis had a higher risk of progression to active MM and a shorter TTP than patients who were PET-negative. In particular, 58% of the patients with a positive PET scan progressed to active myeloma in 2 years with a median TTP of 1.1 years, compared to those with a negative PET scan demonstrating a progression rate of 33% and a median TTP of 4.5 years [18].

2.3. *The Value of ^{18}F-FDG PET/CT in Therapy Assessment*

Due to its ability in distinguishing between active and inactive lesions, ^{18}F-FDG PET/CT is the best imaging tool for therapy response assessment and is considered the gold standard for treatment monitoring in MM [7] (Figure 2). Several studies have highlighted the role of the modality in the evaluation of the metabolic response to therapy in different stages of the treatment protocol, for example during induction treatment as well as after ASCT [9,12,15,19–23].

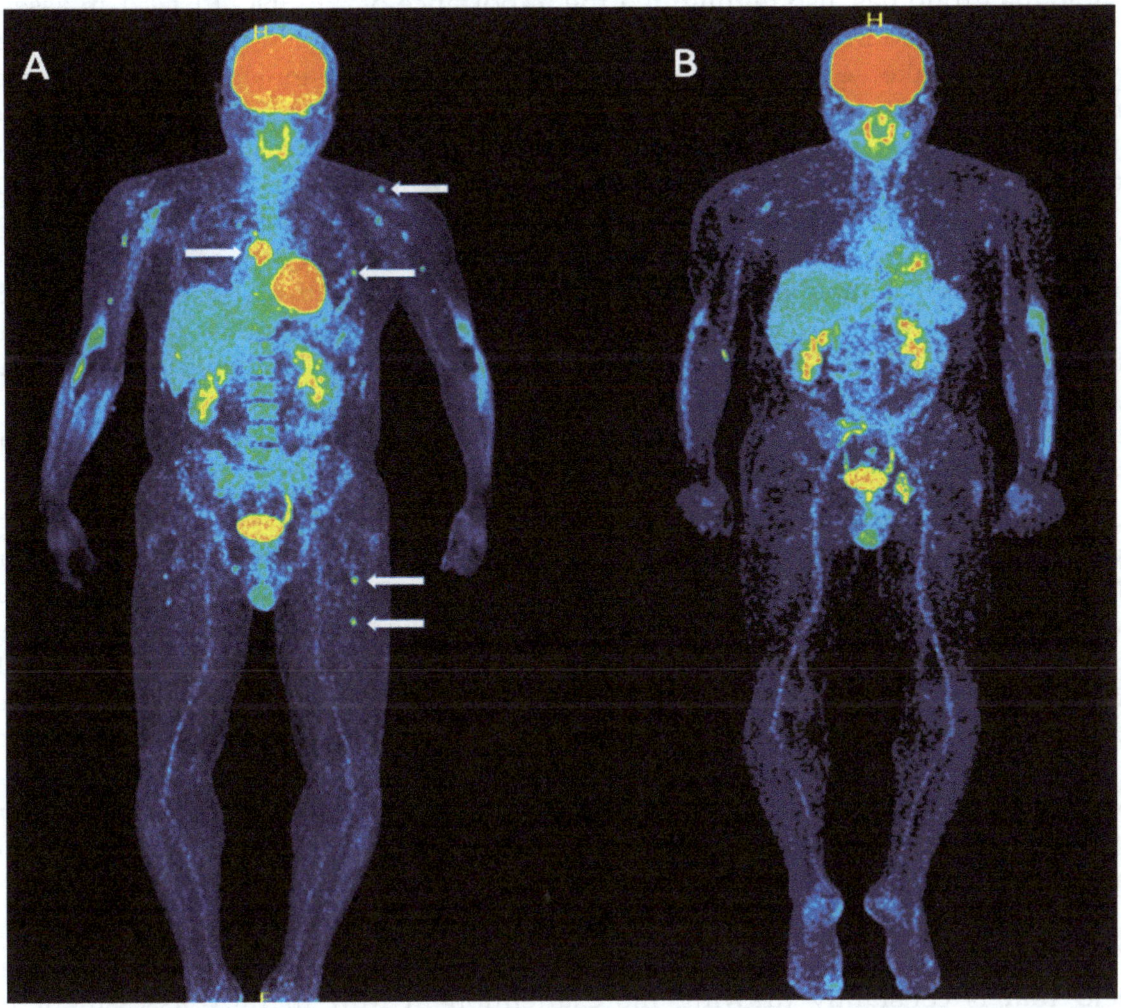

Figure 2. A 39-years old symptomatic MM patient scheduled for HDT and ASCT, undergoing ^{18}F-FDG PET/CT before and after therapy. Maximum intensity projection (MIP) ^{18}F-FDG PET/CT before therapy (**A**) revealed a mixed pattern of ^{18}F-FDG uptake with intense, diffuse uptake in the axial skeleton and multiple, focal bone marrow lesions for example in the sternum, ribs, humerus, scapula and femur (arrows). Follow-up ^{18}F-FDG PET/CT MIP after high-dose chemotherapy and ASCT (**B**) demonstrated a complete remission of both diffuse bone marrow uptake as well as focal MM lesions.

In a study published by the Little Rock group in 2009 involving 239 previously untreated MM patients, it was shown that complete ^{18}F-FDG suppression in focal lesions and EMD after induction treatment and before ASCT conferred superior OS and PFS, and was identified as an independent favorable prognostic variable [9]. A few years later, the same group published a study on a larger cohort involving 302 MM patients studied with PET/CT on day 7 of induction treatment. The authors showed that the persistence of more than three ^{18}F-FDG-avid lesions imparted inferior OS and PFS, suggesting a therapy change in patients with persistent findings on PET/CT early after induction therapy [19]. Most recently, this team published the findings of a trial in 596 patients examined with PET/CT at different time points (day 7 of induction, end of induction, post transplantation, and at maintenance treatment). They demonstrated that patients achieving complete suppression of ^{18}F-FDG activity in focal lesions following treatment at each studied time point had nonsignificant differences in their PFS and OS values than the patients with no lesions at baseline. Importantly, at each time point, patients with no detectable lesions had a significantly superior outcome compared to patients with at least one detectable lesion at that time point, irrespective of whether they had lesions at baseline [22].

The Bologna group has also highlighted the importance of ^{18}F-FDG PET/CT in assessment of response to therapy in MM in different time points. In particular, they have shown that the persistence of severe ^{18}F-FDG uptake—as reflected by the number of focal lesions, SUVmax and presence of EMD—after thalidomide/dexamethasone induction therapy is an early predictor of the worst long-term clinical outcomes. Moreover, a complete response (CR) on PET/CT after ASCT conferred superior PFS and OS in comparison with persistence of ^{18}F-FDG uptake, while the prognostic value of PET/CT was retained also at the time of relapse, with patients positive on PET/CT having a significantly shorter survival compared to those with a negative PET/CT scan [15]. A few years later, they showed in a group of 282 patients that attainment of PET/CT negativity by 3 months after the last cycle of first-line treatment (chemotherapy, novel agents with or without ASCT) significantly influenced both PFS and OS [21]. PET/CT has also been shown effective in response evaluation of patients undergoing allogeneic stem cell transplantation with persistence of EMD being an independent predictor of poor outcome and, on the other hand, achievement of CR on PET/CT after transplantation being associated with a significantly longer OS [23].

The French group (IMAJEM trial) recently evaluated the role of PET/CT after induction treatment (lenalidomide, bortezomib, and dexamethasone) as well as before lenalidomide maintenance in a group of 134 MM patients. The authors showed that normalization of PET/CT after three cycles of induction therapy was associated with improved PFS, and that normalization before maintenance resulted in longer PFS and OS, in comparison to patients without normalization of their PET findings [12]. They could, moreover, show that change in SUV after three cycles of induction therapy was an independent prognostic factor for PFS, rendering SUV a potentially powerful tool for the prediction of long-term outcome in MM [24].

Other groups have also studied ^{18}F-FDG PET/CT in the treatment response evaluation of MM, using different therapeutic agents and protocols. Most of them have confirmed the benefit of applying the modality in the workup of MM patients [25–27].

2.4. *The Value of ^{18}F-FDG PET/CT in Minimal Residual Disease (MRD) Diagnostics*

A field that is constantly drawing more attention in MM therapy assessment is that of standardization and optimization of minimal residual disease (MRD) detection, which is becoming standard diagnostic care. This is driven by the need to improve the definition of disease remission due to the unprecedented rates of CR brought in recent years by the incorporation of novel agents in the treatment of MM patients. It is clear that in MM there is a direct correlation between the depth of response and prolonged survival rates [28]. At present, MRD is detected within the bone marrow, either by multicolor flow cytometry (MFC) or by next generation sequencing technologies [29].

Data on the potential role of ^{18}F-FDG PET/CT in evaluation of the depth of response—beyond the level of conventionally defined CR- are limited but growing. Zamagni et al. retrospectively analyzed 282 MM patients who were evaluated at baseline and during posttreatment follow-up with serial PET/CT scans. They found that the modality could provide a more accurate definition of CR, allowing to stratify patients in conventional CR after up-front therapy into different prognostic subgroups, according to the persistence or absence of ^{18}F-FDG metabolic activity. In particular, the achievement of PET-negativity after treatment was an independent predictor of prolonged PFS and OS for patients with conventionally defined CR [21]. Furthermore, the complementary role of PET/CT and MRD diagnostics with MFC in predicting patient outcome has been supported by some studies. A subanalysis of the IMAJEM trial in 86 patients before maintenance evaluated for both PET/CT and MRD, assessed by MFC, revealed a higher PFS for the group of patients with both a normalized PET/CT and a negative MRD versus patients with either PET positivity and/or MRD positivity before maintenance [12]. In line with these results, the Little Rock group showed in 83 MM patients in CR with available MRD and functional imaging data (in this case PET/CT and/or diffusion weighted MRI) that double-positive and double-negative features defined groups with dismal and excellent PFS, respectively [30]. Most recently, a retrospective study analyzed the prediction of outcome with the combination of ^{18}F-FDG

PET/CT and MRD, assessed by MFC, in 103 patients with newly diagnosed MM. Apart from confirming the benefit—in terms of PFS—linked to the achievement of negativity by MFC and ^{18}F-FDG PET/CT individually, the authors showed that the combination of negativity by both techniques conferred significantly higher PFS than each technique alone, also supporting the potential complementarity between PET/CT and MFC in MRD detection [31].

2.5. Limitations of ^{18}F-FDG PET/CT

Limitations of ^{18}F-FDG PET/CT include its limited availability in comparison to conventional radiological modalities as well as its higher cost. Moreover, the poor sensitivity for the detection of diffuse bone marrow infiltration or skull lesions, due to masking of their activity by the underlying physiological tracer uptake in the brain, is an important drawback. In a report of 227 MM patients the incidence of PET false-negativity was 11% in these patients, a finding attributed to the significantly lower expression of the gene coding for hexokinase-2, which catalyzes the first step of glycolysis [32]. However, this explanation warrants further validation [33]. Further, ^{18}F-FDG, as a glucose analog, is generally restricted in oncological imaging by both false positive (inflammation, post-surgical areas, recent use of chemotherapy, fractures, etc.) and false negative results (hyperglycemia, recent administration of high-dose steroids, etc.). Finally, issues are raised due to the lack of established criteria for image interpretation of ^{18}F-FDG PET/CT scans in MM, resulting in poor interobserver reproducibility in interpreting results. In an attempt to standardize the interpretation of ^{18}F-FDG PET/CT, the Bologna group has recently proposed the Italian Myeloma criteria for PET Use (IMPeTUs) based on the standard Deauville five-point system [34]. These descriptive criteria take into account the number and site of focal lesions, the presence of EMD, as well as the diffuse bone marrow involvement. The first results from the application of IMPeTUs seem to improve the interobserver reproducibility in scan interpretation; however, this needs to be confirmed in further studies.

3. Non ^{18}F-FDG PET Tracers in MM

Due to the limitations of ^{18}F-FDG as an imaging biomarker of MM, several other PET tracers have been proposed and tested in patients with the malignancy. Although some of them have given promising results regarding detection of MM lesions, most studies were performed in rather small patient cohorts and, thus, require validation in further prospective clinical trials. The most important of them will be addressed in the following paragraphs.

3.1. ^{18}F-Choline and ^{11}C-Choline

Choline is a component of phosphatidylcholine and, as such, functions as a substrate for cell membrane biosynthesis. The uptake of radiolabeled choline is increased in proliferating cells because it is involved in membrane metabolism and growth. Choline PET imaging has been traditionally used in the diagnostics of prostate cancer.

The first report of ^{11}C-choline uptake in myeloma lesions was an incidental finding of a solitary plasmacytoma in a patient being re-staged for prostate cancer [35]. Based on this finding, a comparison study of ^{11}C-choline vs. ^{18}F-FDG PET/CT in assessing bone involvement was performed by the Bologna group in a heterogeneous group of 10 MM patients (4 patients at completion of initial therapy, 2 during follow-up and 4 at disease relapse). In 2/10 patients with suspicion of disease relapse, both the ^{11}C-Choline and ^{18}F-FDG PET/CT scans were positive and identified the same number and sites of bone lesions. In 4/10 patients, both techniques were positive, but ^{11}C-choline identified a nonsignificant higher number of lesions than ^{18}F-FDG. Finally, 4 patients were negative with both tracers, a finding consistent with clinical, laboratory and radiological data indicating a CR at the time of imaging [36]. Almost ten years later, another pilot study on choline PET was published on a larger MM patient cohort. Twenty-one patients with suspected progressive or relapsing MM were studied with ^{18}F-choline and ^{18}F-FDG PET/CT. No myeloma lesions were detected in two cases, while uncountable foci were observed in four patients. In the rest, 15 patients with countable bone foci, ^{18}F-choline PET/CT depicted a significantly higher number of lesions than ^{18}F-FDG PET/CT [37]. Further, the performance of ^{18}F-choline and ^{18}F-FDG PET/CT in the detection of skeletal involvement was compared in a case series of five MM patients in a pairwise fashion. Skeletal lesions were detected in all five ^{18}F-choline PET/CT scans compared to four out of five ^{18}F-FDG PET/CT scans. Altogether ^{18}F-choline PET/CT detected a total of 134 bone lesions compared to 64 lesions detected by ^{18}F-FDG PET/CT. Interestingly, the vast majority of the missed lesions in ^{18}F-FDG PET/CT were in the axial skeleton including the skull vault [38].

To summarize, choline PET seems to have a better detection rate of focal lesions than ^{18}F-FDG PET. However, no comparison studies between the two PET tracers in previously untreated MM patients have been performed. A limitation of choline PET is its unfavorable physiological distribution involving increased uptake in the bone marrow and the liver parenchyma potentially masking lesions in these organs; although hepatic lesions are rare in MM and can be reliably detected with MRI, the increased activity in the bone marrow compartment may pose significant diagnostic challenges, in particular in patients showing a diffuse bone marrow infiltration pattern. Moreover, the use of ^{11}C-choline is limited in centres with an on-site cyclotron and radiopharmacy facilities, because of the very short half-life of the radioisotope (20 min).

3.2. ^{11}C-Acetate

^{11}C-acetate is rapidly picked-up by cells and metabolized into acetyl-CoA by the key enzyme acetyl-CoA synthase, which is overexpressed in certain cancer cells [39]. The use of ^{11}C-acetate in MM can be justified by the elevated lipid synthesis in proliferating abnormal plasma cells as reported by studies with myeloma cell lines [40].

Similarly to radiolabeled choline, the first report of ^{11}C-acetate uptake in myeloma lesions was an incidental finding [41]. In total, two comparative studies of ^{11}C-acetate with ^{18}F-FDG have been published thus far. Ho et al. evaluated a heterogeneous group of 35 untreated patients (26 with symptomatic MM, 5 with SMM, and 4 with MGUS), 9 of which undergoing also dual tracer follow-up PET/CT. The authors reported a significantly higher overall sensitivity for symptomatic MM with ^{11}C-acetate than with ^{18}F-FDG (84.6% vs. 57.7%), while the specificity for ^{11}C-acetate and ^{18}F-FDG PET/CT was 100% and, 93.1% respectively. Furthermore, all indolent plasma cell neoplasms (SMM and MUGS) were negative by ^{11}C-acetate PET, whereas 2 cases of MGUS were false-positive by ^{18}F-FDG [42]. A similar study was published a few months later by Lin et al. in 15 untreated MM patients examined with both tracers at diagnosis, 13 of which being evaluated with a repeated dual-tracer examination after completion of induction treatment. They found a higher detection rate for both diffuse and focal myeloma lesions at initial staging using ^{11}C-acetate than ^{18}F-FDG. Moreover, after treatment the diffuse bone marrow ^{11}C-acetate uptake showed a statistically significant difference in SUV_{max} reductions between patients with at least a very good partial response and those with at most a partial response. Such a difference between patients in these two response groups was not observed with ^{18}F-FDG PET/CT [43].

In summary, these preliminary findings imply a potential role for ^{11}C-acetate PET/CT for the evaluation of patients with MM. Nevertheless, practical and logistical considerations are raised due to the fact that the synthesis of the tracer requires technical expertise and an on-site cyclotron.

3.3. ^{11}C-Methionine

^{11}C-Methionine is an aminoacidic PET tracer mainly employed in the diagnosis of central nervous system tumors. The uptake of the tracer primarily reflects its transmembrane transport by the sodium-independent L-transporter into cells. This transport is driven by concentration gradient and is thus influenced by the intracellular metabolism of the amino acid, which in turn reflects proliferation activity [44]. The concept of applying ^{11}C-methionine in MM is mainly based on the knowledge that radiolabeled amino acids show a rapid uptake and metabolic incorporation into newly synthesized immunoglobulins [45]. Moreover, the uptake of 35S-methionine into myeloma cells is higher as compared with other hematopoietic cells [46]. Despite the limited literature on the topic, ^{11}C-methionine PET/CT concordantly appears to perform better than ^{18}F-FDG in detection of myeloma lesions.

Dankerl et al. were the first to apply this PET tracer for imaging of MM in a group of 19 patients with active disease. The authors detected disseminated multifocal ^{11}C-methionine–positive bone marrow lesions in all patients, except two, a finding suggesting widespread dissemination of MM in the hematopoietic bone marrow. The two patients without extensive disease on ^{11}C-methionine PET showed exclusive EMD and monofocal medullary MM, respectively [46]. The first comparative study was published in 2013 by Nakamoto et al. in 20 patients with MM (n = 15) and plasmacytoma (n = 5) who underwent ^{18}F-FDG PET/CT and ^{11}C-methionine PET/CT scans. On a patient basis, two patients were accurately diagnosed only by ^{11}C-methionine PET/CT, while in the remaining 18 patients consistent results were obtained. However, the potential upgrade of staging or restaging was necessary in 6 of 11 positive patients because more abnormal lesions were demonstrated by ^{11}C-methionine PET/CT. The patient-based sensitivity, specificity and accuracy of ^{11}C-methionine PET/CT for restaging were 89%, 100% and 93%, respectively, while those of ^{18}F-FDG PET/CT were 78%, 100% and 86%, respectively [47]. Two years later, Okasaki et al. studied 64 patients with MM or MGUS (21 previously untreated, 43 restaged after treatment) undergoing PET/CT with the tracers ^{11}C-4′-thiothymidine (^{11}C-4DST), ^{11}C-methionine, and ^{18}F-FDG. The main findings of the study were the following: firstly, the number of equivocal lesions observed using ^{18}F-FDG was larger compared to using ^{11}C- methionine or ^{11}C-4DST both before and after therapy. Secondly, ^{11}C- methionine and ^{11}C-4DST were superior to ^{18}F-FDG in clearly detecting skull lesions because of their low physiological accumulation in the brain [48].

The Würzburg group has also highlighted the superiority of ^{11}C-methionine over ^{18}F-FDG for staging and re-staging of both intra- and extramedullary MM lesions [49,50]. These results were further confirmed in both patient- and lesion-based analyses in the largest so far, dual-center study of 78 patients (4 solitary plasmacytoma, 5 SMM, 69 symptomatic MM) published in 2017 [51]. Moreover, the same group has recently performed the first head-to-head comparison of ^{11}C-methionine and ^{11}C-choline for metabolic imaging of MM in 19 patients with a history of MM (n = 18) or solitary bone plasmacytoma (n = 1). ^{11}C-methionine provided advantages over ^{11}C-choline in terms of higher sensitivity by detecting a higher number of intramedullary lesions in approximately 40% of patients, as well as by achieving higher lesion-to-background contrast [52].

Drawbacks of ^{11}C-Methionine PET are considered to be its increased physiological biodistribution in the liver parenchyma and the bone marrow, potentially reducing the detection rate of MM lesions. Moreover, the ^{11}C labeling of the tracer prevents a relatively massive production and distribution of ^{11}C-Methionine [53].

3.4. ^{18}F-Fluorothymidine (^{18}F-FLT)

^{18}F-Fluorothymidine (^{18}F-FLT) is the most studied cellular proliferation PET agent [54]. ^{18}F-FLT is taken up by cells and phosphorylated by thymidine kinase 1, which is upregulated by about tenfold during the S-phase of the cell cycle, producing ^{18}F-FLT monophosphate (^{18}F-FLT-MP), which can then be sequentially phosphorylated to form ^{18}F-FLT diphosphate (^{18}F-FLT-DP) and ^{18}F-FLT triphosphate (^{18}F-FLT-TP). These phosphorylated products are metabolically trapped intracellularly without being incorporated into DNA. The tracer retention within cells reflects, in part, thymidine kinase activity and is often positively correlated with cellular proliferation [55].

The knowledge regarding application and performance of ^{18}F-FLT PET in MM is limited. Agool et al. studied a group of 18 patients with different hematologic disorders, among which were two patients with MM. The authors found that the affected osteolytic areas in these two MM patients demonstrated a low ^{18}F-FLT uptake [56]. In a pilot study on combined ^{18}F-FDG and ^{18}F-FLT PET/CT imaging in 8 myeloma patients (4 patients with symptomatic MM, 4 patients with SMM) the number of myeloma-indicative lesions was significantly higher for ^{18}F-FDG PET/CT than for ^{18}F-FLT

PET/CT. A common finding of the study was a mismatch of focally increased ^{18}F-FDG uptake and reduced ^{18}F-FLT uptake (lower than the surrounding bone marrow) in myeloma lesions. Moreover, ^{18}F-FLT PET/CT was characterized by high background activity in the bone marrow compartment, complicating the evaluation of bone marrow lesions [57].

In conclusion, despite the limited number of patients studied so far, the preliminary results indicate that ^{18}F-FLT does not seem suitable as a single PET tracer in MM diagnostics.

3.5. ^{68}Ga-Pentixafor

Chemokine receptor 4 (CXCR4) is a pleiotropic, G-protein coupled chemokine receptor expressed on hematopoeitic stem and progenitor cells in the bone marrow niche. CXCR4 can mediate the migration as well as the homing process of these cells in the bone marrow in response to its ligand, stromal cell-derived factor 1 (SDF-1) [58]. In MM, CXCR4 is involved in myeloma cell homing, bone marrow retention, angiogenesis and metastasis, while collective evidence from several studies support the pivotal role of CXCR4 in different stages of MM, disease progression, development of therapeutic resistance and MRD, as well as poor prognosis [59–66].

^{68}Ga-pentixafor is a radiolabeled peptide that shows high affinity for CXCR4. The major advantage of the tracer is its potential use in a thera(g)nostic approach in combination with the ^{177}Lu- or ^{90}Y-labeled agent pentixather in progressive MM patients with CXCR4-positive tumor cells, as confirmed by a ^{68}Ga-pentixafor PET scan. Preliminary results of the CXCR4-directed endoradiotherapy with pentixather in three heavily pretreated MM patients were relatively encouraging with low levels of toxicity, good tolerance of the treatment and high initial response rates [67].

Two studies have investigated the diagnostic performance of ^{68}Ga-pentixafor in comparison to ^{18}F-FDG in patients with advanced MM. The initial results in 14 MM patients showed a slight superiority of the novel tracer over ^{18}F-FDG in the relapsed disease setting, with 10/14 patients showing MM manifestations on ^{68}Ga-pentixafor PET, while 9/14 were positive on ^{18}F-FDG PET [68]. The larger second study included 35 patients undergoing ^{68}Ga-pentixafor PET/CT for evaluation of eligibility for endoradiotherapy. In 19 patients, ^{18}F-FDG PET/CT was also available for correlation. ^{68}Ga-pentixafor PET detected CXCR4-positive disease in 23/35 subjects (66%). Importantly, in the 19 patients in whom a comparison to ^{18}F-FDG PET was available, 8/19 (42%) patients had an equal number of lesions with both tracers, in 4/19 (21%) subjects ^{68}Ga-pentixafor PET detected more lesions, while ^{18}F-FDG PET proved superior in 7/19 (37%) of them [69].

Most recently, the first comparative study of ^{18}F-FDG and ^{68}Ga-pentixafor PET/CT in 30 patients with newly diagnosed MM was published. ^{68}Ga-Pentixafor PET/CT had a significantly higher positive rate than ^{18}F-FDG PET/CT in detection of myeloma lesions (93.3% vs. 53.3%). In quantitative analysis, bone marrow uptake values in ^{68}Ga-Pentixafor were positively correlated with end organ damage, staging, and laboratory biomarkers related to tumor burden including serum β2-microglobulin, serum free light chain, and 24-h urine light chain. In contrary, in ^{18}F-FDG PET/CT, only the SUV mean of total bone marrow was positively correlated with serum free light chain and 24-h urine light chain [70]. These results indicate that ^{68}Ga-pentixafor PET might be a promising biomarker in assessing the tumor burden of newly diagnosed MM patients.

3.6. ^{18}F-Sodium Fluoride (^{18}F-NaF)

^{18}F-NaF is a highly sensitive biomarker of bone reconstruction, with potential indications in a wide range of bone disease [71–74]. The uptake of the tracer in bone occurs by chemisorption onto hydroxyapatite, followed by exchange with hydroxyl groups in the hydroxyapatite, resulting in formation of fluoroapatite. The tracer accumulates in nearly all sites of increased new bone formation, reflecting regional blood flow, osteoblastic activity and bone turnover [71,75,76].

An increasing interest has been raised in the last years on the potential application of ^{18}F-NaF PET/CT in MM diagnostics and management. This interest was based, however, on a very small number of studied MM patients without comparison with a robust reference imaging method [77–80].

Despite this initial enthusiasm, subsequent publications demonstrated rather discouraging results. In particular, ^{18}F-NaF PET/CT did not confer any superiority or complementarity to ^{18}F-FDG PET/CT in detection of MM lesions, showing both lower sensitivity and specificity [81–83]. Moreover, ^{18}F-NaF PET/CT does not seem to add significantly to ^{18}F-FDG PET/CT in the treatment response evaluation of MM patients, as shown in a study of 34 patients undergoing high-dose chemotherapy and ASCT [84].

The low sensitivity of ^{18}F-NaF PET/CT in detecting myeloma lesions is mainly attributed to the fact that the tracer indicates osteoblastic activity. However, since the hallmark of MM is the osteolytic lesion, the accumulation of ^{18}F-NaF takes place only in the accompanying, sometimes minimal, reactive osteoblastic changes [85]. Further, being a very sensitive radiopharmaceutical for osteoblastic activity, ^{18}F-NaF accumulates in practically in every site of newly mineralizing bone, irrelevant of its aetiology. This means that any cause of bone reconstruction, such as traumatic or degenerative bone lesions, will lead to tracer accumulation, significantly decreasing its specificity as a myeloma tracer [86].

3.7. ^{18}F-FAZA

One of the reasons leading to an increased metabolic activity detected with ^{18}F-FDG PET/CT is tumor hypoxia. Tumor hypoxia leads to enhanced production of several hypoxia inducible factors, resulting in increased microvessel density (MVD) around the malignant plasma cells [6]. MVD has been proven to be correlated with disease progression in MM [87]. Based on this approach, de Waal et al. applied the PET tracer 1-α-D: -(5-deoxy-5-[^{18}F]-fluoroarabinofuranosyl)-2-nitroimidazole (^{18}F-FAZA), which accumulates in tumor hypoxia. The authors studied 5 patients with relapsed MM with ^{18}F-FDG PET and ^{18}F-FAZA PET. Although all patients had a positive ^{18}F-FDG PET scan, no lesions were demonstrated on ^{18}F-FAZA PET, reflecting a limited performance of this tracer in the workup of MM patients [88].

3.8. ^{89}Zr-Daratumumab

The membrane glycoprotein cluster of differentiation 38 (CD38) is expressed at a high density by almost all myeloma cells, and at relatively low levels on normal hematopoietic cells. CD38 is an established therapeutic target in MM. Daratumumab is an FDA-approved therapeutic monoclonal antibody that binds directly to CD38, offering a clinical benefit in MM patients [89–91]. Recently, daratumumab was radiolabeled with ^{89}Zr through deferoxamine (DFO), producing the PET agent ^{89}Zr-DFO-daratumumab. The results of a Phase I first-in-human ^{89}Zr-DFO-daratumumab PET/CT imaging study in six MM patients demonstrated successful whole-body PET visualization of MM with focal tracer uptake in previously known as well as unknown sites of osseous myeloma, consistent with successful CD38-targeted immunoPET imaging of myeloma in human patients [92]. Although these results warrant validation in further prospective studies, they are highly promising for the usage of this PET antibody in diagnosis and staging of MM. Moreover, it could be applied in terms of a personalized, daratumumab-directed imaging in order to identify those MM patients who would benefit from daratumumab and thus predict the effectiveness of therapy in the context of a thera(g)nostic approach in MM.

4. Conclusions

PET/CT with ^{18}F-FDG is increasingly gaining acceptance in the management of MM patients, and is considered a powerful diagnostic tool for the detection of medullary and extramedullary disease at initial diagnosis, a reliable predictor of survival, as well as the most robust modality for treatment response evaluation in the disease. On the other hand, ^{18}F-FDG carries the limitations of a rather poor sensitivity for the detection of diffuse bone marrow infiltration, a relatively low specificity, and the lack of widely applied, established criteria for image interpretation. These drawbacks have led to the development of several alternative PET tracers for MM detection. Some of these radiotracers have provided promising results—such as ^{18}F-choline and ^{11}C-choline, ^{11}C-acetate, ^{11}C-methionine,

^{68}Ga-pentixafor and ^{89}Zr-Daratumumab—but most studies were performed in small patient cohorts and require validation in further prospective clinical trials.

References

1. Altekruse, S.F.; Kosary, C.L.; Krapcho, M.; Neyman, N.; Aminou, R.; Waldron, W.; Ruhl, J.; Howlader, N.; Tatalovich, Z.; Cho, H.; et al. (Eds.) *SEER Cancer Statistics Review, 1975–2007*; National Cancer Institute: Bethesda, MD, USA, 2009. Available online: http://seer.cancer.gov/csr/1975_2007/index.html (accessed on 5 December 2019).
2. Landgren, O.; Kyle, R.A.; Rajkumar, S.V. From myeloma precursor disease to multiple myeloma: New diagnostic concepts and opportunities for early intervention. *Clin. Cancer Res.* **2011**, *17*, 1243–1252. [CrossRef]
3. Zamagni, E.; Tacchetti, P.; Cavo, M. Imaging in multiple myeloma: How? When? *Blood* **2019**, *133*, 644–651. [CrossRef]
4. Rajkumar, S.V.; Dimopoulos, M.A.; Palumbo, A.; Blade, J.; Merlini, G.; Mateos, M.V.; Kumar, S.; Hillengass, J.; Kastritis, E.; Richardson, P.; et al. International Myeloma Working Group updated criteria for the diagnosis of multiple myeloma. *Lancet Oncol.* **2014**, *15*, e538–e548. [CrossRef]
5. Zamagni, E.; Cavo, M. The role of imaging techniques in the management of multiple myeloma. *Br. J. Haematol.* **2012**, *159*, 499–513. [CrossRef]
6. De Waal, E.G.M.; Glaudemans, A.W.J.M.; Schröder, C.P.; Vellenga, E.; Slart, R.H.J.A. Nuclear medicine imaging of multiple myeloma, particularly in the relapsed setting. *Eur. J. Nucl. Med. Mol. Imaging* **2017**, *44*, 332–341. [CrossRef]
7. Cavo, M.; Terpos, E.; Nanni, C.; Moreau, P.; Lentzsch, S.; Zweegman, S.; Hillengass, J.; Engelhardt, M.; Usmani, S.Z.; Vesole, D.H.; et al. Role of 18F-FDG PET/CT in the diagnosis and management of multiple myeloma and other plasma cell disorders: A consensus statement by the International Myeloma Working Group. *Lancet Oncol.* **2017**, *18*, e206–e217. [CrossRef]
8. Zamagni, E.; Nanni, C.; Patriarca, F.; Englaro, E.; Castellucci, P.; Geatti, O.; Tosi, P.; Tacchetti, P.; Cangini, D.; Perrone, G.; et al. A prospective comparison of 18F-fluorodeoxyglucose positron emission tomography-computed tomography, magnetic resonance imaging and whole-body planar radiographs in the assessment of bone disease in newly diagnosed multiple myeloma. *Haematologica* **2007**, *92*, 50–55. [CrossRef] [PubMed]
9. Bartel, T.B.; Haessler, J.; Brown, T.L.; Shaughnessy, J.D., Jr.; van Rhee, F.; Anaissie, E.; Alpe, T.; Angtuaco, E.; Walker, R.; Epstein, J.; et al. F18-fluorodeoxyglucose positron emission tomography in the context of other imaging techniques and prognostic factors in multiple myeloma. *Blood* **2009**, *114*, 2068–2076. [CrossRef]
10. Van Lammeren-Venema, D.; Regelink, J.C.; Riphagen, I.I.; Zweegman, S.; Hoekstra, O.S.; Zijlstra, J.M. 18F-fluoro-deoxyglucose positron emission tomography in assessment of myeloma-related bone disease: A systematic review. *Cancer* **2012**, *118*, 1971–1981. [CrossRef] [PubMed]
11. Lu, Y.Y.; Chen, J.H.; Lin, W.Y.; Liang, J.A.; Wang, H.Y.; Tsai, S.C.; Kao, C.H. FDG PET or PET/CT for detecting intramedullary and extramedullary lesions in multiple Myeloma: A systematic review and meta-analysis. *Clin. Nucl. Med.* **2012**, *37*, 833–837. [CrossRef] [PubMed]
12. Moreau, P.; Attal, M.; Caillot, D.; Macro, M.; Karlin, L.; Garderet, L.; Facon, T.; Benboubker, L.; Escoffre-Barbe, M.; Stoppa, A.M.; et al. Prospective evaluation of magnetic resonance imaging and [18F]fluorodeoxyglucose positron emission tomography-computed tomography at diagnosis and before maintenance therapy in symptomatic patients with multiple myeloma included in the IFM/DFCI 2009 Trial: Results of the IMAJEM study. *J. Clin. Oncol.* **2017**, *35*, 2911–2918. [CrossRef] [PubMed]
13. Sachpekidis, C.; Mai, E.K.; Goldschmidt, H.; Hillengass, J.; Hose, D.; Pan, L.; Haberkorn, U.; Dimitrakopoulou-Strauss, A. (18)F-FDG dynamic PET/CT in patients with multiple myeloma: Patterns of tracer uptake and correlation with bone marrow plasma cell infiltration rate. *Clin. Nucl. Med.* **2015**, *40*, e300–e307. [CrossRef] [PubMed]

14. Sachpekidis, C.; Hillengass, J.; Goldschmidt, H.; Mosebach, J.; Pan, L.; Schlemmer, H.P.; Haberkorn, U.; Dimitrakopoulou-Strauss, A. Comparison of (18)F-FDG PET/CT and PET/MRI in patients with multiple myeloma. *Am. J. Nucl. Med. Mol. Imaging* **2015**, *5*, 469–478. [PubMed]
15. Zamagni, E.; Patriarca, F.; Nanni, C.; Zannetti, B.; Englaro, E.; Pezzi, A.; Tacchetti, P.; Buttignol, S.; Perrone, G.; Brioli, A.; et al. Prognostic relevance of 18-F FDG PET/CT in newly diagnosed multiple myeloma patients treated with up-front autologous transplantation. *Blood* **2011**, *118*, 5989–5995. [CrossRef]
16. Sachpekidis, C.; Merz, M.; Kopp-Schneider, A.; Jauch, A.; Raab, M.S.; Sauer, S.; Hillengass, J.; Goldschmidt, H.; Dimitrakopoulou-Strauss, A. Quantitative dynamic 18F-fluorodeoxyglucose positron emission tomography/computed tomography before autologous stem cell transplantation predicts survival in multiple myeloma. *Haematologica* **2019**, *104*, e420–e423. [CrossRef]
17. Siontis, B.; Kumar, S.; Dispenzieri, A.; Drake, M.T.; Lacy, M.Q.; Buadi, F.; Dingli, D.; Kapoor, P.; Gonsalves, W.; Gertz, M.A.; et al. Positron emission tomography-computed tomography in the diagnostic evaluation of smoldering multiple myeloma: Identification of patients needing therapy. *Blood Cancer J.* **2015**, *5*, e364. [CrossRef]
18. Zamagni, E.; Nanni, C.; Gay, F.; Pezzi, A.; Patriarca, F.; Bellò, M.; Rambaldi, I.; Tacchetti, P.; Hillengass, J.; Gamberi, B.; et al. 18F-FDG PET/CT focal, but not osteolytic, lesions predict the progression of smoldering myeloma to active disease. *Leukemia* **2016**, *30*, 417–422. [CrossRef]
19. Usmani, S.Z.; Mitchell, A.; Waheed, S.; Crowley, J.; Hoering, A.; Petty, N.; Brown, T.; Bartel, T.; Anaissie, E.; van Rhee, F.; et al. Prognostic implications of serial 18-fluoro-deoxyglucose emission tomography in multiple myeloma treated with total therapy 3. *Blood* **2013**, *121*, 1819–1823. [CrossRef]
20. Nanni, C.; Zamagni, E.; Celli, M.; Caroli, P.; Ambrosini, V.; Tacchetti, P.; Brioli, A.; Zannetti, B.; Pezzi, A.; Pantani, L.; et al. The value of 18F-FDG PET/CT after autologous stem cell transplantation (ASCT) in patients affected by multiple myeloma (MM): Experience with 77 patients. *Clin. Nucl. Med.* **2013**, *38*, e74–e79. [CrossRef]
21. Zamagni, E.; Nanni, C.; Mancuso, K.; Tacchetti, P.; Pezzi, A.; Pantani, L.; Zannetti, B.; Rambaldi, I.; Brioli, A.; Rocchi, S.; et al. PET/CT improves the definition of complete response and allows to detect otherwise unidentifiable skeletal progression in multiple Myeloma. *Clin. Cancer Res.* **2015**, *21*, 4384–4390. [CrossRef]
22. Davies, F.E.; Rosenthal, A.; Rasche, L.; Petty, N.M.; McDonald, J.E.; Ntambi, J.A.; Steward, D.M.; Panozzo, S.B.; van Rhee, F.; Zangari, M.; et al. Treatment to suppression of focal lesions on positron emission tomography-computed tomography is a therapeutic goal in newly diagnosed multiple myeloma. *Haematologica* **2018**, *103*, 1047–1053. [CrossRef] [PubMed]
23. Patriarca, F.; Carobolante, F.; Zamagni, E.; Montefusco, V.; Bruno, B.; Englaro, E.; Nanni, C.; Geatti, O.; Isola, M.; Sperotto, A.; et al. The role of positron emission tomography with 18F-fluorodeoxyglucose integrated with computed tomography in the evaluation of patients with multiple myeloma undergoing allogeneic stem cell transplantation. *Biol. Blood Marrow Transplant.* **2015**, *21*, 1068–1073. [CrossRef] [PubMed]
24. Bailly, C.; Carlier, T.; Jamet, B.; Eugene, T.; Touzeau, C.; Attal, M.; Hulin, C.; Facon, T.; Leleu, X.; Perrot, A.; et al. Interim PET Analysis in First-Line Therapy of Multiple Myeloma: Prognostic Value of ΔSUVmax in the FDG-Avid Patients of the IMAJEM Study. *Clin. Cancer Res.* **2018**, *24*, 5219–5224. [CrossRef] [PubMed]
25. Dimitrakopoulou-Strauss, A.; Hoffmann, M.; Bergner, R.; Uppenkamp, M.; Haberkorn, U.; Strauss, L.G. Prediction of progression-free survival in patients with multiple myeloma following anthracycline-based chemotherapy based on dynamic FDG-PET. *Clin. Nucl. Med.* **2009**, *34*, 576–584. [CrossRef]
26. Elliott, B.M.; Peti, S.; Osman, K.; Scigliano, E.; Lee, D.; Isola, L.; Kostakoglu, L. Combining FDG-PET/CT with laboratory data yields superior results for prediction of relapse in multiple myeloma. *Eur. J. Haematol.* **2011**, *86*, 289–298. [CrossRef]
27. Korde, N.; Roschewski, M.; Zingone, A.; Kwok, M.; Manasanch, E.E.; Bhutani, M.; Tageja, N.; Kazandjian, D.; Mailankody, S.; Wu, P.; et al. Treatment with carfilzomib-lenalidomide-dexamethasone with lenalidomide extension in patients with smoldering or newly diagnosed multiple myeloma. *JAMA Oncol.* **2015**, *1*, 746–754. [CrossRef]
28. Paiva, B.; García-Sanz, R.; San Miguel, J.F. Multiple Myeloma Minimal Residual Disease. In *Plasma Cell Dyscrasias. Cancer Treatment and Research*; Roccaro, A., Ghobrial, I., Eds.; Springer: Cham, Switzerland, 2016; Volume 169, pp. 103–122. [CrossRef]

29. Kumar, S.; Paiva, B.; Anderson, K.C.; Durie, B.; Landgren, O.; Moreau, P.; Munshi, N.; Lonial, S.; Bladé, J.; Mateos, M.V.; et al. International Myeloma Working Group consensus criteria for response and minimal residual disease assessment in multiple myeloma. *Lancet Oncol.* **2016**, *17*, e328–e346. [CrossRef]
30. Rasche, L.; Alapat, D.; Kumar, M.; Gershner, G.; McDonald, J.; Wardell, C.P.; Samant, R.; Van Hemert, R.; Epstein, J.; Williams, A.F.; et al. Combination of flow cytometry and functional imaging for monitoring of residual disease in myeloma. *Leukemia* **2019**, *33*, 1713–1722. [CrossRef]
31. Alonso, R.; Cedena, M.T.; Gómez-Grande, A.; Ríos, R.; Moraleda, J.M.; Cabañas, V.; Moreno, M.J.; López-Jiménez, J.; Martín, F.; Sanz, A.; et al. Imaging and bone marrow assessments improve minimal residual disease prediction in multiple myeloma. *Am. J. Hematol.* **2019**, *94*, 853–861. [CrossRef]
32. Rasche, L.; Angtuaco, E.; McDonald, J.E.; Buros, A.; Stein, C.; Pawlyn, C.; Thanendrarajan, S.; Schinke, C.; Samant, R.; Yaccoby, S.; et al. Low expression of hexokinase-2 is associated with false-negative FDG-positron emission tomography in multiple myeloma. *Blood* **2017**, *130*, 30–34. [CrossRef]
33. Kircher, S.; Stolzenburg, A.; Kortuem, K.M.; Kircher, M.; Da Via, M.; Samnick, S.; Buck, A.; Einsele, H.; Rosenwald, A.; Lapa, C. Hexokinase-2 expression in MET-positive FDG-negative multiple myeloma. *J. Nucl. Med.* **2019**, *60*, 348–352. [CrossRef] [PubMed]
34. Nanni, C.; Versari, A.; Chauvie, S.; Bertone, E.; Bianchi, A.; Rensi, M.; Bellò, M.; Gallamini, A.; Patriarca, F.; Gay, F.; et al. Interpretation criteria for FDG PET/CT in multiple myeloma (IMPeTUs): Final results. IMPeTUs (Italian myeloma criteria for PET USe). *Eur. J. Nucl. Med. Mol. Imaging* **2018**, *45*, 712–719. [CrossRef]
35. Ambrosini, V.; Farsad, M.; Nanni, C.; Schiavina, R.; Rubello, D.; Castellucci, P.; Pasquini, E.; Franchi, R.; Cavo, M.; Fanti, S. Incidental finding of an 11C-choline PET positive solitary plasmacytoma lesion. *Eur. J. Nucl. Med. Mol. Imaging* **2006**, *33*, 1522. [CrossRef] [PubMed]
36. Nanni, C.; Zamagni, E.; Cavo, M.; Rubello, D.; Tacchetti, P.; Pettinato, C.; Farsad, M.; Castellucci, P.; Ambrosini, V.; Montini, G.C.; et al. 11C-choline vs. 18F-FDG PET/ CT in assessing bone involvement in patients with multiple myeloma. *World J. Surg. Oncol.* **2007**, *5*, 68. [CrossRef] [PubMed]
37. Cassou-Mounat, T.; Balogova, S.; Nataf, V.; Calzada, M.; Huchet, V.; Kerrou, K.; Devaux, J.Y.; Mohty, M.; Talbot, J.N.; Garderet, L. 18F-fluorocholine versus 18F-fluorodeoxyglucose for PET/CT imaging in patients with suspected relapsing or progressive multiple myeloma: A pilot study. *Eur. J. Nucl. Med. Mol. Imaging* **2016**, *43*, 1995–2004. [CrossRef] [PubMed]
38. Meckova, Z.; Lambert, L.; Spicka, I.; Kubinyi, J.; Burgetova, A. Is fluorine-18-fluorocholine PET/CT suitable for the detection of skeletal involvement of multiple myeloma? *Hell. J. Nucl. Med.* **2018**, *21*, 167–168. [CrossRef] [PubMed]
39. Grassi, I.; Nanni, C.; Allegri, V.; Morigi, J.J.; Montini, G.C.; Castellucci, P.; Fanti, S. The clinical use of PET with (11)C-acetate. *Am. J. Nucl. Med. Mol. Imaging* **2012**, *2*, 33–47.
40. Khoo, S.H.; Al-Rubeai, M. Metabolic characterization of a hyper-productive state in an antibody producing NS0 myeloma cell line. *Metab. Eng.* **2009**, *11*, 199–211. [CrossRef]
41. Lee, S.M.; Kim, T.S.; Lee, J.W.; Kwon, H.W.; Kim, Y.I.; Kang, S.H.; Kim, S.K. Incidental finding of an ^{11}C-acetate PET-positive multiple myeloma. *Ann. Nucl. Med.* **2010**, *24*, 41–44. [CrossRef]
42. Ho, C.L.; Chen, S.; Leung, Y.L.; Cheng, T.; Wong, K.N.; Cheung, S.K.; Liang, R.; Chim, C.S. ^{11}C-Acetate PET/CT for metabolic characterization of multiple myeloma: A comparative study with 18F-FDG PET/CT. *J. Nucl. Med.* **2014**, *55*, 749–752. [CrossRef]
43. Lin, C.; Ho, C.L.; Ng, S.H.; Wang, P.N.; Huang, Y.; Lin, Y.C.; Tang, T.C.; Tsai, S.F.; Rahmouni, A.; Yen, T.C. (11)C-Acetate as a new biomarker for PET/CT in patients with multiple myeloma: Initial staging and postinduction response assessment. *Eur. J. Nucl. Med. Mol. Imaging* **2014**, *41*, 41–49. [CrossRef] [PubMed]
44. Glaudemans, A.W.; Enting, R.H.; Heesters, M.A.; Dierckx, R.A.; van Rheenen, R.W.; Walenkamp, A.M.; Slart, R.H. Value of ^{11}C-methionine PET in imaging brain tumours and metastases. *Eur. J. Nucl. Med. Mol. Imaging* **2013**, *40*, 615–635. [CrossRef] [PubMed]
45. Hammerton, K.; Cooper, D.A.; Duckett, M.; Penny, R. Biosynthesis of immunoglobulin in human immunoproliferative diseases. I. Kinetics of synthesis and secretion of immunoglobulin and protein by bone marrow cells in myeloma. *J. Immunol.* **1978**, *121*, 409–417. [PubMed]
46. Dankerl, A.; Liebisch, P.; Glatting, G.; Friesen, C.; Blumstein, N.M.; Kocot, D.; Wendl, C.; Bunjes, D.; Reske, S.N. Multiple Myeloma: Molecular Imaging with C-Methionine PET/CT—Initial Experience. *Radiology* **2007**, *242*, 498–508. [CrossRef] [PubMed]

47. Nakamoto, Y.; Kurihara, K.; Nishizawa, M.; Yamashita, K.; Nakatani, K.; Kondo, T.; Takaori-Kondo, A.; Togashi, K. Clinical value of ^{11}C-methionine PET/CT in patients with plasma cell malignancy: Comparison with ^{18}F-FDG PET/CT. *Eur. J. Nucl. Med. Mol. Imaging* **2013**, *40*, 708–715. [CrossRef] [PubMed]
48. Okasaki, M.; Kubota, K.; Minamimoto, R.; Miyata, Y.; Morooka, M.; Ito, K.; Ishiwata, K.; Toyohara, J.; Inoue, T.; Hirai, R.; et al. Comparison of (11)C-4′-thiothymidine, (11)C-methionine, and (18)F-FDG PET/CT for the detection of active lesions of multiple myeloma. *Ann. Nucl. Med.* **2015**, *29*, 224–232. [CrossRef] [PubMed]
49. Lapa, C.; Knop, S.; Schreder, M.; Rudelius, M.; Knott, M.; Jörg, G.; Samnick, S.; Herrmann, K.; Buck, A.K.; Einsele, H.; et al. 11C-Methionine-PET in Multiple Myeloma: Correlation with Clinical Parameters and Bone Marrow Involvement. *Theranostics* **2016**, *6*, 254–261. [CrossRef]
50. Lapa, C.; Schreder, M.; Lückerath, K.; Samnick, S.; Rudelius, M.; Buck, A.K.; Kortüm, K.M.; Einsele, H.; Rosenwald, A.; Knop, S. [11 C]Methionine emerges as a new biomarker for tracking active myeloma lesions. *Br. J. Haematol.* **2018**, *181*, 701–703. [CrossRef]
51. Lapa, C.; Garcia-Velloso, M.J.; Lückerath, K.; Samnick, S.; Schreder, M.; Otero, P.R.; Schmid, J.S.; Herrmann, K.; Knop, S.; Buck, A.K.; et al. 11C-Methionine-PET in Multiple Myeloma: A Combined Study from Two Different Institutions. *Theranostics* **2017**, *7*, 2956–2964. [CrossRef]
52. Lapa, C.; Kircher, M.; Da Via, M.; Schreder, M.; Rasche, L.; Kortüm, K.M.; Einsele, H.; Buck, A.K.; Hänscheid, H.; Samnick, S. Comparison of 11C-Choline and 11C-Methionine PET/CT in Multiple Myeloma. *Clin. Nucl. Med.* **2019**, *44*, 620–624. [CrossRef]
53. Nanni, C. PET/CT with Standard Non-FDG Tracers in Multiple Myeloma. In *Molecular Imaging in Multiple Myeloma*; Nanni, C., Fanti, S., Zanoni, L., Eds.; Springer: Cham, Switzerland, 2019; pp. 93–98.
54. Peck, M.; Pollack, H.A.; Friesen, A.; Muzi, M.; Shoner, S.C.; Shankland, E.G.; Fink, J.R.; Armstrong, J.O.; Link, J.M.; Krohn, K.A. Applications of PET imaging with the proliferation marker [18F]-FLT. *Q. J. Nucl. Med. Mol. Imaging* **2015**, *59*, 95–104. [PubMed]
55. Lodge, M.A.; Holdhoff, M.; Leal, J.P.; Bag, A.K.; Nabors, L.B.; Mintz, A.; Lesser, G.J.; Mankoff, D.A.; Desai, A.S.; Mountz, J.M.; et al. Repeatability of 18F-FLT PET in a multicenter study of patients with high-grade glioma. *J. Nucl. Med.* **2017**, *58*, 393–398. [CrossRef] [PubMed]
56. Agool, A.; Slart, R.H.; Kluin, P.M.; de Wolf, J.T.; Dierckx, R.A.; Vellenga, E. F-18 FLT PET: A noninvasive diagnostic tool for visualization of the bone marrow compartment in patients with aplastic anemia: A pilot study. *Clin. Nucl. Med.* **2011**, *36*, 286–289. [CrossRef] [PubMed]
57. Sachpekidis, C.; Goldschmidt, H.; Kopka, K.; Kopp-Schneider, A.; Dimitrakopoulou-Strauss, A. Assessment of glucose metabolism and cellular proliferation in multiple myeloma: A first report on combined 18F-FDG and 18F-FLT PET/CT imaging. *EJNMMI Res.* **2018**, *8*, 28. [CrossRef] [PubMed]
58. Zou, Y.R.; Kottmann, A.H.; Kuroda, M.; Taniuchi, I.; Littman, D.R. Function of the chemokine receptor CXCR4 in haematopoiesis and in cerebellar development. *Nature* **1998**, *393*, 595–599. [CrossRef] [PubMed]
59. Alsayed, Y.; Ngo, H.; Runnels, J.; Leleu, X.; Singha, U.K.; Pitsillides, C.M.; Spencer, J.A.; Kimlinger, T.; Ghobrial, J.M.; Jia, X.; et al. Mechanisms of regulation of CXCR4/SDF-1 (CXCL12)–dependent migration and homing in multiple myeloma. *Blood* **2007**, *109*, 2708–2717. [CrossRef] [PubMed]
60. Paiva, B.; Corchete, L.A.; Vidriales, M.B.; Puig, N.; Maiso, P.; Rodriguez, I.; Alignani, D.; Burgos, L.; Sanchez, M.L.; Barcena, P.; et al. Phenotypic and genomic analysis of multiple myeloma minimal residual disease tumor cells: A new model to understand chemoresistance. *Blood* **2016**, *127*, 1896–1906. [CrossRef]
61. Peled, A.; Klein, S.; Beider, K.; Burger, J.A.; Abraham, M. Role of CXCL12 and CXCR4 in the pathogenesis of hematological malignancies. *Cytokine* **2018**, *109*, 11–16. [CrossRef]
62. Chatterjee, S.; Behnam Azad, B.; Nimmagadda, S. The intricate role of CXCR4 in cancer. *Adv. Cancer Res.* **2014**, *124*, 31–82. [CrossRef]
63. Guo, F.; Wang, Y.; Liu, J.; Mok, S.C.; Xue, F.; Zhang, W. CXCL12/CXCR4: A symbiotic bridge linking cancer cells and their stromal neighbors in oncogenic communication networks. *Oncogene* **2016**, *35*, 816–826. [CrossRef]
64. Liu, S.H.; Gu, Y.; Pascual, B.; Yan, Z.; Hallin, M.; Zhang, C.; Fan, C.; Wang, W.; Lam, J.; Spilker, M.E.; et al. A novel CXCR4 antagonist IgG1 antibody (PF-06747143) for the treatment of hematologic malignancies. *Blood Adv.* **2017**, *1*, 1088–1100. [CrossRef] [PubMed]
65. Coniglio, S.J. Role of Tumor-Derived Chemokines in Osteolytic Bone Metastasis. *Front Endocrinol.* **2018**, *9*, 313. [CrossRef] [PubMed]

66. Ullah, T.R. The role of CXCR4 in multiple myeloma: Cells' journey from bone marrow to beyond. *J. Bone Oncol.* **2019**, *17*, 100253. [CrossRef] [PubMed]
67. Herrmann, K.; Schottelius, M.; Lapa, C.; Osl, T.; Poschenrieder, A.; Hänscheid, H.; Lückerath, K.; Schreder, M.; Bluemel, C.; Knott, M.; et al. First-in-Human Experience of CXCR4-Directed Endoradiotherapy with 177Lu- and 90Y-Labeled Pentixather in Advanced-Stage Multiple Myeloma with Extensive Intra- and Extramedullary Disease. *J. Nucl. Med.* **2016**, *57*, 248–251. [CrossRef]
68. Philipp-Abbrederis, K.; Herrmann, K.; Knop, S.; Schottelius, M.; Eiber, M.; Lückerath, K.; Pietschmann, E.; Habringer, S.; Gerngroß, C.; Franke, K.; et al. In Vivo molecular imaging of chemokine receptor CXCR4 expression in patients with advanced multiple myeloma. *EMBO Mol. Med.* **2015**, *7*, 477–487. [CrossRef]
69. Lapa, C.; Schreder, M.; Schirbel, A.; Samnick, S.; Kortüm, K.M.; Herrmann, K.; Kropf, S.; Einsele, H.; Buck, A.K.; Wester, H.J.; et al. [68Ga]Pentixafor-PET/CT for imaging of chemokine receptor CXCR4 expression in multiple myeloma-Comparison to [18F]FDG and laboratory values. *Theranostics* **2017**, *7*, 205–212. [CrossRef]
70. Pan, Q.; Cao, X.; Luo, Y.; Li, J.; Feng, J.; Li, F. Chemokine receptor-4 targeted PET/CT with 68Ga-Pentixafor in assessment of newly diagnosed multiple myeloma: Comparison to 18F-FDG PET/CT. *Eur. J. Nucl. Med. Mol. Imaging* **2019**. [CrossRef]
71. Czernin, J.; Satyamurthy, N.; Schiepers, C. Molecular mechanisms of bone 18F-NaF deposition. *J. Nucl. Med.* **2010**, *51*, 1826–1829. [CrossRef]
72. Segall, G.; Delbeke, D.; Stabin, M.G.; Even-Sapir, E.; Fair, J.; Sajdak, R.; Smith, G.T. SNM. SNM practice guideline for sodium 18F-fluoride PET/CT bone scans 1.0. *J. Nucl. Med.* **2010**, *51*, 1813–1820. [CrossRef]
73. Beheshti, M.; Mottaghy, F.M.; Payche, F.; Behrendt, F.F.; Van den Wyngaert, T.; Fogelman, I.; Strobel, K.; Celli, M.; Fanti, S.; Giammarile, F.; et al. (18)F-NaF PET/CT: EANM procedure guidelines for bone imaging. *Eur. J. Nucl. Med. Mol. Imaging* **2015**, *42*, 1767–1777. [CrossRef]
74. Hillner, B.E.; Siegel, B.A.; Hanna, L.; Duan, F.; Quinn, B.; Shields, A.F. 18F-fluoride PET used for treatment monitoring of systemic cancer therapy: Results from the National Oncologic PET Registry. *J. Nucl. Med.* **2015**, *56*, 222–228. [CrossRef] [PubMed]
75. Hawkins, R.A.; Choi, Y.; Huang, S.C.; Hoh, C.K.; Dahlbom, M.; Schiepers, C.; Satyamurthy, N.; Barrio, J.R.; Phelps, M.E. Evaluation of the skeletal kinetics of fluorine-18-fluoride ion with PET. *J. Nucl. Med.* **1992**, *33*, 633–642. [PubMed]
76. Grant, F.D.; Fahey, F.H.; Packard, A.B.; Davis, R.T.; Alavi, A.; Treves, S.T. Skeletal PET with 18 F-fluoride: Applying new technology to an old tracer. *J. Nucl. Med.* **2008**, *49*, 68–78. [CrossRef] [PubMed]
77. Kurdziel, K.A.; Shih, J.H.; Apolo, A.B.; Lindenberg, L.; Mena, E.; McKinney, Y.Y.; Adler, S.S.; Turkbey, B.; Dahut, W.; Gulley, J.L.; et al. The kinetics and reproducibility of 18F-sodium fluoride for oncology using current PET camera technology. *J. Nucl. Med.* **2012**, *53*, 1175–1184. [CrossRef] [PubMed]
78. Nishiyama, Y.; Tateishi, U.; Shizukuishi, K.; Shishikura, A.; Yamazaki, E.; Shibata, H.; Yoneyama, T.; Ishigatsubo, Y.; Inoue, T. Role of 18F-fluoride PET/CT in the assessment of multiple myeloma: Initial experience. *Ann. Nucl. Med.* **2013**, *27*, 78–83. [CrossRef] [PubMed]
79. Xu, F.; Liu, F.; Pastakia, B. Different lesions revealed by 18F-FDG PET/CT and 18F-NaF PET/CT in patients with multiple myeloma. *Clin. Nucl. Med.* **2014**, *39*, e407–e409. [CrossRef] [PubMed]
80. Oral, A.; Yazici, B.; Ömür, Ö.; Comert, M.; Saydam, G. 18F-FDG and 18F-NaF PET/CT Findings of a Multiple Myeloma Patient With Thyroid Cartilage Involvement. *Clin. Nucl. Med.* **2015**, *40*, 873–876. [CrossRef]
81. Sachpekidis, C.; Goldschmidt, H.; Hose, D.; Pan, L.; Cheng, C.; Kopka, K.; Haberkorn, U.; Dimitrakopoulou-Strauss, A. PET/CT studies of multiple myeloma using (18) F-FDG and (18) F-NaF: Comparison of distribution patterns and tracers' pharmacokinetics. *Eur. J. Nucl. Med. Mol. Imaging* **2014**, *41*, 1343–1353. [CrossRef]
82. Ak, İ.; Onner, H.; Akay, O.M. Is there any complimentary role of F-18 NaF PET/CT in detecting of osseous involvement of multiple myeloma? A comparative study for F-18 FDG PET/CT and F-18 FDG NaF PET/CT. *Ann. Hematol.* **2015**, *94*, 1567–1575. [CrossRef]
83. Sachpekidis, C.; Hillengass, J.; Goldschmidt, H.; Anwar, H.; Haberkorn, U.; Dimitrakopoulou-Strauss, A. Quantitative analysis of 18F-NaF dynamic PET/CT cannot differentiate malignant from benign lesions in multiple myeloma. *Am. J. Nucl. Med. Mol. Imaging* **2017**, *7*, 148–156.

84. Sachpekidis, C.; Hillengass, J.; Goldschmidt, H.; Wagner, B.; Haberkorn, U.; Kopka, K.; Dimitrakopoulou-Strauss, A. Treatment response evaluation with 18F-FDG PET/CT and 18F-NaF PET/CT in multiple myeloma patients undergoing high-dose chemotherapy and autologous stem cell transplantation. *Eur. J. Nucl. Med. Mol. Imaging* **2017**, *44*, 50–62. [CrossRef] [PubMed]
85. Even-Sapir, E.; Mishani, E.; Flusser, G.; Metser, U. 18F-Fluoride positron emission tomography and positron emission tomography/computed tomography. *Semin. Nucl. Med.* **2007**, *37*, 462–469. [CrossRef] [PubMed]
86. Dimitrakopoulou-Strauss, A. PET-CT in der nuklearmedizinischen Diagnostik des multiplen Myeloms [PET-CT for nuclear medicine diagnostics of multiple myeloma]. *Radiologe* **2014**, *54*, 564–571. [CrossRef] [PubMed]
87. Rajkumar, S.V.; Mesa, R.A.; Fonseca, R.; Schroeder, G.; Plevak, M.F.; Dispenzieri, A.; Lacy, M.Q.; Lust, J.A.; Witzig, T.E.; Gertz, M.A.; et al. Bone marrow angiogenesis in 400 patients with monoclonal gammopathy of undetermined significance, multiple myeloma, and primary amyloidosis. *Clin. Cancer Res.* **2002**, *8*, 2210–2216. [PubMed]
88. De Waal, E.G.; Slart, R.H.; Leene, M.J.; Kluin, P.M.; Vellenga, E. 18F-FDG PET increases visibility of bone lesions in relapsed multiple myeloma: Is this hypoxia-driven? *Clin. Nucl. Med.* **2015**, *40*, 291–296. [CrossRef] [PubMed]
89. Dimopoulos, M.A.; Oriol, A.; Nahi, H.; San-Miguel, J.; Bahlis, N.J.; Usmani, S.Z.; Rabin, N.; Orlowski, R.Z.; Komarnicki, M.; Suzuki, K.; et al. Daratumumab, Lenalidomide, and Dexamethasone for Multiple Myeloma. *N. Engl. J. Med.* **2016**, *375*, 1319–1331. [CrossRef] [PubMed]
90. Facon, T.; Kumar, S.; Plesner, T.; Orlowski, R.Z.; Moreau, P.; Bahlis, N.; Basu, S.; Nahi, H.; Hulin, C.; Quach, H.; et al. Daratumumab plus Lenalidomide and Dexamethasone for Untreated Myeloma. *N. Engl. J. Med.* **2019**, *380*, 2104–2115. [CrossRef]
91. Moreau, P.; Attal, M.; Hulin, C.; Arnulf, B.; Belhadj, K.; Benboubker, L.; Béné, M.C.; Broijl, A.; Caillon, H.; Caillot, D.; et al. Bortezomib, thalidomide, and dexamethasone with or without daratumumab before and after autologous stem-cell transplantation for newly diagnosed multiple myeloma (CASSIOPEIA): A randomised, open-label, phase 3 study. *Lancet* **2019**, *394*, 29–38. [CrossRef]
92. Ulaner, G.; Sobol, N.; O'Donoghue, J.; Burnazi, E.; Staton, K.; Weber, W.; Lyashchenko, S.; Lewis, J.; Landgren, C.O. Preclinical development and First-in-human imaging of 89Zr-Daratumumab for CD38 targeted imaging of myeloma. *J. Nucl. Med.* **2019**, *60*, 203.

8

Radiosynthesis and Biological Investigation of a Novel Fluorine-18 Labeled Benzoimidazotriazine-Based Radioligand for the Imaging of Phosphodiesterase 2A with Positron Emission Tomography

Rien Ritawidya [1,2,*], Barbara Wenzel [1], Rodrigo Teodoro [1], Magali Toussaint [1], Mathias Kranz [3,4], Winnie Deuther-Conrad [1], Sladjana Dukic-Stefanovic [1], Friedrich-Alexander Ludwig [1], Matthias Scheunemann [1] and Peter Brust [1]

1 Helmholtz-Zentrum Dresden-Rossendorf, Institute of Radiopharmaceutical Cancer Research, Research Site Leipzig, Department of Neuroradiopharmaceuticals, 04318 Leipzig, Germany; b.wenzel@hzdr.de (B.W.); r.teodoro@hzdr.de (R.T.); m.toussaint@hzdr.de (M.T.); w.deuther-conrad@hzdr.de (W.D.-C.); s.dukic-stefanovic@hzdr.de (S.D.-S.); f.ludwig@hzdr.de (F.-A.L.); m.scheunemann@hzdr.de (M.S.); p.brust@hzdr.de (P.B.)

2 Center for Radioisotope and Radiopharmaceutical Technology, National Nuclear Energy Agency (BATAN), Puspiptek Area, Serpong, South Tangerang 15314, Indonesia

3 Tromsø PET Center, University Hospital of North Norway, 9009 Tromsø, Norway; Mathias.Kranz@unn.no

4 Nuclear Medicine and Radiation Biology Research Group, The Arctic University of Norway, 9009 Tromsø, Norway

* Correspondence: r.ritawidya@hzdr.de or rienrita@batan.go.id

Abstract: A specific radioligand for the imaging of cyclic nucleotide phosphodiesterase 2A (PDE2A) via positron emission tomography (PET) would be helpful for research on the physiology and disease-related changes in the expression of this enzyme in the brain. In this report, the radiosynthesis of a novel PDE2A radioligand and the subsequent biological evaluation were described. Our prospective compound 1-(2-chloro-5-methoxy phenyl)-8-(2-fluoropyridin-4-yl)-3-methylbenzo[e]imidazo[5,1-c][1,2,4]triazine, benzoimidazotriazine (**BIT1**) (IC_{50} PDE2A = 3.33 nM; 16-fold selectivity over PDE10A) was fluorine-18 labeled via aromatic nucleophilic substitution of the corresponding nitro precursor using the $K[^{18}F]F-K_{2.2.2}$-carbonate complex system. The new radioligand $[^{18}F]$**BIT1** was obtained with a high radiochemical yield (54 ± 2%, n = 3), a high radiochemical purity (≥99%), and high molar activities (155–175 GBq/μmol, n = 3). In vitro autoradiography on pig brain cryosections exhibited a heterogeneous spatial distribution of $[^{18}F]$**BIT1** corresponding to the known pattern of expression of PDE2A. The investigation of in vivo metabolism of $[^{18}F]$**BIT1** in a mouse revealed sufficient metabolic stability. PET studies in mouse exhibited a moderate brain uptake of $[^{18}F]$**BIT1** with a maximum standardized uptake value of ~0.7 at 5 min p.i. However, in vivo blocking studies revealed a non-target specific binding of $[^{18}F]$**BIT1**. Therefore, further structural modifications are needed to improve target selectivity.

Keywords: cyclic nucleotide phosphodiesterase; PDE2A radioligand; nitro-precursor; fluorine-18; in vitro autoradiography; PET imaging

1. Introduction

The cyclic nucleotide phosphodiesterases (PDEs) are a superfamily of enzymes catalyzing the hydrolysis of the intracellular secondary messengers, cyclic adenosine monophosphate (cAMP) and cyclic guanosine monophosphate (cGMP) [1–3]. These secondary messengers are involved in a great variety of cellular functions associated with normal and pathophysiological processes in the brain and periphery [3–6].

The 11 family members of PDEs are encoded by 21 genes and classified by their substrate specificity [3,7]. PDE 4, 7, and 8 are only cAMP-specific, PDE 5, 6, and 9 are cGMP-specific, and the remaining PDE 1, 2, 3, 10, and 11 hydrolyze both substrates [3,6,7].

The dual-substrate enzyme PDE2A is abundantly expressed in brain, in particular, in caudate, nucleus accumbens, cortex, hippocampus [3,8,9], amygdala [10,11], substantia nigra, as well as olfactory tubercle [11,12], while the expression in the midbrain, hindbrain, and cerebellum is comparatively low [8,11,12]. This specific distribution indicates a role of PDE2A in the modulation of complex neuronal processes, such as learning, concentration, memory, emotion, depression, anxiety, and CNS related disorder [10,13,14]. The pharmacological inhibition of PDE2A has been evaluated in preclinical studies, thus suggesting PDE2A inhibitors as a potential treatment for neurodegenerative diseases, such as Alzheimer's disease, schizophrenia, and dementia [15,16]. PDE2A inhibition has the potential to prolong the duration of cAMP- and cGMP-dependent signaling pathways, eventually improving neural plasticity and memory function [3,13,17].

Positron emission tomography (PET) is a molecular imaging modality that enables the visualization, characterization, and measurement of molecular targets and biochemical processes in living systems [18]. Accordingly, a PDE2A specific radiotracer would allow quantification of PDE2A expression, as well as disease-related changes thereof.

The so far most developed PDE2A radioligands are shown in Figure 1. The first highly potent PDE2A compound $[^{18}F]$**B-23** (IC_{50} hPDE2A = 1 nM; IC_{50} rPDE10A = 11 nM) was developed by Janssen Pharmaceutica NV (Beerse, Belgium) [10,19]. Biodistribution and microPET imaging studies in rats demonstrated high uptake of activity in the striatum; however, brain-penetrating radio-metabolites limited further evaluation. Pfizer Inc. (New York, NY, USA) also reported on a highly affine PDE2A radioligand, $[^{18}F]$**PF-05270430** (IC_{50} hPDE2A = 0.5 nM; IC_{50} hPDE10A >3000 nM) [10,20], which has been evaluated in monkeys [20] and translated to clinical trials [21,22]. $[^{18}F]$**PF-05270430** showed high target-specific accumulation in the putamen, caudate, and nucleus-accumbens, as well as good metabolic stability and a favorable kinetic profile, pointing out $[^{18}F]$**PF-05270430** as a promising PDE2A PET ligand [21]. However, using the cerebellum as a reference region, the estimated binding potential of $[^{18}F]$**PF-05270430** was low, and the authors concluded that further studies are required to validate the suitability of the cerebellum as a reference region [21].

In parallel to Pfizer, our group developed further PDE2A radioligands on the basis of pyridoimidazotriazine. The recently published compounds $[^{18}F]$**TA3** (IC_{50} PDE2A = 11.4 nM; IC_{50} PDE10A = 318 nM) and $[^{18}F]$**TA4** (IC_{50} PDE2A = 7.3 nM; IC_{50} PDE10A = 913 nM) (Figure 1) were characterized by high potency and selectivity towards PDE2A [24]. Notably, both radiotracers were found to be suitable radioligands for in vitro imaging of PDE2A; however, in vivo metabolism studies revealed a high fraction of polar radio-metabolites in the brain limiting their use for in vivo PDE2A imaging. The latest radioligand out of this series, $[^{18}F]$**TA5** ((IC_{50} PDE2A = 3.0 nM; IC_{50} PDE10A >1000 nM, Figure 1), exhibited the highest potency towards PDE2A and selectivity over PDE10A. However, autoradiographic studies of $[^{18}F]$**TA5** showed a homogenous and non-displaceable binding in rat and pig brain cryosections, indicating an insufficient specificity of this radioligand [25]. In addition, $[^{18}F]$**TA5** is degraded extremely fast in the mouse. Therefore, we decided to perform further structural modifications to develop fluorine-18 labeled PET tracers with improved metabolic stability for the molecular imaging of PDE2A.

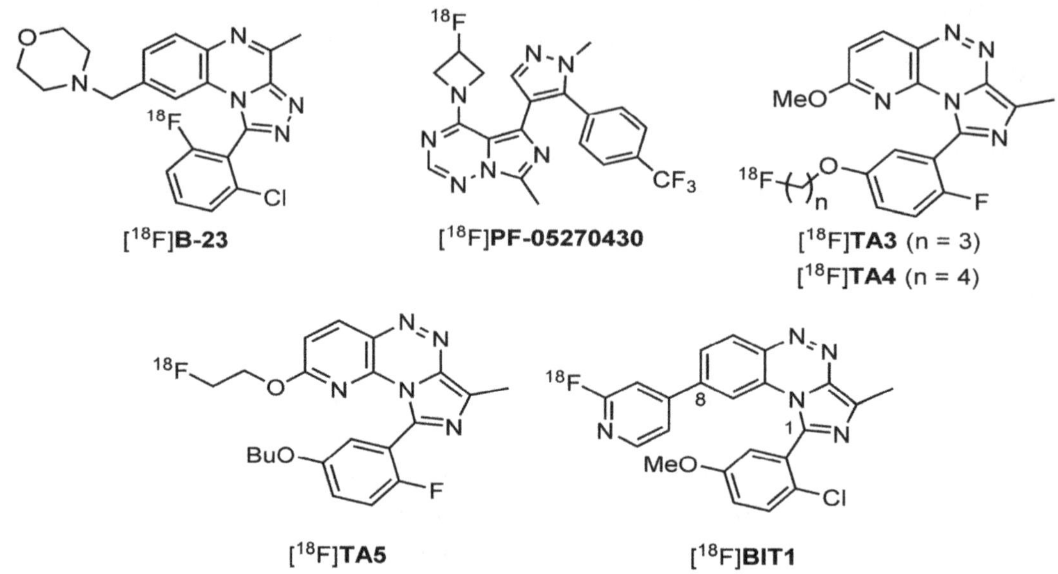

Figure 1. Selected phosphodiesterase 2A (PDE2A) PET radioligands [10,19,20,23–25].

In our continuous effort to develop fluorine-18 labeled PET tracers dedicated to molecular imaging of PDE2A, we selected the benzoimidazotriazine (BIT) scaffold (Figure 1) as lead structure by replacing the pyrido ring of the **TA** compounds with a benzo ring [26,27]. As a first result, we very recently reported on the synthesis and inhibitory potency of nine new fluorinated derivatives based on this BIT scaffold [28]. In order to increase the metabolic stability of the corresponding PDE2A radioligands, the fluorine was introduced by substituting a fluoropyridine ring at the benzene moiety. Out of this series, derivative **BIT1** (Figure 1) was selected as the most suitable candidate for ^{18}F-labeling and biological investigation (IC_{50} PDE2A = 3.33 nM; 16-fold selectivity over PDE10A) [28].

Herein, we reported on the development and the evaluation of [^{18}F]**BIT1**, including the synthesis of the corresponding nitro precursor, the manual radiosynthesis, and the transfer to an automated synthesis module, and the subsequent in vitro and in vivo investigations.

2. Results and Discussion

2.1. Precursor Synthesis and Radiochemistry

2.1.1. Synthesis of the Labeling Precursor 5

The synthesis of the reference compound **BIT1** has been reported previously [28]. For an efficient radiosynthesis of [^{18}F]**BIT1**, we selected the nitro precursor **5** because of its higher reactivity to nucleophilic aromatic substitutions in comparison to a bromo-substituted precursor [29,30]. As depicted in Scheme 1, **5** was prepared in four steps starting from the BIT key intermediate **1 [28]**. Firstly, Miyaura borylation of **1** with bis(pinacolato)diboron, using potassium acetate and [Pd(dppf)Cl_2] as base and catalyst, afforded the pinacol boronic ester **2** in a satisfactory yield of 85% [31]. By palladium-catalyzed Suzuki coupling with 4-bromo-2-nitropyridine, compound **3** was obtained in 63% yield. This 4-bromo-2-nitropyridine was synthesized according to a slightly modified procedure, already described in the literature [32]. Thereafter, the bromination at 1-position of the imidazole ring using *N*-bromo-succinimide (NBS) afforded compound **4** in an excellent yield of 97%. Finally, the subsequent Suzuki coupling with 2-chloro-5-methoxy-phenyl boronic acid gave the nitro precursor **5** in 68% yield (NMR spectrums of precursor **5** see in the Supplementary Materials).

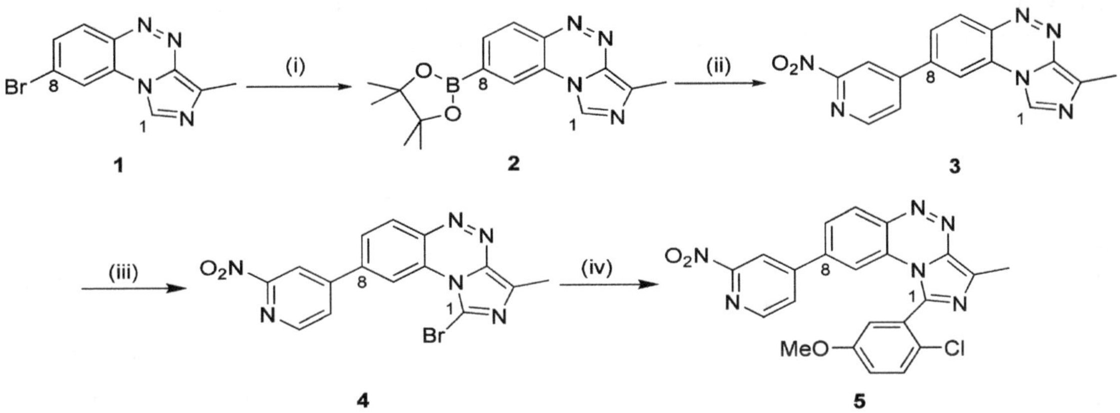

Scheme 1. Synthesis of precursor **5**. Reagents and conditions: (i) Bis(pinacolato)diboron [Pd(dppf)Cl_2], KOAc, 2-methyltetrahydrofuran (2-MeTHF), 100 °C (6 h), 85 °C (12 h), 85%; (ii) 4-bromo-2-nitropyridine, K_2CO_3, Pd(PPh_3)$_4$, 1,2-dimethoxyethane, 63%; (iii) N-bromo-succinimide (NBS), acetonitrile (MeCN), room temperature (RT), 4–6 h, 97%; (iv) 2-chloro-5-methoxy-phenyl-1-yl-boronic acid, K_2CO_3, [Pd(PPh_3)$_4$], 1,4-dioxane/H_2O (4:1), reflux, 1–2 d, 68%.

2.1.2. Radiosynthesis and Characterization of [^{18}F]**BIT1**

Manual Radiosynthesis

The new PDE2A radioligand [^{18}F]**BIT1** was prepared by heteroaromatic nucleophilic substitution of **5** using a classical anhydrous K[^{18}F]F-$K_{2.2.2}$ carbonate complex. The radiolabeling process of [^{18}F]**BIT1** was carried out under thermal heating applying a constant amount of 1.0 mg of precursor **5** by using different (i) polar aprotic solvents dimethylsulfoxide (DMSO), *N,N*-dimethylformamide (DMF), and acetonitrile (MeCN), (ii) temperatures, and (iii) reaction times.

As shown in Figure 2, after 5 min (min) reaction time, a radiochemical yield (RCY) of ~57% was obtained when DMF was used at 150 °C. According to radio-TLC, besides [^{18}F]fluoride, three radioactive by-products were observed, which accounted for 10% of total radioactivity. When the temperature was reduced to 120 °C, an increase of the RCY up to 93% was observed at this early time point. However, the RCY decreased with increasing the reaction time, indicating a decomposition of [^{18}F]**BIT1** under these conditions. The highest RCY in DMF (~94%) was achieved when the reaction temperature was further reduced to 100 °C. At this temperature, the product remained stable over 20 min reaction time. By contrast, almost no radiofluorination could be observed when MeCN was used (RCY ≤1%). With DMSO as a solvent, high RCYs (>85%) were obtained at 150 °C and 120 °C, which remained constant up to 20 min reaction time in contrast to the findings with DMF. A further decrease to 100 °C resulted in an increase of the RCY (>95%) after 10 min of reaction time. The precursor **5** was stable throughout the time of analysis, as proven by HPLC (data not shown). Based on these results, DMSO was selected for the production of [^{18}F]**BIT1**.

Due to the similarity of the chromatographic behavior of the nitro precursor and the corresponding ^{18}F-radiotracer, the use of a low amount of precursor is beneficial for subsequent isolation of the radiotracer via semi-preparative HPLC [33,34]. Accordingly, the further reduction of the amount of the nitro precursor **5** up to 0.5 mg was investigated, achieving an excellent RCY of ≥95% (DMSO, 100 °C, 5 min reaction time). The selection of a suitable column for semi-preparative HPLC was also somewhat crucial in order to have a separation of the radiotracer and its nitro precursor in a reasonable time [33]. According to our previous experiences [33], a slightly polar C18 phase turned out to be most appropriate for the isolation of [^{18}F]**BIT1** using a mixture of MeCN/water and ammonium acetate as a buffer.

[^{18}F]**BIT1** was successfully isolated under the aforementioned conditions and further purified by solid-phase extraction (SPE). After formulation in 0.9% saline containing 10% ethanol, [^{18}F]**BIT1** was obtained with an RCY of 38% (decay corrected to the end of the bombardment, EOB), and molar activities in the range of 38 GBq/μmol (at the end of synthesis, EOS).

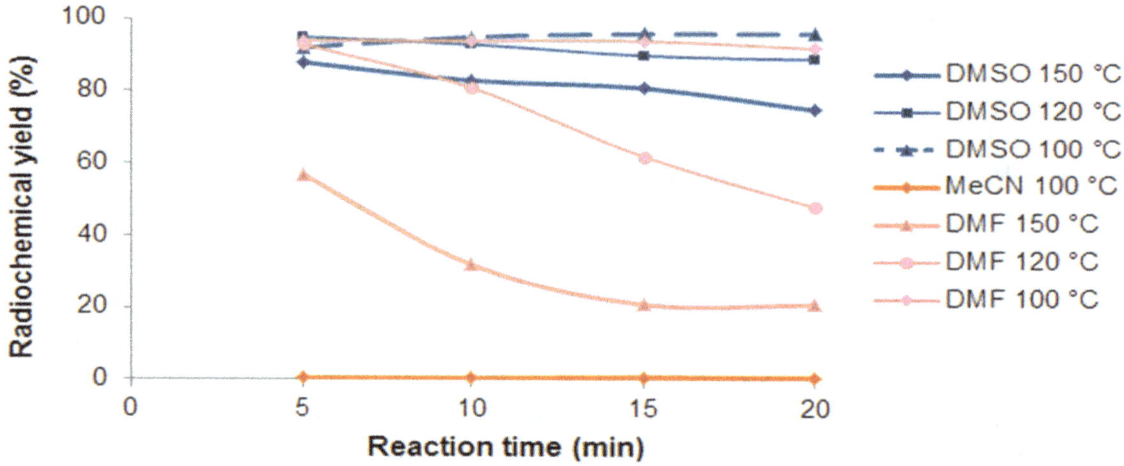

Figure 2. The radiochemical yield of [^{18}F]**BIT1** depending on reaction time, temperature, and solvent. (Conditions: K[^{18}F]F-$K_{2.2.2}$, thermal heating, 1.0 mg of **5**). BIT, benzoimidazotriazine.

Automated Radiosynthesis of [^{18}F]**BIT1**

By using the most appropriate conditions of the manual procedure, the automated radiosynthesis of [^{18}F]**BIT1** (Scheme 2) was established using a TRACERlab FX2 N synthesis module (GE Healthcare, Waukesha, WI, USA). The detailed configuration is shown in theexperimental part. Briefly, the [^{18}F]F^- was firstly trapped on an anion exchange cartridge and then eluted into the reactor using an aqueous potassium carbonate solution. The reaction took place with the [^{18}F]F^-/$K_{2.2.2.}$/K_2CO_3 system and the nitro precursor **5** (0.5 mg) in DMSO at 100 °C for 5 min. After the isolation of [^{18}F]**BIT1** via semi-preparative RP-HPLC (Figure 3A), the product was purified via SPE on an RP cartridge and formulated in sterile isotonic saline containing 10% of EtOH. The total synthesis time of [^{18}F]**BIT1** was approximately 75 min. Analytical radio- and UV-HPLC of the final product, spiked with the non-labeled reference compound **BIT1**, confirmed the identity of [^{18}F]**BIT1** (Figure 3B). Finally, the radiotracer was obtained with a radiochemical purity of ≥99%, an RCY of 54 ± 2% (EOB, n = 3), and molar activities in the range of 155–175 GBq/μmol (EOS, n = 3).

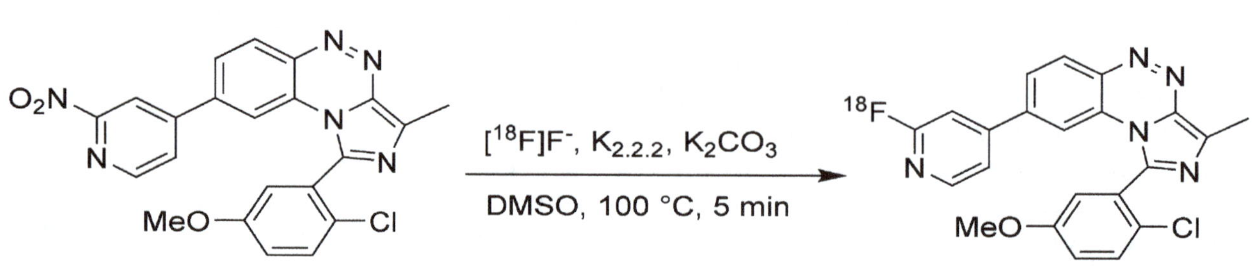

Scheme 2. ^{18}F-labeling of [^{18}F]**BIT1**.

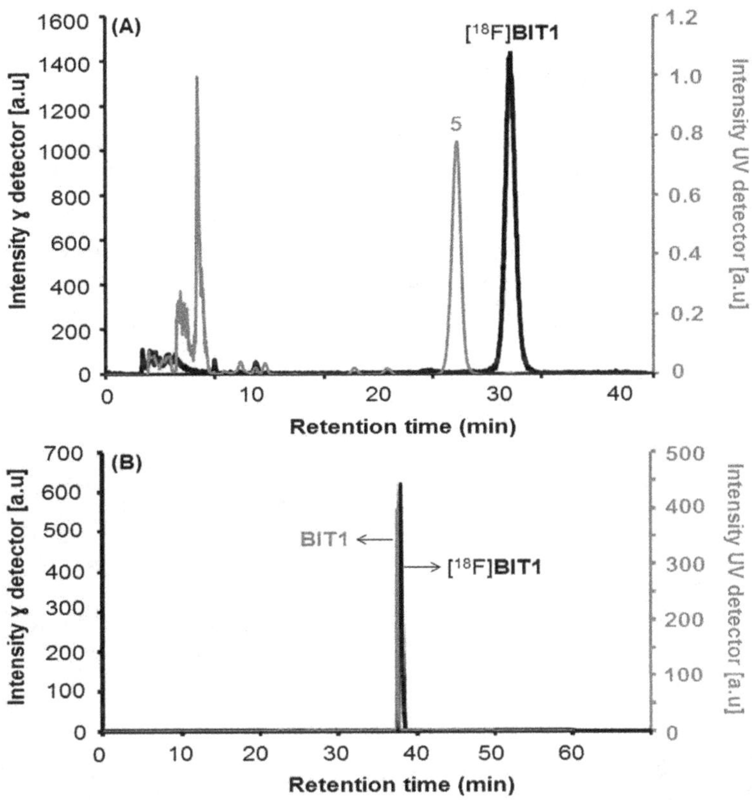

Figure 3. (**A**) Semi-preparative radio- and UV-HPLC chromatograms of [^{18}F]**BIT1** (conditions: Reprosil-Pur C18-AQ, 250 × 10 mm, 46% MeCN/20 mM NH_4OAc_{aq}., 5.5 mL/min); (**B**) Analytical radio- and UV-HPLC chromatograms of the final product of [^{18}F]**BIT1** spiked with the non-radioactive reference **BIT1** (conditions: Reprosil-Pur C18-AQ, 250 × 4.6 mm, gradient system with eluent mixture of MeCN/20 mM NH_4OAc_{aq}., 1.0 mL/min).

In vitro Stability and Lipophilicity of [^{18}F]**BIT1**

The radioligand [^{18}F]**BIT1** was stable (radiochemical purity ≥99%) in phosphate-buffered saline (PBS), pig plasma, *n*-octanol, as well as in the saline formulation containing 10% ethanol at 40 °C for up to 1 h. The lipophilicity was determined by the shake-flask method in the *n*-octanol/PBS system. With a $logD_{7.4}$ value of 1.81 ± 0.05, [^{18}F]**BIT1** falls within the range of radiotracers with optimal brain passive diffusion [35–37]. However, the calculated coefficient distribution value (ACD/Labs, Version 12.0, Advanced Chemistry Development, Inc.) displayed value of 4.03. The significant deviations between the calculation and experimental methods were observed in particular when the pattern of connectivity and non-bonded intramolecular interactions are not included in the applied database [38–41]. Moreover, the big discrepancy between the experimental and the calculated $logD_{7.4}$ value was already observed for our PDE2 tracer [^{18}F]**TA5** and has been previously discussed [25]. It is assumed that the experimentally determined higher hydrophilicity of [^{18}F]**TA5** might be due to the solvation effect related to hydrogen bonding and ionization of the radioligand in the aqueous buffered system [25,35]. Whereas with the software-based determination, this effect may be underestimated [25]. Therefore, the calculated logD value is often higher than the experimentally determined value [25,35]. Since **TA5** and **BIT1** are rather structurally similar, we assume the apparent strong discrepancy of logD for [^{18}F]**BIT1** might also be caused by the same reasons as those for [^{18}F]**TA5**.

2.2. *In Vitro and In Vivo Characterization of [^{18}F]***BIT1**

2.2.1. In Vitro Autoradiography of [^{18}F]**BIT1**

To investigate the distribution of binding sites of [^{18}F]**BIT1** in the brain, in vitro autoradiographic studies using cryosections of pig brain were performed. As depicted in Figure 4B, the distribution pattern of [^{18}F]**BIT1** corresponds to the known spatial distribution of PDE2A with a high density of binding sites in the caudate nucleus (Cd), nucleus accumbens (Acb), cortex (Cx), and hippocampus (Hip) (Nissl staining of the corresponding slice is shown in Figure 4A). However, [^{18}F]**BIT1** also binds to the non-PDE2A specific regions cerebellum (Cb) and thalamus (Th), indicating binding of [^{18}F]**BIT1** to other targets.

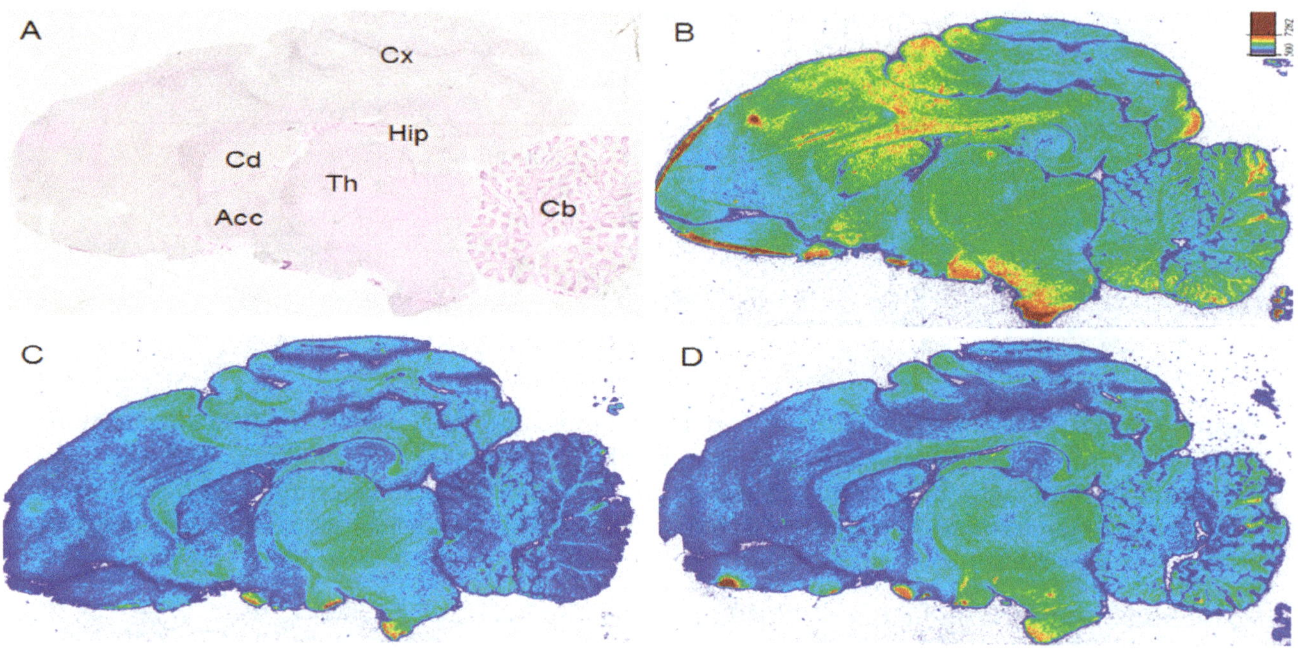

Figure 4. In vitro autoradiography of [^{18}F]**BIT1** in pig brain slices, (**A**) Nissl staining, (**B**) Total binding of 1.72 nM of [^{18}F]**BIT1**, (**C**) Blocking studies (10 µM of **TA1**), (**D**) Self-blocking (10 µM of **BIT1**). Abbreviations: (Acb: nucleus accumbens; Cb: cerebellum; Cd: nucleus caudatus; Cx: cortex; Hip: hippocampus; Th: thalamus).

To verify these findings, blocking studies with 10 µM of **TA1** (a potent PDE2 ligand) [42] (Figure 4C) and **BIT1** (Figure 4D) were performed. The decrease of [^{18}F]**BIT1** binding of ~50% and ~30% in PDE2A specific regions Cd and Acb, respectively, observed for both **TA1** and **BIT1** indicated in vitro specificity of the radiotracer. However, the simultaneous decrease of [^{18}F]**BIT1** binding in the range of 20–30% in Cb by **TA1**, as well as **BIT1**, suggested further non-specific binding of the radiotracer. We hypothesized the high non-specific binding of [^{18}F]**BIT1** could be related to the moderate selectivity of **BIT1** over PDE10A. Accordingly, these results limited the suitability of [^{18}F]**BIT1** for in vitro molecular imaging of PDE2A.

2.2.2. In Vivo Metabolism of [^{18}F]**BIT1**

The in vivo metabolism of [^{18}F]**BIT1** was investigated in plasma and brain homogenate obtained from mice at 30 min p.i.. Prior to the analysis with RP-HPLC, the samples were treated with a mixture of MeCN/H_2O (4:1, v/v) to precipitate the proteins. The recovery of radioactivity in plasma and brain samples was 96% and 99%, respectively. Intact tracer accounted for 43% and 78% of total activity in plasma and brain, respectively, indicating higher metabolic stability of [^{18}F]**BIT1** in comparison to our previous PDE2A radioligands [^{18}F]**TA3**, [^{18}F]**TA4**, and [^{18}F]**TA5** **[23]**. As shown in the chromatograms

(Figure 5), the two radio-metabolites ([^{18}F]**M1** and [^{18}F]**M2**) found in the brain were also observed in the corresponding plasma sample, indicating their ability to penetrate the blood-brain barrier. For further clarification, samples obtained as previously described in our in vitro metabolism study with **BIT1** using mouse liver microsomes [28] were investigated similarly by HPLC, but with UV detection (Figure 5C). On the basis of the in vitro metabolites **M1** and **M2**, both elucidated by LC-MS in the mentioned study, we can conclude about the brain penetrating radio-metabolites [^{18}F]**M1** and [^{18}F]**M2** as products of *N*-oxidation or *C*-hydroxylation. Besides, some of the more polar radio-metabolites detected in plasma could only tentatively be assigned as formed by mono-oxygenation, di-oxygenation, reduction, and demethylation, but were not investigated further.

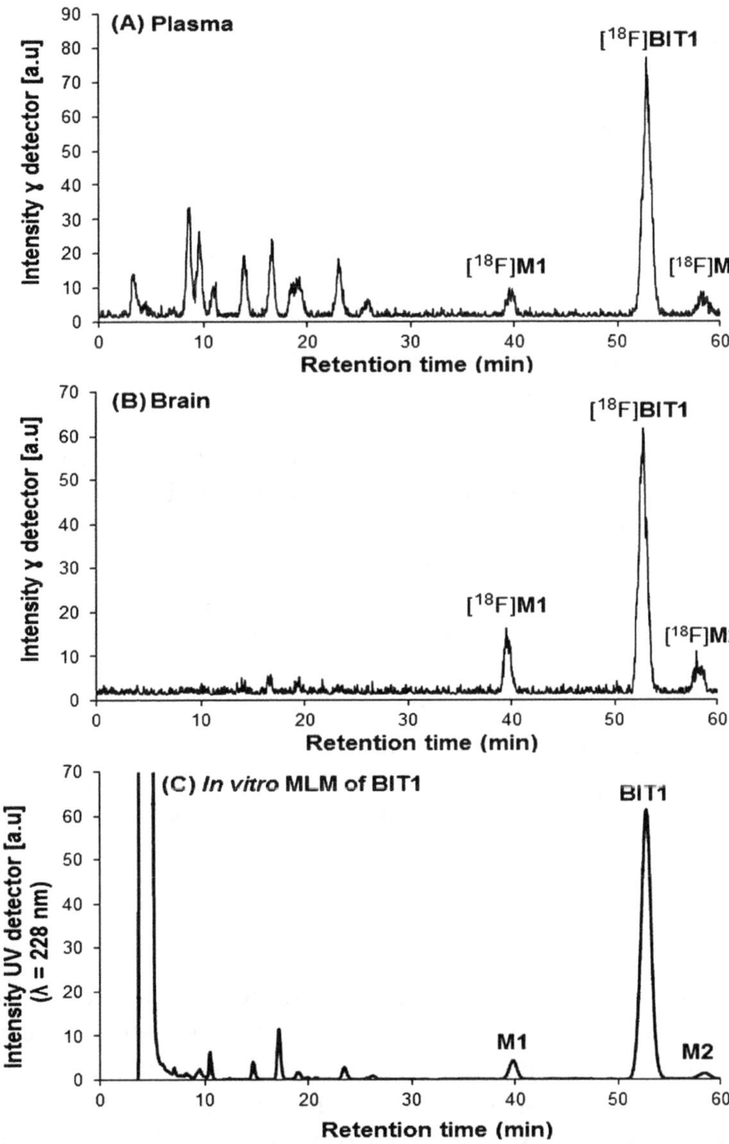

Figure 5. Representative analytical HPLC chromatogram: (**A**) plasma and (**B**) brain samples at 30 min p.i of [^{18}F]**BIT1** in a CD-1 mouse; (**C**) sample from incubation of **BIT1** with mouse liver microsomes (MLM) in the presence of NADPH for 90 min at 37 °C (UV detection: 228 nm; axis of retention time was adjusted). Conditions: isocratic system, column: Reprosil-Pur C18-AQ, 250 × 4.6 mm; eluent: 42% MeCN in 20 mM $NH_4OAc_{aq.}$, flow: 1.0 mL/min.

2.3. *In Vivo PET-MRI Studies of [^{18}F]**BIT1***

Dynamic PET-MRI studies were performed in female CD-1 mice after intravenous administration of [^{18}F]**BIT1**. As reflected by the time-activity curves (TACs) shown in Figure 6, the radioactivity uptake in the whole brain, striatum, and cerebellum reached standardized uptake values (SUVs) of about 0.7 at 5 min p.i., indicating blood-brain barrier penetration. Since there is no difference in the TACs between the whole brain, striatum, and cerebellum, [^{18}F]**BIT1** is assumed to possess low specific binding also in vivo.

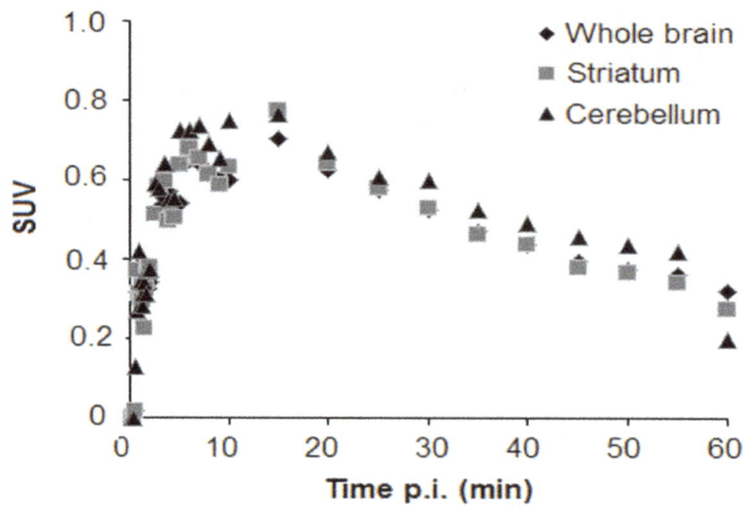

Figure 6. Averaged time-activity curves of [^{18}F]**BIT1** in CD-1 mice (n = 2) with standard uptake values (SUV) in the whole brain, striatum, and cerebellum.

To further investigate this hypothesis, blocking studies were performed by concomitant injection of **TA1** and [^{18}F]**BIT1**. However, since no significant reduction of radioactivity uptake in the PDE2A-specific region striatum was detectable (data not shown), the high non-specific binding of [^{18}F]**BIT1** already observed in vitro was confirmed.

Overall, the herein reported potential PDE2A radioligand, selected from a new class of 8-pyridinyl-BIT compounds, demonstrated sufficient blood-brain barrier (BBB) permeability. However, [^{18}F]**BIT1** was found to be insufficient for in vivo imaging of PDE2A with PET. Further structural modifications are needed to obtain PDE2A selective radioligands for in vitro and in vivo research. Extensive structure-activity relationship (SAR) studies could lead to the improvement of the selectivity and specificity of compounds. In particular, modifications of the set substituents at 1- and 8-positions of the BIT scaffold might result in additive as well as nonadditive effects in compound potency [43].

3. Materials and Methods

3.1. General Methods

All chemicals were purchased from commercial sources and used without further purification. Solvents were dried before used if required. Air and moisture-sensitive reactions were carried out under argon atmosphere. Room temperature (RT) refers to 20–25 °C. Reaction mixtures were monitored by thin-layer chromatography (TLC) using pre-coated TLC-plates POLYGRAM® SIL G/UV254 (Macherey-Nagel GmbH & Co. KG, Düren, Germany). The spots were detected under UV light at λ 254 nm and 365 nm. For the purification of final products, flash chromatography was performed with silica gel 40–63 μm (Merck KGaA, Darmstadt, Germany). Radio-TLC was performed on Polygram SIL G/UV$_{254}$ plates (Macherey-Nagel GmbH & Co. KG, Düren, Germany) pre-coated plates with a mixture of chloroform/methanol (10:1, v/v) as eluent. The radio-TLC plates were exposed to storage phosphor screens (BAS-IP MS 2025, FUJIFILM Co., Tokyo, Japan) and recorded using the AmershamTyphoon RGB Biomolecular Imager (GE Healthcare Life Sciences, Freiburg, Germany), and the images were quantified with ImageQuant TL8.1 software (GE Healthcare Life Sciences, Freiburg, Germany).

NMR spectra (^{1}H and ^{13}C) were recorded on Mercury 300/Mercury 400 (Varian, Palo Alto, CA, USA) or Fourier 300/Avance DRX 400 Bruker (Billerica, MA, USA) instruments. Residual solvent proton (^{1}H) and carbon (^{13}C) resonances were used as internal standards for ^{1}H-NMR ($CDCl_3$, $\delta_H = 7.26$; DMSO-d_6, $\delta_H = 2.50$) and ^{13}C-NMR ($CDCl_3$, $\delta_C = 77.16$; DMSO-d_6, $\delta_C = 39.52$). The chemical shifts (δ) were reported in ppm as follows: s, singlet; d, doublet; t, triplet; m, multiplet, and the coupling constants (J) are reported in Hz. Mass spectra were recorded on an ESQUIRE 3000 Plus (ESI, low resolution) and a 7 T APEX II (ESI, high resolution) (Bruker Daltonics, Bruker Corporation, Billerica, MA, USA).

For semi-preparative HPLC, the following conditions were used. Column: Reprosil-Pur C18-AQ, 250 × 10 mm, particle size: 10 μm; eluent: 46% MeCN/20 mM $NH_4OAc_{aq.}$; flow: 5.5 mL/min; ambient temperature; UV detection at 254 nm. The semi-preparative HPLC separations in the manual radiosynthesis were performed on a JASCO LC-2000 system, using a PU-2080-20 pump, an UV/VIS-2075 detector coupled with a radioactivity HPLC flow monitor (Gabi Star, raytest Isotopenmessgeräte GmbH, Straubenhardt, Germany) and a fraction collector (Advantec CHF-122SC, Dublin, CA, USA). Data recording was performed with the Galaxie chromatography software (Agilent Technologies, Santa Clara, USA).

Analytical chromatographic separations were performed on a JASCO LC-2000 system, incorporating a PU-2080*Plus* pump, AS-2055*Plus* auto-injector (100 μL sample loop), and a UV-2070 *Plus* detector coupled with a gamma radioactivity HPLC detector (Gabi Star, raytest Isotopenmessgeräte GmbH, Straubenhardt, Germany). Data analysis was performed with the Galaxie chromatography software (Agilent Technologies, Santa Clara, USA) using the chromatogram obtained at 254 nm. A Reprosil-Pur C18-AQ column (250 × 4.6 mm; 5 μm; Dr. Maisch HPLC GmbH, Ammerbuch-Entringen, Germany) with MeCN/20 mM $NH_4OAc_{aq.}$ (pH 6.8) as eluent mixture and a flow of 1.0 mL/min was used (gradient: eluent A 10% MeCN/20 mM $NH_4OAc_{aq.}$; eluent B 90% MeCN/20 mM $NH_4OAc_{aq.}$; 0–10 min 100% A, 10–40 min up to 100% B, 40–45 min 100% B, 45–50 min up to 100% A, 50–60 min 100% A; isocratic system 42% MeCN/20 mM $NH_4OAc_{aq.}$; flow: 1.0 mL/min; ambient temperature).

The molar activities were determined on the basis of a calibration curve (0.1–6 μg of **BIT1**) performed under isocratic HPLC conditions (46% MeCN/20 mM $NH_4OAc_{aq.}$) using chromatograms obtained at 228 nm as the maximum of UV absorbance of compound **BIT1**.

No-carrier-added (n.c.a.) [^{18}F]fluoride ($t_{1/2}$ = 109.8 min) was produced by irradiation of [^{18}O]H_2O (Hyox 18 enriched water, Rotem Industries Ltd., Arava, Israel) via [^{18}O(p,n)^{18}F] nuclear reaction by irradiation of on a Cyclone® 18/9 (iba RadioPharma Solutions, Louvain-la-Neuve, Belgium).

Remote-controlled automated syntheses were performed using a TRACERlab FX2 N synthesizer (GE Healthcare, USA) equipped with a N810.3FT.18 pump (KNF Neuburger GmbH, Freiburg, Germany), a BlueShadow UV detector 10D (KNAUER GmbH, Berlin, Germany), NaI(Tl)- counter, and the TRACERlab FX Software.

3.2. Precursor Synthesis and Radiochemistry

The final compounds described in this manuscript meet the purity requirement (>95%) determined by UV-HPLC.

3.2.1. Synthesis of Precursor

3-Methyl-8-(4,4,5,5-tetramethyl-1,3,2-dioxaborolan-2-yl)benzo[e]imidazo[5,1-c][1,2,4]triazine (**2**)

A mixture of bromo derivative **1** [28] (1.32 g, 5 mmol), potassium acetate (1.1 g, 11.2 mmol), and bis(pinacolato)diboron (1.3 g, 5.11 mmol) in 2-MeTHF (20 mL) was degassed with argon for 10 min. After the addition of Pd(dppf)Cl_2 (0.055 g, 0.075 mmol), the mixture was refluxed at 100 °C for 6 h and at 85 °C for 12 h. Upon completion of the reaction (monitored by TLC), CH_2Cl_2 (25 mL) was added, and the reaction mixture was stirred for 1 h. The solid was filtered off, and the filtrate was evaporated. The dark brown semi-solid residue (2.5 g) was dissolved in MTBE (60 mL) and filtered through a short silica gel column (H: 3 cm × D: 2 cm). Heptane (30 mL) was added to the eluate, followed by concentration to a volume of approximately 20 mL. The precipitated solid was filtered and dissolved in MTBE (120 mL), and the solution obtained was filtered again through a short silica gel column (H: 2 cm × D: 2 cm). The yellow eluate was concentrated (→ ~15 mL) and treated with *n*-heptane (30 mL). The solid obtained was filtered and dried under reduced pressure to afford a yellow solid **2** (1.32 g, 85%). TLC [$CHCl_3$/MeCN (10:1)]: $R_f = 0.26$ (strong tailing). ^1H NMR (400 MHz, $CDCl_3$) $\delta_H = 8.57$ (s, 1H), 8.41 (d, J = 8.0 Hz, 1H), 8.25 (s, 1H), 8.05 (dd, J = 8.0, 1.1 Hz, 1H), 2.89 (s, 3H), 1.40 (s, 13H).

3-Methyl-8-(2-nitropyridin-4-5 yl)benzo[e]imidazo[5,1-c][1,2,4]triazine (**3**)

A mixture of boronic ester **2** (470 mg, 1.5 mmol, 1 eq) and 4-bromo-2-nitropyridine (243 mg, 1.2 mmol) in 1,2-dimethoxyethane (6 mL) and an aqueous solution of K_2CO_3 (2 M, 1.75 mL, 3.5 mmol) was degassed with argon for 20 min. $Pd(PPh_3)_4$ (50 mg, 0.043 mmol) was added, and the reaction mixture was heated at 95 °C for 1 h and 88 °C for 14 h. Upon full conversion of starting material (monitored by TLC), the solvent was evaporated, and the residue was partitioned between water (30 mL) and $CHCl_3$ (50 mL). After separation of the organic layer, the aqueous layer was extracted with $CHCl_3$/MeCN (8:1, 6 × 30) and $CHCl_3$ (5 × 30 mL). The combined organic layers were dried over Na_2CO_3, and the solvent was evaporated to leave a solid residue (370 mg). The residue was refluxed in MeCN (50 mL) for 5 min, and after cooling to 0–2 °C, the product was filtered and dried to give **3** as yellow solid (233 mg, 63%). TLC [$CHCl_3$/MeOH/30% NH_3 (10:1:0.1)]: $R_f = 0.35$. ^1H NMR (300 MHz, DMSO-d6) $\delta_H = 9.26$ (s, 1H), 8.96 (dd, J = 2.0, 0.5 Hz, 1H), 8.85 (dt, J = 5.1, 0.8 Hz, 1H), 8.82–8.80 (m, 1H), 8.52 (dd, J = 8.7, 1.5 Hz, 1H), 8.42 (dd, J = 5.1, 1.7 Hz, 1H), 8.28 (dd, J = 8.5, 2.0 Hz, 1H), 2.78 (d, J = 1.7 Hz, 3H). ^{13}C NMR (75 MHz, DMSO-d6) $\delta_C = 157.67$, 149.59, 149.28, 138.82, 138.14, 136.18, 135.67, 130.31, 127.22, 127.17, 126.02, 122.45, 115.55, 114.35, 12.18.

1-Brom-3-methyl-8-(2-nitropyridin-4-yl)benzo[e]imidazo[5,1-c][1,2,4]triazine (**4**)

N-Bromosuccinimide (NBS) (48 mg, 1.58 eq) was added to a suspension of compound **3** (52 mg, 1 eq) in 2.5 mL MeCN. The reaction mixture was protected from light and stirred at RT for 1–2 d. After the complete conversion of starting material (monitored by TLC), the mixture was partitioned between $CHCl_3$ (15 mL) and water (15 mL). The organic layer was washed with aqueous $NaHCO_3$ (5%, 15 mL) and Na_2SO_3 (5%, 15 mL). The aqueous layer was extracted again with $CHCl_3$ (4x5 mL). The combined organic layers were dried (Na_2SO_4) and evaporated. The crude product was purified by column chromatography ($CHCl_3$/MeOH, 20:1) to afford compound **4** as a yellow solid (64 mg, 97%). TLC [$CHCl_3$/MeOH (20:1)]: $R_f = 0.59$. ^1H NMR (400 MHz, $CDCl_3$) $\delta_H = 9.31$ (d, *J* = 1.8 Hz, 1H), 8.84 (d, *J* = 5.0 Hz, 1H), 8.65 (d, *J* = 8.4 Hz, 1H), 8.59 (d, *J* = 1.6 Hz, 1H), 8.04–7.98 (m, 2H), 2.90 (s, 3H).

1-(2-Chloro-5-methoxyphenyl)-3-methyl-8-(2-nitropyridin-4-yl)benzo[e]imidazo[5,1-c][1,2,4]triazine (**5**)

Brominated compound **4** (43 mg, 0.112 mmol, 1 eq), 2-chloro-5-methoxyphenyl boronic acid (27 mg, 0.145 mmol, 1.29 eq), and K_2CO_3 (44 mg, 0.318 mmol, 2.8 eq) were combined in a mixture of 1,4-dioxane and H_2O (4:1). Under argon atmosphere, [$Pd(PPh_3)_4$] (13 mg, 10 mol%) was added. After refluxing at 101–105 °C for 3 h, the reaction mixture was stirred at RT for 16 h. Afterward, the residue was partitioned between $CHCl_3$ (20 mL) and water (20 mL). The organic layer was washed with water (20 mL) and brine (20 mL). The aqueous layer was extracted with $CHCl_3$ (3 × 10 mL), and the combined organic layers were dried over Na_2SO_4, and the solvent was evaporated under reduced pressure. The crude product was purified by column chromatography using a gradient system (*n*-hexane/ethyl acetate from 1:1 to 1:3) to get the corresponding precursor **5** as a yellow solid (34 mg, 68%). TLC [*n*-hexane/ethyl acetate (1:2)]: $R_f = 0.38$. ^1H NMR (400 MHz, $CDCl_3$) $\delta_H = 8.71$ (dd, *J* = 5.0, 0.6 Hz, 1H), 8.60 (d, *J* = 8.4 Hz, 1H), 8.15 (dd, *J* = 1.6, 0.6 Hz, 1H), 7.95 (dd, *J* = 8.4, 1.9 Hz, 1H), 7.77 (dd, *J* = 5.0, 1.6 Hz, 1H), 7.67–7.64 (m, 1H), 7.58 (d, *J* = 1.9 Hz, 1H), 7.24–7.20 (m, 2H), 3.87 (s, 3H), 3.00 (s, 3H). ^{13}C NMR (101 MHz, $CDCl_3$) $\delta_C = 159.24$, 157.85, 150.52, 149.96, 140.32, 138.66, 137.53, 137.22, 136.47, 131.76, 131.27, 131.11, 126.50, 125.79, 125.61, 124.31, 118.59, 117.99, 115.77, 114.21, 56.06, 12.94. ESI (+): *m/z* = 447.10 (calcd. 447.10 for $C_{22}H_{16}ClN_6O_3^+$ $[M + H]^+$).

3.2.2. In Vitro Metabolism of **BIT1**

BIT1 was incubated with mouse liver microsomes in the presence of NADPH, including positive and negative controls, for 90 min at 37 °C, as previously described [28]. Obtained samples were investigated by analytical HPLC with an isocratic system (42% MeCN/20 mM NH_4OAc_{aq}; flow rate of 1.0 mL/min) and UV detection (228 nm).

3.2.3. Radiochemistry

Manual Radiosynthesis

No carrier added [^{18}F]fluoride in 1.5 mL water and was trapped on a Chromafix® 30 PS-HCO_3^- cartridge (Macherey-Nagel GmbH & Co. KG, Düren, Germany). The activity was eluted with 300 μL of an aqueous solution of potassium carbonate solution (K_2CO_3, 1.8 mg, 13 μmol) into a 4 mL V-vial, and Kryptofix$_{2.2.2}$. ($K_{2.2.2}$) (11 mg, 29 μmol) in 1.0 mL MeCN was added. The aqueous [^{18}F]fluoride was azeotropically dried under vacuum and nitrogen flow within 7–10 min using a single-mode microwave (75 W, at 50–60 °C, power cycling mode). Two aliquots of MeCN (2 × 1.0 mL) were added during the drying procedure, and the final complex was dissolved in 500 μL of solvent (DMSO, DMF, and MeCN) ready for labeling. Thereafter, 0.5–1.0 mg of precursor in 500 μL labeling solvent was added, and the ^{18}F-labeling was performed at different temperatures (100 °C, 120 °C, and 150 °C). To analyze the reaction mixture and to determine radiochemical yields, samples were taken for radio-HPLC and radio-TLC at different time points (5, 10, 15, and 20 min).

After cooling to <30 °C, the reaction mixture was diluted with 1.0 mL water and 2.0 mL of MeCN/H_2O (1:1) and directly applied to an isocratic semi-preparative RP-HPLC for isolation of [^{18}F]**BIT1** (46% MeCN/20 mM $NH_4OAc_{aq.}$, 5.5 mL/min, Reprosil-Pur C18-AQ column, 250 × 10 mm; 10 μm; Dr. Maisch HPLC GmbH, Ammerbuch-Entringen, Germany). The collected radiotracer fraction was diluted with 35 mL water to perform purification by sorption on a Sep-Pak® C18 light cartridge (Waters, Milford, MA, USA) and successive elution with 0.75 mL of ethanol.

Automated Radiosynthesis of [^{18}F]**BIT1**

The automated radiosynthesis was performed in a TRACERlab FX2 N synthesis module (GE Healthcare, Waukesha, WI, USA). About 2–4.5 GBq of aqueous n.c.a [^{18}F]fluoride was trapped on a Chromafix® 30 PS-HCO_3^- cartridge (Figure 7, Macherey-Nagel GmbH & Co. KG, Düren, Germany, entry 1) and eluted with K_2CO_3 (1.8 mg, 13 μmol, entry 2) in 400 μL water. Kryptofix $K_{2.2.2}$ (11 mg, 29 μmol, in 1.0 mL MeCN, entry 3) was directly added. Afterward, azeotropic drying was performed at 60 °C and 85 °C under a vacuum. Thereafter, 0.5 mg of **5** in 1.0 mL DMSO (entry 4) was transferred to the reactor, and subsequently, the reaction was performed at 100 °C for 5 min. After cooling the reactor to 30 °C, 1.0 mL of H_2O and 2.0 mL of MeCN/H_2O (1:1) (entry 5) were added and transferred into the injection vial (entry 6). The semi-preparative HPLC was performed using a Reprosil-Pur C-18 AQ column (250 × 10 mm; 10 μM) using 46% MeCN in aqueous 20 mM ammonium acetate at a flow rate of 5.5 mL/min (entry 7). The [^{18}F]**BIT1** fraction was pooled in 35 mL H_2O (entry 8) and then loaded on a preconditioned Sep-Pak® C18 light cartridge (Waters, Milford, MA, USA, entry 9), and washed with 2.0 mL of H_2O (entry 10). Afterward, the trapped [^{18}F]**BIT1** was eluted with 1.2 mL EtOH (entry 11) into the product vial (entry 12). The product was transferred out of the hot cell, and the solvent was reduced under a gentle argon stream at 70 °C to a final volume of 10–50 μL. Afterward, the radiotracer was diluted in isotonic saline to obtain a final product containing 10% of EtOH (v/v). The identity of the final product was confirmed using radioanalytical HPLC.

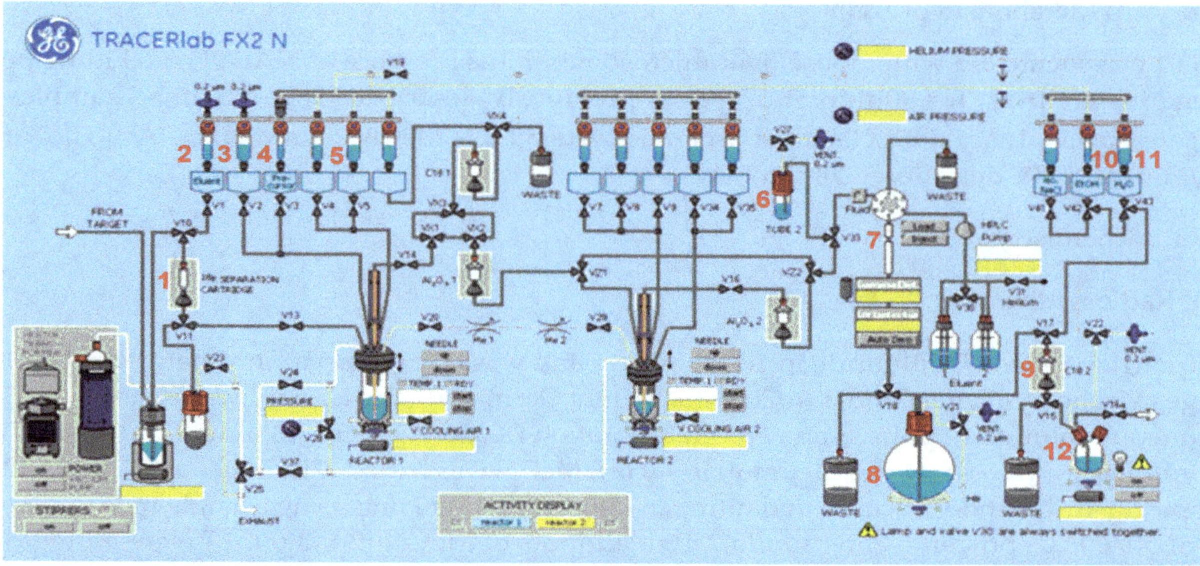

Figure 7. Scheme of the synthesis module TRACERlab FX2 N for the radiosynthesis of [^{18}F]**BIT1**. (1) Chromafix® 30 PS-HCO_3−, (2) K_2CO_3 (1.8 mg in 400 µL water), (3) $K_{2.2.2.}$ (11 mg, 29 µmol in 1.0 mL MeCN), (4) precursor (0.5 mg of **5** in 1.0 mL DMSO), (5) 1.0 mL H_2O and 2.0 mL MeCN/H_2O (1:1), (6) injection vial, (7) Reprosil-Pur C18-AQ column (46% MeCN/20mM $NH_4OAc_{aq.}$, flow 5.5 mL/min), (8) 35 mL water, (9) Sep-Pak® C18 light, (10) 2.0 mL water, (11) 1.2 mL EtOH, (12) product vial.

The molar activity of [^{18}F]**BIT1** was determined by analytical HPLC (isocratic mode: 46% MeCN/20 5mM $NH_4OAc_{aq.}$, Reprosil-Pur C18-AQ column 250 × 4.6 mm, flow rate: 1.0 mL/min). The UV/Vis detection was carried out at 228 nm as the absorption maximum of **BIT1**.

Determination of Stability

In vitro stability of [^{18}F]**BIT1** was investigated by incubation of the radioligand in phosphate-buffered saline (PBS, pH 7.4), *n*-octanol, and pig plasma at 40 °C for 60 min (~5 MBq of the radioligand was added to 500 µL of each medium). Samples were taken at 30 and 60 min and analyzed by radio-TLC and radio-HPLC.

Determination of log D

The lipophilicity of [^{18}F]**BIT1** was determined by partitioning between *n*-octanol and phosphate-buffered saline (PBS, pH 7.4) at ambient temperature using the conventional shake-flask method. An aliquot of 10 µL of the formulated solution containing ~500 kBq of [^{18}F]**BIT1** was added to a tube containing 6 mL of the *n*-octanol/PBS-mixture (1:1, v/v, four-fold determination). The tubes were shaken for 20 min using a mechanical shaker (HS250 basic, IKA Labortechnik GmbH & Co. KG, Staufen, Germany) followed by centrifugation (5000 rpm for 5 min) and separation of the phases. Aliquots of 1 mL of the organic and the aqueous phase were taken, and the activity was measured using an automated gamma counter (1480 WIZARD, Fa. Perkin Elmer, Waltham, MA, USA). The distribution coefficient (D) was calculated as [activity (cpm/mL) in *n*-octanol]/[(activity (cpm/mL) in PBS], specified as the decadic logarithm (logD).

3.3. Animal Studies

All experimental work, including animals, was conducted in accordance with the national legislation on the use of animals for research (Tierschutzgesetz (TierSchG), Tierschutz-Versuchstierverordnung (TierSchVersV)) and was approved by the responsible research ethics committee (TVV 18/18, DD24.1-5131/446/19, Landesdirektion Sachsen, 20th June 2018). Female CD-1 mice, 10–12 weeks, were obtained from the Medizinisch-Experimentelles Zentrum at Universität Leipzig.

For the time of the experiments, the animals were kept in a dedicated climatic chamber with free access to water and food under a 12:12 h dark:light cycle at a constant temperature of 24 °C. Piglet brains were obtained from anesthetized and euthanized juvenile female German landrace pigs (Lehr- und Versuchsgut Oberholz, Universität Leipzig).

3.3.1. In Vitro Autoradiography of [^{18}F]**BIT1**

Pig brain cryosections (16 μm; Microm HM560 Cryostat, FischerScientific GmbH, Schwerte, Germany) were thawed, dried in a stream of cold air, and preincubated for 10 min with buffer (50 mM TRIS-HCl, pH 7.4, 120 mM NaCl, 5 mM KCl, 2 mM $MgCl_2$) at room temperature. Afterward, brain sections were incubated with 1.72 nM of [^{18}F]**BIT1** in the buffer for 60 min at room temperature. The sections were then washed twice with ice-cold 50 mM TRIS-HCl (pH 7.4), dipped in ice-cold deionized water, dried in a stream of cold air, and exposed for 60 min to an image plate. The analysis was performed using an image plate scanner (HD-CR 35; Duerr NDT GmbH, Bietigheim Bissingen, Germany). Non-specific binding was determined using 10 μM **TA1** and **BIT1** as blocking compounds.

3.3.2. In Vivo Metabolism of [^{18}F]**BIT1**

[^{18}F]**BIT1** (~19 MBq) was injected in female CD-1 mice (10–12 weeks old) via the tail vein. Brain and blood samples were obtained at 30 min p.i., plasma separated by centrifugation (14,000 rpm, 1 min), and brain homogenized in ~1 mL isotonic saline on ice (10 strokes of a PTFE plunge at 1000 rpm) in borosilicate glass.

Protein precipitation of plasma and brain samples was performed in duplicate with ice-cold $MeCN/H_2O$ (8:2, v/v), which was added to the samples (sample/solvent, 1:4, v/v). The samples were vortexed for 1 min, followed by resting on ice for 10 min. Afterward, the samples were centrifuged for 5 min at 10,000 g. Supernatants were collected, and 100 μL ice-cold $MeCN/H_2O$ (8:2, v/v) was added to the pellets for the second extraction, applying the same treatment as before. The combined supernatants were concentrated at 70 °C under nitrogen stream until a remaining volume of 100 μL and subsequently quantified by analytical radio-HPLC with an isocratic system (42% MeCN/20 mM $NH_4OAc_{aq.}$; flow rate: 1.0 mL/min). The activity recovery was determined by measuring the radioactivity of aliquots taken from supernatants and the pellets using a gamma counter.

*3.4. PET-MRI Studies of [^{18}F]**BIT1***

PET/MRI scans were performed using a preclinical PET/MRI system (nanoScan, Mediso Medical Imaging Systems, Budapest, Hungary). Animals were anesthetized with a mixture of air/isoflurane (2.0%, 200 mL/min) (Anesthesia Unit U-410, agntho's, Lidingö, Sweden), and their body temperature maintained at 37 °C with a thermal bed system. [^{18}F]**BIT1** (2 MBq, A_m: 155 GBq/μmol, EOS) was injected via the tail vein, either without (baseline study, n = 2) or with **TA1** (2 mg/kg, DMSO/NaCl (1:25); blocking study, n = 2). A dynamic 60-min PET scan was started 20 sec before radioligand injection. The list-mode data were reconstructed into 33 frames (12 × 10 sec, 6 × 30 sec, 5 × 1 min, 10 × 5 min) with 3D-ordered subset expectation maximization, 4 iterations, and 6 subsets, using an energy window of 400 to 600 KeV and coincidence mode of 1–5. After the PET scan, an MRI scan was performed for anatomical orientation and attenuation correction on a 1T magnet using a T1-weighted gradient-echo sequence (TR = 15 ms, TE = 2.6 ms). The data analysis was done with PMOD (PMOD Technologies Ltd., Zurich, Switzerland, v. 3.6), and an atlas-based method was used to obtain SUV time-activity curves for the striatum, cerebellum, and the whole brain.

4. Conclusions

In our efforts to develop a specific radioligand for PET imaging of PDE2A in the brain on the basis of a benzoimidazotriazine scaffold, we successfully prepared the novel PDE2A radioligand [^{18}F]**BIT1** with a high radiochemical yield, radiochemical purity, as well as molar activity. Our findings showed that this class of compound demonstrated good brain penetration and sufficient in vivo metabolic stability. However, [^{18}F]**BIT1** was not suitable for the molecular imaging of PDE2A in the brain because of a high non-specific binding. Further structural modifications are required to obtain more satisfactory PDE2A specific radioligands.

Author Contributions: B.W., M.S., and P.B. designed the study; M.S. and R.R. designed and performed organic syntheses; B.W., R.R., and R.T. performed radiosynthesis; W.D.-C., B.W., R.T., F.-A.L., and R.R. performed in vivo metabolism studies; S.D.-S., W.D.-C., and P.B. performed in vitro autoradiographic studies; M.T., M.K., W.D.-C., and P.B. designed and performed PET-MR studies; R.R., B.W., R.T., M.T., M.K., W.D.-C., S.D.-S, F.-A.L., M.S., and P.B. wrote the paper. All authors read and approved the final manuscript.

Acknowledgments: This work was financially supported by the Deutsche Forschungsgemeinschaft (DFG), Project Number: SCHE 1825/3-1. We further thank the Research and Innovation in Science and Technology Project (RISET-Pro), the Ministry of Research, Technology, and Higher Education, Republic of Indonesia, World Bank Loan No. 8245-ID, for supporting the Ph.D. thesis of Rien Ritawidya, the staff of the Institute of Analytical Chemistry (University of Leipzig) for measuring NMR and LR/HR-MS spectra, Karsten Franke and Steffen Fischer for the production of [^{18}F]fluoride, and Tina Spalholz for technical assistance.

References

1. Helal, C.J.; Arnold, E.P.; Boyden, T.L.; Chang, C.; Chappie, T.A.; Fennell, K.F.; Forman, M.D.; Hajos, M.; Harms, J.F.; Hoffman, W.E.; et al. Application of structure-based design and parallel chemistry to identify a potent, selective, and brain penetrant phosphodiesterase 2A inhibitor. *J. Med. Chem.* **2017**, *60*, 5673–5698. [CrossRef] [PubMed]
2. Zhu, J.; Yang, Q.; Dai, D.; Huang, Q. X-ray crystal structure of phosphodiesterase 2 in complex with a highly selective, nanomolar inhibitor reveals a binding-induced pocket important for selectivity. *J. Am. Chem. Soc.* **2013**, *135*, 11708–11711. [CrossRef] [PubMed]
3. Wu, Y.; Li, Z.; Huang, Y.-Y.; Wu, D.; Luo, H.-B. Novel phosphodiesterase inhibitors for cognitive improvement in Alzheimer's disease. *J. Med. Chem.* **2018**, *61*, 5467–5483. [CrossRef] [PubMed]
4. Svensson, F.; Bender, A.; Bailey, D. Fragment-based drug discovery of phosphodiesterase inhibitors. *J. Med. Chem.* **2018**, *61*, 1415–1424. [CrossRef] [PubMed]
5. Jäger, R.; Schwede, F.; Genieser, H.-G.; Koesling, D.; Russwurm, M. Activation of PDE2 and PDE5 by specific GAF ligands: Delayed activation of PDE5. *Br. J. Pharmacol.* **2010**, *161*, 1645–1660. [CrossRef] [PubMed]
6. Maurice, D.H.; Ke, H.; Ahmad, F.; Wang, Y.; Chung, J.; Manganiello, V.C. Advances in targeting cyclic nucleotide phosphodiesterases. *Nat. Rev. Drug Discov.* **2014**, *13*, 290–314. [CrossRef]
7. Conti, M.; Beavo, J. Biochemistry and physiology of cyclic nucleotide phosphodiesterases: Essential components in cyclic nucleotide signaling. *Annu. Rev. Biochem.* **2007**, *76*, 481–511. [CrossRef]
8. Lakics, V.; Karran, E.H.; Boess, F.G. Quantitative comparison of phosphodiesterase mRNA distribution in human brain and peripheral tissues. *Neuropharmacology* **2010**, *59*, 367–374. [CrossRef]
9. Menniti, F.S.; Faraci, W.S.; Schmidt, C.J. Phosphodiesterases in the CNS: Targets for drug development. *Nat. Rev. Drug Discov.* **2006**, *5*, 660–670. [CrossRef]
10. Gomez, L.; Breitenbucher, J.G. PDE2 inhibition: Potential for the treatment of cognitive disorders. *Bioorganic Med. Chem. Lett.* **2013**, *23*, 6522–6527. [CrossRef]
11. Stephenson, D.T.; Coskran, T.M.; Wilhelms, M.B.; Adamowicz, W.O.; O'Donnell, M.M.; Muravnick, K.B.; Menniti, F.S.; Kleiman, R.J.; Morton, D. Immunohistochemical localization of phosphodiesterase 2A in multiple mammalian species. *J. Histochem. Cytochem.* **2009**, *57*, 933–949. [CrossRef] [PubMed]
12. Stephenson, D.T.; Coskran, T.M.; Kelly, M.P.; Kleiman, R.J.; Morton, D.; O'Neill, S.M.; Schmidt, C.J.; Weinberg, R.J.; Menniti, F.S. The distribution of phosphodiesterase 2A in the rat brain. *Neuroscience* **2012**, *226*, 145–155. [CrossRef] [PubMed]
13. Gomez, L.; Massari, M.E.; Vickers, T.; Freestone, G.; Vernier, W.; Ly, K.; Xu, R.; McCarrick, M.; Marrone, T.; Metz, M.; et al. Design and synthesis of novel and selective phosphodiesterase 2 (PDE2a) inhibitors for the treatment of memory disorders. *J. Med. Chem.* **2017**, *60*, 2037–2051. [CrossRef] [PubMed]

14. Sierksma, A.S.R.; Rutten, K.; Sydlik, S.; Rostamian, S.; Steinbusch, H.W.M.; van den Hove, D.L.A.; Prickaerts, J. Chronic phosphodiesterase type 2 inhibition improves memory in the APPswe/PS1dE9 mouse model of Alzheimer's disease. *Neuropharmacology* **2013**, *64*, 124–136. [CrossRef] [PubMed]
15. Umar, T.; Hoda, N. Selective inhibitors of phosphodiesterases: Therapeutic promise for neurodegenerative disorders. *Med. Chem. Commun.* **2015**, *6*, 2063–2080. [CrossRef]
16. Mikami, S.; Sasaki, S.; Asano, Y.; Ujikawa, O.; Fukumoto, S.; Nakashima, K.; Oki, H.; Kamiguchi, N.; Imada, H.; Iwashita, H.; et al. Discovery of an orally bioavailable, brain-penetrating, in vivo active phosphodiesterase 2A inhibitor lead series for the treatment of cognitive disorders. *J. Med. Chem.* **2017**, *60*, 7658–7676. [CrossRef]
17. Reneerkens, O.A.H.; Rutten, K.; Steinbusch, H.W.M.; Blokland, A.; Prickaerts, J. Selective phosphodiesterase inhibitors: A promising target for cognition enhancement. *Psychopharmacology* **2009**, *202*, 419–443. [CrossRef]
18. Brust, P.; van den Hoff, J.; Steinbach, J. Development of ^{18}F-labeled radiotracers for neuroreceptor imaging with positron emission tomography. *Neurosci. Bull.* **2014**, *30*, 777–811. [CrossRef]
19. Andrés-Gil, J.I.; Rombouts, F.J.R.; Trabanco, A.A.; Vanhoof, G.C.P.; De Angelis, M.; Buijnsters, P.J.J.A.; Guillemont, J.E.G.; Bormans, G.M.R.; Celen, S.J.L.; Vliegen, M. 1-aryl-4-methyl-[1,2,4]triazolo[4,3-a]quinoxaline Derivatives. Patent No. WO 2013/000924 A1, 3 January 2013.
20. Zhang, L.; Villalobos, A.; Beck, E.M.; Bocan, T.; Chappie, T.A.; Chen, L.; Grimwood, S.; Heck, S.D.; Helal, C.J.; Hou, X.; et al. Design and selection parameters to accelerate the discovery of novel central nervous system positron emission tomography (PET) ligands and their application in the development of a novel phosphodiesterase 2A PET ligand. *J. Med. Chem.* **2013**, *56*, 4568–4579. [CrossRef]
21. Naganawa, M.; Waterhouse, R.N.; Nabulsi, N.; Lin, S.-F.; Labaree, D.; Ropchan, J.; Tarabar, S.; DeMartinis, N.; Ogden, A.; Banerjee, A.; et al. First-in-human assessment of the novel PDE2A PET radiotracer ^{18}F-PF-05270430. *J. Nucl. Med.* **2016**, *57*, 1388–1395. [CrossRef]
22. Naganawa, M.; Nabulsi, N.; Waterhouse, R.; Lin, S.-F.; Zhang, L.; Cass, T.; Ropchan, J.; McCarthy, T.; Huang, Y.; Carson, R. Human PET studies [^{18}F]PF-05270430, a PET radiotracer for imaging phosphodiesterase-2A. *J. Nucl. Med.* **2013**, *54*, 201.
23. Schröder, S.; Wenzel, B.; Deuther-Conrad, W.; Scheunemann, M.; Brust, P. Novel radioligands for cyclic nucleotide phosphodiesterase imaging with positron emission tomography: An update on developments since 2012. *Molecules* **2016**, *21*, 650. [CrossRef] [PubMed]
24. Schröder, S.; Wenzel, B.; Deuther-Conrad, W.; Teodoro, R.; Egerland, U.; Kranz, M.; Scheunemann, M.; Höfgen, N.; Steinbach, J.; Brust, P. Synthesis, ^{18}F-radiolabelling and biological characterization of novel fluoroalkylated triazine derivatives for in vivo imaging of phosphodiesterase 2A in brain via positron emission tomography. *Molecules* **2015**, *20*, 9591–9615. [CrossRef] [PubMed]
25. Schröder, S.; Wenzel, B.; Deuther-Conrad, W.; Teodoro, R.; Kranz, M.; Scheunemann, M.; Egerland, U.; Höfgen, N.; Briel, D.; Steinbach, J.; et al. Investigation of an ^{18}F-labelled imidazopyridotriazine for molecular imaging of cyclic nucleotide phosphodiesterase 2A. *Molecules* **2018**, *23*, 556. [CrossRef]
26. Stange, H.; Langen, B.; Egerland, U.; Hoefgen, N.; Priebs, M.; Malamas, M.S.; Erdei, J.J.; Ni, Y. Imidazo[5,1-c][1,2,4]benzotriazine Derivatives as Inhibitors of Phosphodiesterases. Patent US 2010/0120763 A1, 13 May 2010.
27. Malamas, M.S.; Stange, H.; Schindler, R.; Lankau, H.-J.; Grunwald, C.; Langen, B.; Egerland, U.; Hage, T.; Ni, Y.; Erdei, J.; et al. Novel triazines as potent and selective phosphodiesterase 10A inhibitors. *Bioorganic Med. Chem. Lett.* **2012**, *22*, 5876–5884. [CrossRef]
28. Ritawidya, R.; Ludwig, F.-A.; Briel, D.; Brust, P.; Scheunemann, M. Synthesis and in vitro evaluation of 8-pyridinyl-substituted benzo[e]imidazo[2,1-c][1,2,4]triazines as phosphodiesterase 2A inhibitors. *Molecules* **2019**, *24*, 2791. [CrossRef]
29. Dolci, L.; Dolle, F.; Valette, H.; Vaufrey, F.; Fuseau, C.; Bottlaender, M.; Crouzel, C. Synthesis of a fluorine-18 labeled derivative of epibatidine for in vivo nicotinic acetylcholine receptor PET imaging. *Bioorganic Med. Chem.* **1999**, *7*, 467–479. [CrossRef]
30. Wagner, S.; Teodoro, R.; Deuther-Conrad, W.; Kranz, M.; Scheunemann, M.; Fischer, S.; Wenzel, B.; Egerland, U.; Hoefgen, N.; Steinbach, J.; et al. Radiosynthesis and biological evaluation of the new PDE10A radioligand [^{18}F]AQ28A. *J. Label. Compd. Radiopharm.* **2017**, *60*, 36–48. [CrossRef]
31. Ishiyama, T.; Murata, M.; Miyaura, N. Palladium(0)-catalyzed cross-coupling reaction of alkoxydiboron with haloarenes: A direct procedure for arylboronic esters. *J. Org. Chem.* **1995**, *60*, 7508–7510. [CrossRef]
32. Wiley, R.H.; Hartman, J.L. Oxidation of aminopyridines to nitropyridines. *J. Am. Chem. Soc.* **1951**, *73*, 494.

33. Wenzel, B.; Günther, R.; Brust, P.; Steinbach, J. A fluoro versus a nitro derivative-a high-performance liquid chromatography study of two basic analytes with different reversed phases and silica phases as basis for the separation of a positron emission tomography radiotracer. *J. Chromatogr. A* **2013**, *1311*, 98–105. [CrossRef] [PubMed]
34. Lindemann, M.; Hinz, S.; Deuther-Conrad, W.; Namasivayam, V.; Dukic-Stefanovic, S.; Teodoro, R.; Toussaint, M.; Kranz, M.; Juhl, C.; Steinbach, J.; et al. Radiosynthesis and in vivo evaluation of a fluorine-18 labeled pyrazine based radioligand for PET imaging of the adenosine A_{2B} receptor. *Bioorganic Med. Chem.* **2018**, *26*, 4650–4663. [CrossRef] [PubMed]
35. Waterhouse, R.N. Determination of lipophilicity and its use as a predictor of blood–brain barrier penetration of molecular imaging agents. *Mol. Imaging Biol.* **2003**, *5*, 376–389. [CrossRef] [PubMed]
36. Pike, V.W. PET radiotracers: Crossing the blood-brain barrier and surviving metabolism. *Trends Pharmacol. Sci.* **2009**, *30*, 431–440. [CrossRef] [PubMed]
37. van de Waterbeemd, H.; Camenisch, G.; Folkers, G.; Chretien, J.R.; Raevsky, O.A. Estimation of blood-brain barrier crossing of drugs using molecular size and shape, and H-bonding descriptors. *J. Drug Target.* **1998**, *6*, 151–165. [CrossRef] [PubMed]
38. Testa, B.; Crivori, P.; Reist, M.; Carrupt, P.-A. The influence of lipophilicity on the pharmacokinetic behavior of drugs: Concepts and examples. *Perspect. Drug Discov. Des.* **2000**, *19*, 179–211. [CrossRef]
39. Bodor, N.; Gabanyi, Z.; Wong, C.-K. A new method for the estimation of partition coefficient. *J. Am. Chem. Soc.* **1989**, *111*, 3783–3786. [CrossRef]
40. Donovan, S.F.; Pescatore, M.C. Method for measuring the logarithm of the octanol–water partition coefficient by using short octadecyl–poly(vinyl alcohol) high-performance liquid chromatography columns. *J. Chromatogr. A* **2002**, *952*, 47–61. [CrossRef]
41. Vraka, C.; Nics, L.; Wagner, K.-H.; Hacker, M.; Wadsak, W.; Mitterhauser, M. LogP, a yesterday's value? *Nucl. Med. Biol.* **2017**, *50*, 1–10. [CrossRef]
42. Stange, H.; Langen, B.; Egerland, U.; Hoefgen, N.; Priebs, M.; Malamas, M.S.; Erdei, J.; Ni, Y. Triazine Derivatives as Inhibitors of Phosphodiesterases. Patent No. WO 2010/054253 A1, 14 May 2010.
43. Gomez, L.; Xu, R.; Sinko, W.; Selfridge, B.; Vernier, W.; Ly, K.; Truong, R.; Metz, M.; Marrone, T.; Sebring, K.; et al. Mathematical and Structural characterization of strong nonadditive structure-activity relationship caused by protein conformational changes. *J. Med. Chem.* **2018**, *61*, 7754–7766. [CrossRef]

9

Preclinical Incorporation Dosimetry of $[^{18}F]$FACH—A Novel ^{18}F-Labeled MCT1/MCT4 Lactate Transporter Inhibitor for Imaging Cancer Metabolism with PET

Bernhard Sattler [1,*,†], Mathias Kranz [2,3,4,†], Barbara Wenzel [2], Nalin T. Jain [2], Rareş-Petru Moldovan [2], Magali Toussaint [2], Winnie Deuther-Conrad [2], Friedrich-Alexander Ludwig [2], Rodrigo Teodoro [2], Tatjana Sattler [5], Masoud Sadeghzadeh [2,‡], Osama Sabri [1,‡] and Peter Brust [2,‡]

1 Department of Nuclear Medicine, University Hospital Leipzig, 04103 Leipzig, Germany; osama.sabri@medizin.uni-leipzig.de
2 Helmholtz-Zentrum Dresden-Rossendorf, Institute of Radiopharmaceutical Cancer Research, Department of Neuroradiopharmaceuticals, 04318 Leipzig, Germany; mathias.kranz@unn.no (M.K.); m.sadeghzadeh@hzdr.de (M.S.); nalintjain@gmail.com (N.T.J.); b.wenzel@hzdr.de (B.W.); r.moldovan@hzdr.de (R.-P.M.); m.toussaint@hzdr.de (M.T.); w.deuther-conrad@hzdr.de (W.D.-C.); f.ludwig@hzdr.de (F.-A.L.); r.teodoro@hzdr.de (R.T.); p.brust@hzdr.de (P.B.)
3 Tromsø PET Center, University Hospital of North Norway, 9009 Tromsø, Norway
4 Nuclear Medicine and Radiation Biology Research Group, The Arctic University of Norway, 9009 Tromsø, Norway
5 Department of Claw Animals, University of Leipzig, 04103 Leipzig, Germany; tasat@vetmed.uni-leipzig.de
* Correspondence: bernhard.sattler@medizin.uni-leipzig.de
† These authors contributed equally to this work.
‡ These authors contributed equally to this work.

Academic Editors: Anne Roivainen and Xiang-Guo Li

Abstract: Overexpression of monocarboxylate transporters (MCTs) has been shown for a variety of human cancers (e.g., colon, brain, breast, and kidney) and inhibition resulted in intracellular lactate accumulation, acidosis, and cell death. Thus, MCTs are promising targets to investigate tumor cancer metabolism with positron emission tomography (PET). Here, the organ doses (ODs) and the effective dose (ED) of the first ^{18}F-labeled MCT1/MCT4 inhibitor were estimated in juvenile pigs. Whole-body dosimetry was performed in three piglets (age: ~6 weeks, weight: ~13–15 kg). The animals were anesthetized and subjected to sequential hybrid Positron Emission Tomography and Computed Tomography (PET/CT) up to 5 h after an intravenous (iv) injection of 156 ± 54 MBq $[^{18}F]$FACH. All relevant organs were defined by volumes of interest. Exponential curves were fitted to the time–activity data. Time and mass scales were adapted to the human order of magnitude and the ODs calculated using the ICRP 89 adult male phantom with OLINDA 2.1. The ED was calculated using tissue weighting factors as published in Publication 103 of the International Commission of Radiation Protection (ICRP103). The highest organ dose was received by the urinary bladder (62.6 ± 28.9 µSv/MBq), followed by the gall bladder (50.4 ± 37.5 µSv/MBq) and the pancreas (30.5 ± 27.3 µSv/MBq). The highest contribution to the ED was by the urinary bladder (2.5 ± 1.1 µSv/MBq), followed by the red marrow (1.7 ± 0.3 µSv/MBq) and the stomach (1.3 ± 0.4 µSv/MBq). According to this preclinical analysis, the ED to humans is 12.4 µSv/MBq when applying the ICRP103 tissue weighting factors. Taking into account that preclinical dosimetry underestimates the dose to humans by up to 40%, the conversion factor applied for estimation of the ED to humans would rise to 20.6 µSv/MBq. In this case, the ED to humans upon an iv application of ~300 MBq $[^{18}F]$FACH would be about 6.2 mSv. This risk assessment encourages the translation of $[^{18}F]$FACH into clinical study phases and the further investigation of its potential as a clinical tool for cancer imaging with PET.

Keywords: preclinical radiopharmaceutical dosimetry; image-based internal dosimetry; OLINDA; MCT1/MCT4 lactate transporter inhibitor; [^{18}F]FACH; radiation safety

1. Introduction

Aerobic glycolysis is a common feature of cancer physiology. Even under adequate oxygenation, cancer cells generate energy mainly via the cytosolic conversion of glucose into pyruvate and not via the downstream mitochondrial respiratory chain, known as the Warburg effect [1]. Due to the conversion of pyruvate to lactate, this phenomenon results in intracellularly high concentrations of lactate along with a decrease in the pH. Consequently, to avoid apoptosis caused by an acidic environment in the cytoplasm, cancer cells facilitate the proton-coupled efflux of pyruvate and lactate [2,3] by the transmembrane monocarboxylate transporters (MCTs). Upregulation of several MCTs was observed in different cancer types [4–8] and pharmacological inhibition of MCT1/MCT4 impairs cancer cell proliferation and tumor growth [9]. Increased expression of MCT1 and MCT4 in brain malignancies is assumed to be linked to the pathogenesis of glioblastoma in particular [8]. Accordingly, MCT1 and MCT4 are interesting targets for inhibitor-based molecular imaging and pharmacological treatment of this aggressive form of glioma.

Recently, [^{18}F]FLac, [^{18}F]FP, and an ^{11}C-labeled coumarin analog were developed as radiotracers to monitor MCT1 with positron emission tomography (PET). However, defluorination, nonspecific binding, and insufficient affinity hamper the applicability of these tracers [10,11]. Recently, with [^{18}F]FACH, a fluorinated analog of α-cyano-4-hydroxycinnamic acid (α-CHC) [6] ((*E*)-2-cyano-3-{4-[(3-[^{18}F]fluoropropyl)(propyl)amino]-2-methoxyphenyl}acrylic acid), a novel radiolabeled MCT1/4 inhibitor was developed by our group. The inhibitory potency of FACH ($IC_{50,\,MCT1}$ = 11 nM; $IC_{50,\,MCT4}$ = 6.5 nM) indicates the suitability of [^{18}F]FACH for in vivo molecular imaging of MCT1/MCT4 with PET [12,13].

For the clinical translation of newly developed radiopharmaceuticals, a safety and tolerability assessment is mandatory. One integral part of the assessment is the preclinical radiation dose assessment to estimate the radiation exposure caused by systemic, i.e., intravenous (iv), application of the radiotracer. For the estimation of organ doses (ODs) and the effective dose (ED), the pharmacokinetics and tissue distribution of the tracer have to be determined. The activity concentration in the different organs and tissues is required to determine time-integrated activity concentrations (TIAC) and finally calculate the region-specific numbers of disintegration (NOD). As recently shown, our approach to perform respective PET imaging studies combined with CT or Magnet Resonance Imaging (MRI) in a small number of piglets is suitable to generate pharmacokinetic data for dosimetric calculations [14–17]. With this fully imaging-based approach [18], the total number of animals used for dosimetry studies can be reduced to a minimum and the acquired data can be re-used for further research questions. It is important to note that when using animals for dose estimation in humans, an interspecies scaling has to be applied [19]. However, as also shown by our previous studies [14–16], preclinical dosimetry underestimates the ED in humans by up to 40% independent of the species and size of the test animal, and the radiation dose assessment has to be adapted accordingly.

Herein, we present the results of a preclinical dosimetry study of the newly developed MCT1/MCT4-specific radioligand [^{18}F]FACH performed in juvenile pigs with a clinical PET/CT system and report on the estimation of the ED in humans as required for approval of application of the new radiopharmaceutical in clinical studies.

2. Results

The radiation safety of the newly developed MCT1/MCT4-specific radioligand [^{18}F]FACH was preclinically investigated. Following intravenous injection of 156 ± 54 MBq (0.63 ± 0.49 μg) of the radiopharmaceutical, no adverse effects were observed based on vital sign monitoring, and three piglets were subjected to sequential PET/CT up to 252 min post injection (p.i.). Afterwards, volumes of interest (VOIs) of the various organs were manually defined using the respective whole-body CT dataset for anatomical orientation. The estimated TIACs were extrapolated to the human entity (Equation (2)), followed by estimation of the organ doses with OLINDA 2.1 and calculation of the effective dose using tissue weighting factors as published in Publication 103 of the International Commission of Radiation Protection (ICRP103) [20]. Finally, it can be concluded that [^{18}F]FACH is safe with respect to the radiation risk that is caused by its systemic application for PET studies. This supports and encourages the translation of this newly developed radiopharmaceutical to clinical study phases.

The TIAC courses in organs allow for determination of the fraction of administered activity, also referred to as percent of injected dose (%ID), in the particular region, followed by calculation of the NOD by integration over time applied at mono-, bi-, or tri-exponentially fitted TIACs. Figure 1 shows six examples of the exponential fits of the fractions of activity (%ID) in different organs over time (all scaled to human dimensions). The fits of all organs of the three investigated animals as well as the exact exponential equations of the fits can be found in the Supplementary Materials (Figures S1–S3).

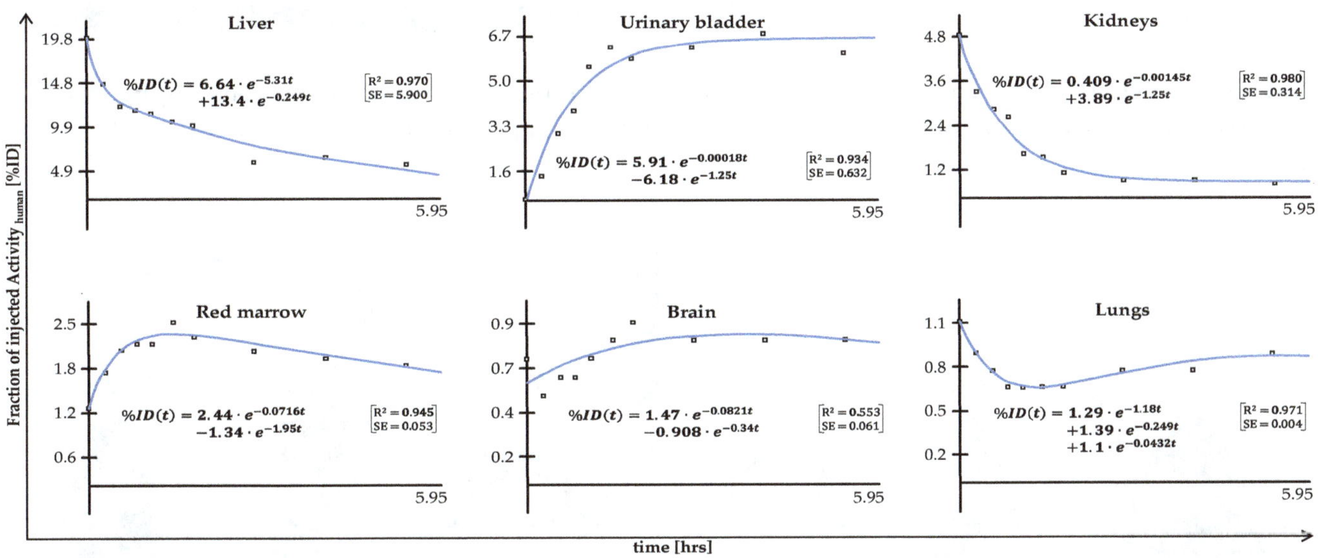

Figure 1. Examples of the mono-, bi-, or tri-exponential fits, including exponential fit equations and parameters of fit goodness (R-squared and squared error) of the human scale time–activity data using the EXM-Module of OLINDA. All fits are presented in the Supplementary Materials (Figures S1–S3).

In Figure 2, the distribution of activity in one representative animal at different times p.i. of [^{18}F]FACH is presented, showing a high uptake in the liver, pancreas, small intestines, and spleen. The rapid uptake in the liver and later also in the gall bladder indicates hepatobiliary excretion. Early accumulation in the bone structures might be related to defluorination. At later time points, activity also accumulated in the gall bladder and the urinary bladder.

An example of manually delineated VOIs using the PET or CT information to extract the accumulated amount of activity in the respective organ is presented in Figure 3. All biodistribution data, including TIACs for all organs, are available in the Supplementary Materials (Tables S1–S4; Figure S1).

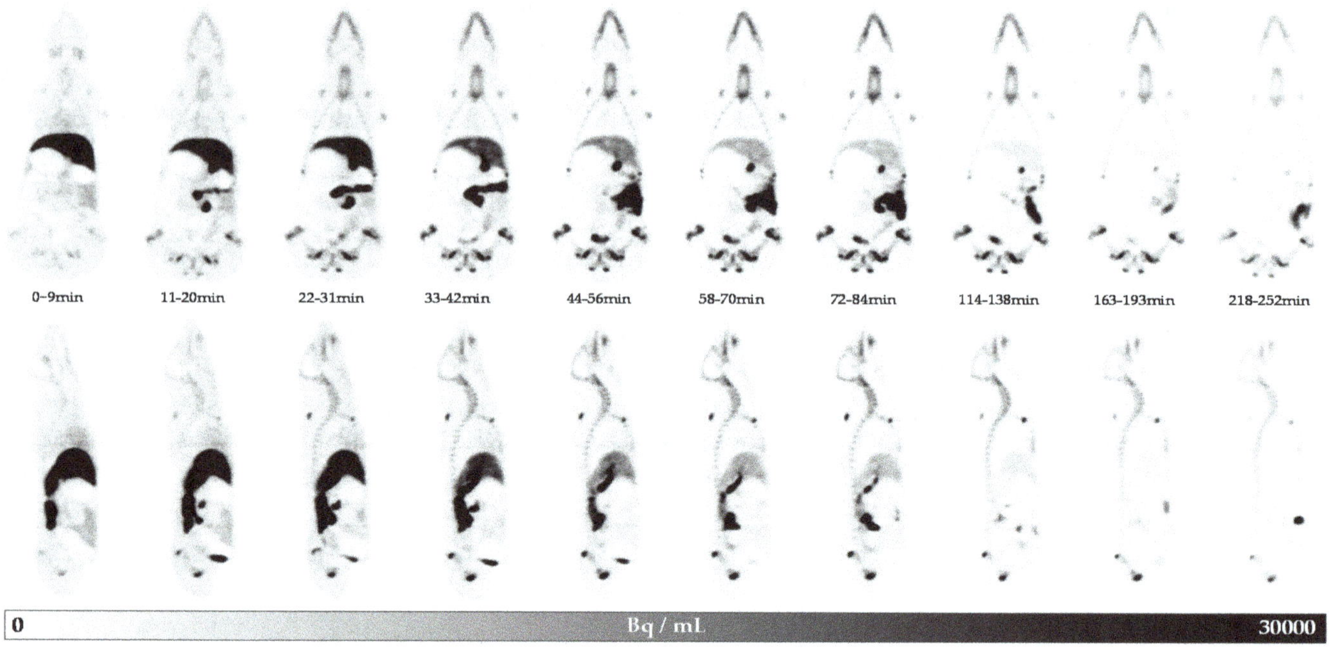

Figure 2. Whole body dynamic positron emission tomography (PET) images in coronal (upper row) and sagittal (lower row) views of pig 1 after intravenous (iv) application of 191 MBq [^{18}F]FACH.

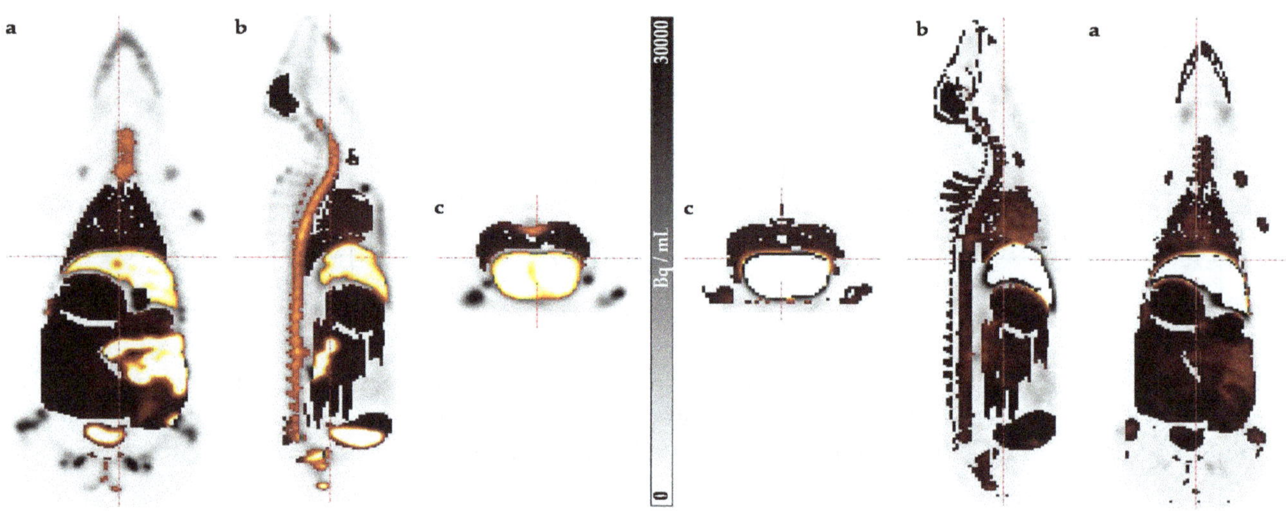

Figure 3. PET image with volumes of interest (VOIs) superimposed in (**a**) coronal, (**b**) sagittal, and (**c**) transversal views. The left panel, pig 1, obtained at 42 min post injection (p.i.), shows the organs except for the peripheral bone, whereas the right panel, pig 2, obtained at 56 min. p.i., shows all delineated organs. (The gray scale in the middle refers to the original quantitative PET data, not to the colored VOI structures).

Based on the biokinetic data extracted from the VOI analysis in piglets and the following extrapolation to the human entity (Equations (3) and (4)), the ODs and the ED were estimated for the adult male model. The resulting mean values obtained for 24 organs are presented in Table 1.

Table 1. Complete results of the dose assessment of the three investigated piglets using OLINDA 2.1 (mean value ± standard deviation (SD)).

Target Organ	OD in mSv/MBq	ED Contr. in ± mSv/MBq	ED Contr. in mSv/MBq	SD in ± mSv/MBq
Adrenals	1.42×10^{-2}	5.69×10^{-4}	1.31×10^{-4}	4.73×10^{-6}
Brain	4.69×10^{-3}	8.09×10^{-4}	4.69×10^{-5}	8.09×10^{-6}
Esophagus	9.03×10^{-3}	1.21×10^{-3}	3.61×10^{-4}	4.86×10^{-5}
Eyes	6.91×10^{-3}	1.68×10^{-3}	0.00	0.00
Gall Bladder Wall	5.04×10^{-2}	3.75×10^{-2}	4.65×10^{-4}	3.47×10^{-4}
Left Colon	1.37×10^{-2}	2.91×10^{-3}	6.63×10^{-4}	1.41×10^{-4}
Small Intestine	1.84×10^{-2}	8.44×10^{-3}	1.71×10^{-4}	7.81×10^{-5}
Stomach Wall	1.09×10^{-2}	3.07×10^{-3}	1.31×10^{-3}	3.64×10^{-4}
Right Colon	2.40×10^{-2}	7.40×10^{-3}	1.16×10^{-3}	3.62×10^{-4}
Rectum	1.38×10^{-2}	1.15×10^{-3}	3.18×10^{-4}	2.60×10^{-5}
Heart Wall	9.46×10^{-3}	7.51×10^{-4}	8.72×10^{-5}	6.72×10^{-6}
Kidneys	2.62×10^{-2}	2.19×10^{-3}	2.42×10^{-4}	2.00×10^{-5}
Liver	2.33×10^{-2}	1.36×10^{-2}	9.34×10^{-4}	5.46×10^{-4}
Lungs	7.88×10^{-3}	2.27×10^{-4}	9.46×10^{-4}	2.72×10^{-5}
Pancreas	3.05×10^{-2}	2.73×10^{-2}	2.81×10^{-4}	2.52×10^{-4}
Prostate	1.30×10^{-2}	2.85×10^{-3}	6.01×10^{-5}	1.32×10^{-5}
Salivary Glands	7.90×10^{-3}	2.11×10^{-3}	7.90×10^{-5}	2.11×10^{-5}
Red Marrow	1.39×10^{-2}	2.19×10^{-3}	1.67×10^{-3}	2.63×10^{-4}
Osteogenic Cells	2.12×10^{-2}	1.88×10^{-3}	2.12×10^{-4}	1.88×10^{-5}
Spleen	9.08×10^{-3}	1.14×10^{-3}	8.37×10^{-5}	1.04×10^{-5}
Testes	8.45×10^{-3}	2.21×10^{-3}	3.38×10^{-4}	8.87×10^{-5}
Thymus	8.33×10^{-3}	1.73×10^{-3}	7.69×10^{-5}	1.59×10^{-5}
Thyroid	7.08×10^{-3}	8.70×10^{-4}	2.83×10^{-4}	3.49×10^{-5}
Urinary Bladder Wall	6.26×10^{-2}	2.89×10^{-2}	2.50×10^{-3}	1.15×10^{-3}
Total Body	9.76×10^{-3}	1.53×10^{-3}	0.00	0.00
ED			**12.4×10^{-2}**	

OD = organ equivalent dose; ED contr. = effective dose contribution.

Here, the effective dose (E) represents the tissue-weighted sum of the equivalent doses in all specified tissues and organs of the body (Equation (1)), where H_T is the equivalent dose in the respective tissue or organ, T, and w_T is the tissue weighting factor [20].

$$E = \sum_T w_T \times H_T \left[\frac{mSv}{MBq}\right] \tag{1}$$

The highest OD was received by the urinary bladder (62.6 ± 28.9 μSv/MBq), followed by the gall bladder (50.4 ± 37.5 μSv/MBq), the pancreas (30.5 ± 27.3 μSv/MBq), the kidneys (26.2 ± 2.2 μSv/MBq), the right colon (24.0 ± 7.4 μSv/MBq), and the liver (23.3 ± 13.6 μSv/MBq). When involving the tissue weighting factor w_T, which weights the organ equivalent dose in a tissue or organ to represent the relative contribution of that tissue or organ to the total health risk resulting from uniform irradiation of the body, this ranking changes: the highest contribution to the ED is by the urinary bladder (2.5 ± 1.1 μSv/MBq), followed by the red marrow (1.7 ± 0.3 μSv/MBq), the stomach (1.3 ± 0.4 μSv/MBq), the right colon (1.2 ± 0.4 μSv/MBq), the lungs (0.9 ± 0.05 μSv/MBq), and the liver (0.1 ± 0.05 μSv/MBq). The ED was found to be 12.4 μSv/MBq. According to this preclinically obtained data, a standard injection in humans of 300 MBq [^{18}F]FACH for PET in three-dimensional (3D) mode would result in an ED of about 3.7 mSv. As known from other studies [21], preclinical incorporation dose estimates underrate the ED to humans by up to 40% [14–16]. Taking this into account, the conversion factor to estimate the ED to humans undergoing a clinical PET investigation using [^{18}F]FACH would rise to 20.6 μSv/MBq and finally result in an ED of about 6.2 mSv/300 MBq of administered [^{18}F]FACH.

In comparison to ED values determined for other clinically applied diagnostic radiotracers [21], this risk assessment encourages the translation of [^{18}F]FACH into clinical study phases and the further investigation of its potential as a clinical tool for PET imaging of MCT1/MCT4 in different pathologies, including oncological diseases.

3. Discussion

Due to metabolic reprogramming, highly proliferating cancer cells utilize large amounts of glucose and convert the glucose carbon mainly to lactate to support their anabolic requirements [22–24]. Given the availability of suitable radiolabeled agents, non-invasive molecular imaging by PET enables the investigation of cancer-related alterations in the metabolism of cells. For example, the enhanced uptake of glucose in cancer cells can be monitored by [^{18}F]fluoro-deoxyglucose ([^{18}F]FDG), a substrate of the glucose transporters (GLUT) overexpressed in cancer cells that has been clinically used for more than three decades for diagnosis, staging, and treatment monitoring in oncology [25,26]. Monocarboxylate transporters (MCTs), which mediate the proton-coupled transport of small carboxylic acids such as lactate, the end product of aerobic glycolysis, are also known to be overexpressed in different cancers [27,28]. Accordingly, ^{11}C- or ^{18}F-labeled substrates of MCTs such as [^{18}F]lactate and [^{11}C]pyruvate have already been developed and evaluated regarding their potential to image the expression of MCTs in tumors using PET [10,29,30]. Besides, highly affine and small molecule inhibitors of MCTs designed for targeted cancer therapies also bear the potential for the development of respective imaging agents. In this context, our group has recently reported on the development and evaluation of [^{18}F]FACH as a new MCT-targeting imaging agent possessing high inhibitory potency towards MCT1 and MCT4 [12,13]. For further assessment of the suitability of this radiopharmaceutical in clinical settings, a preclinical dosimetry study is necessary to estimate the doses delivered to humans to ensure the safe usage of [^{18}F]FACH.

According to the data obtained in this study, the overall dose estimate and vital signs monitoring confirm the radiation safety and tolerability of [^{18}F]FACH and support the translation of [^{18}F]FACH to further clinical study phases.

As found for other low-molecular-weight ^{18}F-labeled tracers, which were investigated by our group in recent years (Table 2), the organs involved in the renal as well as the hepatobiliary excretion received the highest ODs. Due to the high initial uptake of activity in the liver, although decreasing over time, the surrounding tissues, such as lung, pancreas, and kidney tissues, are exposed to comparatively high doses and thus belong to the organs contributing mainly to the ED. Furthermore, the increasing concentration in urine results in the high OD and subsequently ED of the urinary bladder wall. Notably, besides being excretory organs, the liver and kidneys are also target organs due to a high expression of MCT1/MCT4 [31–35].

Table 2. Dosimetry results of different PET radiopharmaceuticals preclinically estimated using piglet biokinetic data.

Tracer	Target/Organ	Preclinical (µSv/MBq)	Reference
[^{18}F]FACH	MCT1/4/brain tumor	12.4	this study
[^{18}F]DBT10	α7 receptor/brain tumor	13.7	[22]
(S)-(−)-[^{18}F]fluspidine (R)-(+)-[^{18}F]fluspidine	σ receptor/brain	12.9 14.0	[15]
(−)-[^{18}F]flubatine (+)-[^{18}F]flubatine	α4β2 receptor/brain	14.7 14.3	[16] [14]

A limitation of this preclinical study is that the piglets did not void during the entire imaging phase, which results in a simplification of the data analysis. As the voiding bladder model implemented in the OLINDA software cannot be applied, the dose estimation for the wall of the urinary bladder is purely imaging based and uses data based on a continuously filling bladder over the imaging time (see Figure 1). Therefore, to reduce the dose to this dose-limiting organ in humans, participants of clinical studies should be instructed to void the bladder before and immediately after each imaging session.

Another limitation of this study is related to the increasing uptake of activity in the bones. Anatomically, high amounts of the red marrow are found not only in the backbone, sternum, and pelvis but also in the epiphyseal plates of the peripheral bone of juvenile piglets, because bone growth is not yet complete. Hence, target-specific accumulation of activity due to physiological expression of MCTs in erythrocytes produced by the red bone marrow [36,37] may contribute to comparatively high ODs and finally explain the high ED contribution of bone marrow. In addition, accumulation of [^{18}F]fluoride is indicated by the radio-chromatographic analysis of plasma samples obtained during the PET imaging study (data are not shown).

Furthermore, a limitation of preclinical dosimetry studies is that the animals usually have to be anesthetized. Depending on the target of the tracer under investigation, anesthesia will have an influence on biodistribution and biokinetics. In this study, however, the anesthesia should have had a rather secondary influence. First and foremost, the anesthesia as described does not affect MCT1/MCT4 transporter inhibitors. It does act in the central nervous system (mainly the brain). With our protocol, we maintained a rather shallow anesthesia so that the animals respired spontaneously. Thus, the alterations of the biodistribution and biokinetics of [^{18}F]FACH by this anesthesia should have had a rather small influence on the dosimetry result. We expect a slight general deceleration of the metabolism, particularly that of the gastro-intestinal tract, just as while sleeping very deeply. However, animal anesthesia is generally necessary to render preclinical incorporation dosimetry possible. Although it is a well-known limitation of preclinical dosimetry studies, it does not invalidate their results. Moreover, alongside the other limitations of preclinical dosimetry described, it will be part of the comparison once clinical data have been acquired and be involved in the (up)scaling of preclinical ED results for the assessment of the ED to humans by a particular radiotracer.

4. Materials and Methods

4.1. *Synthesis of [^{18}F]FACH*

The radiosynthesis of [^{18}F]FACH has recently been published [38]. Briefly, [^{18}F]FACH is produced via a one-step radiosynthesis approach by using a mesylate precursor bearing an unprotected carboxylic acid function and the Kryptofix 2.2.2/K_2CO_3/[^{18}F]F-complex system. Isolation of [^{18}F]FACH was performed by semi-preparative HPLC (Reprosil-Pur C18-AQ column, 250 × 10 mm, 10 μm, 50% CH_3CN/20 mM NH_4HCO_2 (aq.), pH = 4–4.5, flow 3.5 mL/min). The tracer (chemical structure shown in Figure 4) was finally purified via solid-phase extraction (Sep-Pak® C18 light cartridge) and formulated in 10% EtOH/saline solution with molar activities in the range of 50–120 GBq/μmol (n = 8, at the end of synthesis) using starting activities of 1–3 GBq.

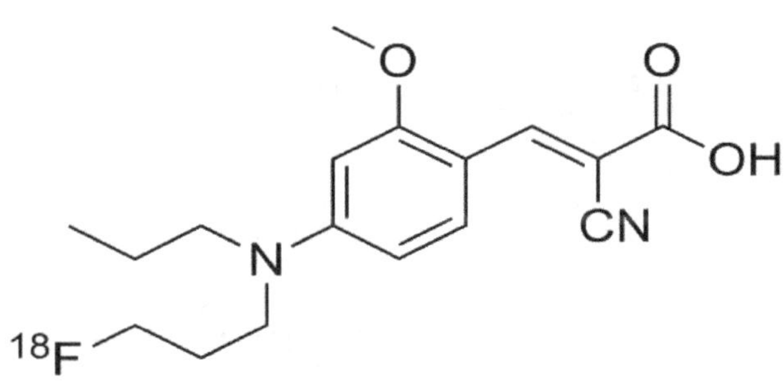

Figure 4. Chemical structure of [^{18}F]FACH.

4.2. *Preclinical Dosimetry Studies—In Vivo PET/CT Imaging in Pigs*

All animal experiments were approved by the responsible institutional and federal state authorities (Landesdirektion Leipzig; TVV 18/18, Reference Number DD24.1-5131/446/19).

Three piglets (age: ~6 weeks, weight: ~13–15 kg) were fasted on the day of imaging and received an intranuscular. injection of 1 mL azaperone and 4 mL ketamine to introduce anesthesia. After 15 min, 2 mL of ketamine and 1 mL of midazolam (5 mg/mL) were iv injected (ear vein, V. auricularis), followed by 5 mL of G40, 3 mL of ketamine, and 1.5 mL of midazolam in 50 mL of NaCl 0.9% with an infusion pump at a flow rate of 37.5 mL/h to maintain the narcosis throughout the entire investigation time. During narcosis, the animals maintained spontaneous respiration and no mandatory ventilation was applied. The subjects were sequentially imaged after an iv injection (contralateral ear vein) of 156 ± 54 MBq [^{18}F]FACH (0.63 ± 0.49 μg) in a PET/CT system (Biograph16, SIEMENS, Erlangen, Germany). The piglets were positioned prone with legs alongside the body on a custom-made plastic trough including a piglet head-holder (Figure 5). The PET acquisition was divided into a sequential (4 × 9 min, 3 × 12 min) and a static part (1 × 24 min, 1 × 30 min, 1 × 36 min), each of which was preceded by a low-dose CT to acquire structural data for attenuation correction (AC) and anatomical orientation (Figure 6). Post mortem, the urine was collected by bladder punctuation, weighted, and divided into three 1 mL samples for activity measurements in a gamma-counter (Packard Cobra II 5003 Auto Gamma Counting System, GMI, Ramsey, MN, USA).

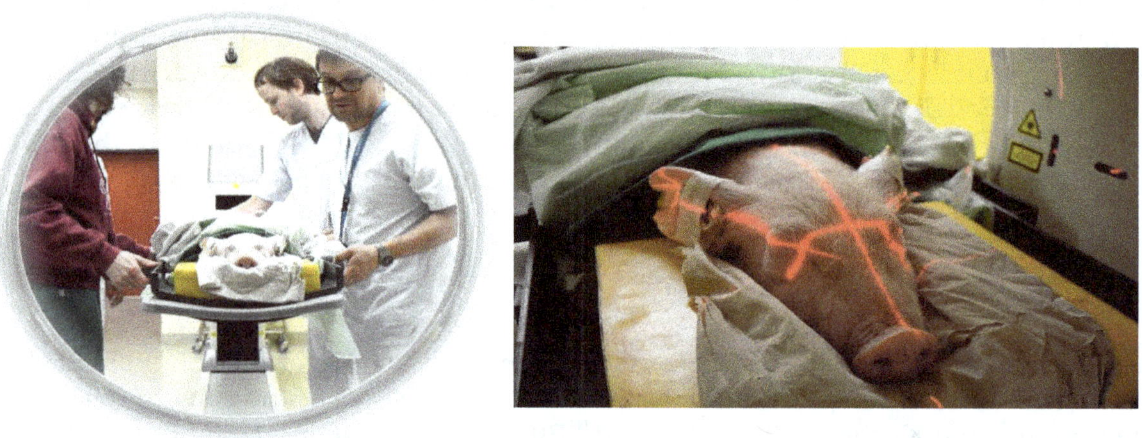

Figure 5. The animals were placed in a plastic trough and a special head rest to guarantee reproducible positioning and avoid the movement of artefacts.

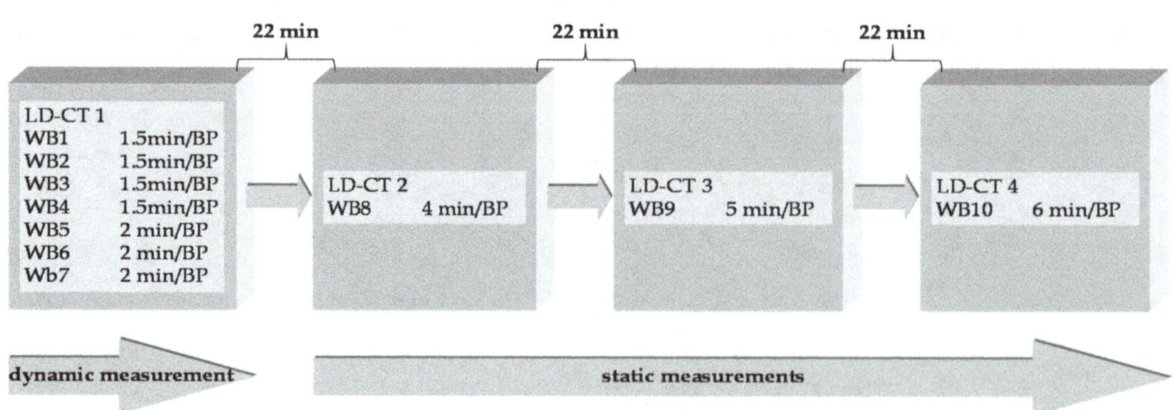

Figure 6. PET/CT imaging protocol comprising a dynamic and static part with increasing duration per bed position (BP) to compensate for decay and, thus, decreasing count statistics, preceded by a low-dose CT (LD-CT) for attenuation correction and anatomical orientation, respectively. Positioning of the animal in the PET field of view.

PET data reconstruction was done using low-dose CT attenuation correction (AC) and an iterative OSEM algorithm with 4 iterations and 8 subsets. As the PET/CT system is in daily clinical use, it is periodically subjected to detector normalization and activity calibration. Furthermore, all peripheral activity-measuring devices to be used for the investigation (dose calibrator, gamma counter) are cross-calibrated in terms of timing and a radioactivity adjustment.

4.3. Image Analysis

The image data were analyzed with ROVER (ABX, Radeberg, Germany; v. 3.0.46h). The organs were identified and manually delineated using 3D volumes of interest (VOI). The CT data were used for anatomical orientation and for image registration with the PET data. Relevant source organs like brain, gall bladder, large intestine, small intestine, stomach, heart, kidneys, liver, lungs, pancreas, red marrow (backbone, pelvis, sternum), spleen, thyroid, testes, skeleton (bone), and the urinary bladder were delineated and the time–activity data transformed into percentage of injected dose ($\%ID_{organ}$) with Equation (2).

$$\%ID_{organ_t} = \frac{A_{organ_t} \times c_{scant}}{A_{0t}} \; [\%] \tag{2}$$

where A_{organ_t} is the activity in the organ at the time t; c_{scant} is a calibration factor representing the theoretical body activity (derived from a whole body mask of a volume that equals the body dimentions of the animal) decay corrected to t and divided by the imaged body activity in each image frame at the time t, and A_{0t} is the injected activity decay corrected to t_0.

4.4. Incorporation Dosimetry

The dose calculation has been described by our group in detail before [14–16]. Briefly, due to differences in weight, size, and metabolic rates between the animal species and the human volunteers, it is necessary to map the preclinical extracted biodistribution data to human circumstances. Thus, the animal biokinetic data (time scale and $\%ID$ values) were adapted to the human circumstances according to [22] to fit the human weight, size, and metabolic rates (Equations (3) and (4)).

$$t_{human} = t_{animal}\left[\frac{m_{human}}{m_{animal}}\right]^{0.25} \tag{3}$$

$$[\%ID]/organ_{human} = [\%ID]/g_{animal} \times \frac{m_{TB_{animal}}[g]}{m_{TB_{human}}[g]} \times m_{organ_{human}}[g] \tag{4}$$

The TIACs were estimated by exponential fitting and the dosimetry estimation was performed using OLINDA/EXM software (v. 2.1). Finally, organ doses (OD) were estimated and multiplied by tissue weighting factors as published in ICRP103 [20].

5. Conclusions

By extrapolation of the preclinical dosimetry data obtained in piglets, the effective dose as a measure of the overall radiation risk upon iv application of about 300 MBq [^{18}F]FACH to humans is estimated to be 3.7 mSv. However, as frequently observed for other PET tracers, the preclinical dosimetry underestimates the ED to humans by up to 40%. Accordingly, we conclude that the ED to humans by [^{18}F]FACH can be expected to be about 20.6 μSv/MBq. With a systemic application of 300 MBq, PET imaging with [^{18}F]FACH would yield an effective dose of about 6.2 mSv to human subjects. This value is well within the range of other ^{18}F-labeled radiopharmaceuticals. Despite the study-specific overestimation of the contributions of bone and the urinary bladder to the ED, this risk assessment encourages the transference of [^{18}F]FACH from preclinical to clinical study phases to further assess the suitability of this new radiopharmaceutical for PET imaging of oncological diseases.

Author Contributions: B.S., M.K., M.S., P.B., W.D.-C., and O.S. conceived and designed the experiments; M.K., W.D.-C., M.T., N.T.J., C.D., T.S., and B.S. performed the experiments; B.S., M.K., N.T.J., and O.S. analyzed the data; B.S., M.K., M.S., T.S., W.D.-C., O.S., and P.B. drafted the manuscript; M.S., R.-P.M., and P.B. designed the molecule and performed the organic chemistry; M.S., B.W., and R.T. performed the radiosynthesis; B.W., M.S., R.T., and F.-A.L. performed the metabolite analysis; T.S. handled the animals, conducted and maintained their anesthesia, and took all the blood and urine samples. All authors have read and agreed to the published version of the manuscript.

Acknowledgments: We are very thankful to K. Franke, A. Mansel, and S. Fischer for providing [^{18}F]fluoride.

References

1. Warburg, O. On the origin of cancer cells. *Science* **1956**, *123*, 309–314. [CrossRef] [PubMed]
2. Ponisovskiy, M.R. Warburg effect mechanism as the target for theoretical substantiation of a new potential cancer treatment. *Crit. Rev. Eukaryot. Gene Expr.* **2011**, *21*, 13–28. [CrossRef] [PubMed]
3. Koppenol, W.H.; Bounds, P.L.; Dang, C.V. Otto Warburg's contributions to current concepts of cancer metabolism. *Nat. Rev. Cancer* **2011**, *11*, 325. [CrossRef] [PubMed]
4. Halestrap, A.P. The SLC16 gene family–structure, role and regulation in health and disease. *Mol. Asp. Med.* **2013**, *34*, 337–349. [CrossRef]
5. Pinheiro, C.; Longatto-Filho, A.; Azevedo-Silva, J.; Casal, M.; Schmitt, F.C.; Baltazar, F. Role of monocarboxylate transporters in human cancers: State of the art. *J. Bioenerg. Biomembr.* **2012**, *44*, 127–139. [CrossRef]
6. Gurrapu, S.; Jonnalagadda, S.K.; Alam, M.A.; Nelson, G.L.; Sneve, M.G.; Drewes, L.R.; Mereddy, V.R. Monocarboxylate transporter 1 inhibitors as potential anticancer agents. *ACS Med. Chem. Lett.* **2015**, *6*, 558–561. [CrossRef]
7. Fang, J.; Quinones, Q.J.; Holman, T.L.; Morowitz, M.J.; Wang, Q.; Zhao, H.; Sivo, F.; Maris, J.M.; Wahl, M.L. The H+-linked monocarboxylate transporter (MCT1/SLC16A1): A potential therapeutic target for high-risk neuroblastoma. *Mol. Pharmacol.* **2006**, *70*, 2108–2115. [CrossRef]
8. Park, S.J.; Smith, C.P.; Wilbur, R.R.; Cain, C.P.; Kallu, S.R.; Valasapalli, S.; Sahoo, A.; Guda, M.R.; Tsung, A.J.; Velpula, K.K. An overview of MCT1 and MCT4 in GBM: Small molecule transporters with large implications. *Am. J. Cancer Res.* **2018**, *8*, 1967.
9. Payen, V.L.; Mina, E.; van Hée, V.F.; Porporato, P.E.; Sonveaux, P. Monocarboxylate transporters in cancer. *Mol. Metab.* **2020**, *33*, 48–66. [CrossRef]
10. van Hée, V.F.; Labar, D.; Dehon, G.; Grasso, D.; Grégoire, V.; Muccioli, G.G.; Frédérick, R.; Sonveaux, P. Radiosynthesis and validation of (±)-[^{18}F]-3-fluoro-2-hydroxypropionate ([^{18}F]-FLac) as a PET tracer of lactate to monitor MCT1-dependent lactate uptake in tumors. *Oncotarget* **2017**, *8*, 24415. [CrossRef]
11. Tateishi, H.; Tsuji, A.B.; Kato, K.; Sudo, H.; Sugyo, A.; Hanakawa, T.; Zhang, M.-R.; Saga, T.; Arano, Y.; Higashi, T. Synthesis and evaluation of ^{11}C-labeled coumarin analog as an imaging probe for detecting monocarboxylate transporters expression. *Bioorganic Med. Chem. Lett.* **2017**, *27*, 4893–4897. [CrossRef] [PubMed]
12. Sadeghzadeh, M.; Moldovan, R.-P.; Fischer, S.; Wenzel, B.; Ludwig, F.-A.; Teodoro, R.; Deuther-Conrad, W.; Jonnalagadda, S.; Jonnalagadda, S.K.; Gudelis, E.; et al. Development and radiosynthesis of the first ^{18}F-labeled inhibitor of monocarboxylate transporters (MCTs). *J. Label. Comp. Radiopharm.* **2019**, *62*, 411–424. [CrossRef] [PubMed]
13. Sadeghzadeh, M.; Moldovan, R.-P.; Wenzel, B.; Kranz, M.; Deuther-Conrad, W.; Toussaint, M.; Fischer, S.; Ludwig, F.-A.; Teodoro, R.; Jonnalagadda, S.K.; et al. Development of the first ^{18}F-labeled MCT1/MCT4 lactate transport inhibitor: Radiosynthesis and preliminary in vivo evaluation in mice. *J. Label. Comp. Radiopharm.* **2019**, *62*, S59–S60. [CrossRef] [PubMed]
14. Kranz, M.; Sattler, B.; Tiepolt, S.; Wilke, S.; Deuther-Conrad, W.; Donat, C.K.; Fischer, S.; Patt, M.; Schildan, A.; Patt, J. Radiation dosimetry of the $\alpha 4 \beta 2$ nicotinic receptor ligand (+)-[^{18}F] flubatine, comparing preclinical PET/MRI and PET/CT to first-in-human PET/CT results. *EJNMMI Phys.* **2016**, *3*, 25. [CrossRef] [PubMed]

15. Kranz, M.; Sattler, B.; Wüst, N.; Deuther-Conrad, W.; Patt, M.; Meyer, P.; Fischer, S.; Donat, C.; Wünsch, B.; Hesse, S. Evaluation of the enantiomer specific biokinetics and radiation doses of [^{18}F] fluspidine—A new tracer in clinical translation for imaging of σ1 receptors. *Molecules* **2016**, *21*, 1164. [CrossRef] [PubMed]
16. Sattler, B.; Kranz, M.; Starke, A.; Wilke, S.; Donat, C.K.; Deuther-Conrad, W.; Patt, M.; Schildan, A.; Patt, J.; Smits, R. Internal Dose assessment of (–)-^{18}F-flubatine, comparing animal model datasets of mice and piglets with first-in-human results. *J. Nucl. Med.* **2014**, *55*, 1885–1892. [CrossRef]
17. Stabin, M.G.; Siegel, J.A. RADAR dose estimate report: A compendium of radiopharmaceutical dose estimates based on OLINDA/EXM version 2.0. *J. Nucl. Med.* **2018**, *59*, 154–160. [CrossRef]
18. McParland, B.J. *Nuclear Medicine Radiation Dosimetry: Advanced Theoretical Principles*; Springer: London, UK, 2010; ISBN 978-184-882-1262.
19. Stabin, M.G. *Fundamentals of Nuclear Medicine Dosimetry*; Springer: New York, NY, USA, 2008; ISBN 978-038-774-5794.
20. Valentin, J. *The 2007 Recommendations of the International Commission on Radiological Protection*; Elsevier: Oxford, UK, 2007; Volume 37, pp. 1–133. [CrossRef]
21. Zanotti-Fregonara, P.; Lammertsma, A.A.; Innis, R.B. Suggested pathway to assess radiation safety of 18 F-labeled PET tracers for first-in-human studies. *Eur. J. Nucl. Med. Mol. Imaging* **2013**, *40*, 1781–1783. [CrossRef]
22. Kranz, M.; Sattler, B.; Deuther-Conrad, W.; Teodoro, R.; Donat, C.; Wenzel, B.; Scheunemann, M.; Patt, M.; Sabri, O.; Brust, P. Preclinical dose assessment and biodistribution of [^{18}F]DBT10, a new $\alpha7$ nicotinic acetylcholine receptor ($\alpha7$-nAChR) imaging ligand. *J. Nucl. Med.* **2014**, *55*, 1143.
23. Tennant, D.A.; Durán, R.V.; Gottlieb, E. Targeting metabolic transformation for cancer therapy. *Nat. Rev. Cancer* **2010**, *10*, 267–277. [CrossRef]
24. Ward, P.S.; Thompson, C.B. Metabolic reprogramming: A cancer hallmark even warburg did not anticipate. *Cancer Cell* **2012**, *21*, 297–308. [CrossRef] [PubMed]
25. O'Neill, H.; Malik, V.; Johnston, C.; Reynolds, J.V.; O'Sullivan, J. Can the efficacy of ^{18}FFDG-PET/CT in clinical oncology be enhanced by screening biomolecular profiles? *Pharmaceuticals (Basel)* **2019**, *12*, 16. [CrossRef] [PubMed]
26. Endo, K.; Oriuchi, N.; Higuchi, T.; Iida, Y.; Hanaoka, H.; Miyakubo, M.; Ishikita, T.; Koyama, K. PET and PET/CT using ^{18}F-FDG in the diagnosis and management of cancer patients. *Int. J. Clin. Oncol.* **2006**, *11*, 286–296. [CrossRef] [PubMed]
27. Payen, V.L.; Hsu, M.Y.; Rädecke, K.S.; Wyart, E.; Vazeille, T.; Bouzin, C.; Porporato, P.E.; Sonveaux, P. Monocarboxylate transporter MCT1 promotes tumor metastasis independently of its activity as a lactate transporter. *Cancer Res.* **2017**, *77*, 5591–5601. [CrossRef]
28. Jones, R.S.; Morris, M.E. Monocarboxylate transporters: Therapeutic targets and prognostic factors in disease. *Clin. Pharmacol. Ther.* **2016**, *100*, 454–463. [CrossRef]
29. Herrero, P.; Dence, C.S.; Coggan, A.R.; Kisrieva-Ware, Z.; Eisenbeis, P.; Gropler, R.J. L-3-^{11}C-lactate as a PET tracer of myocardial lactate metabolism: A feasibility study. *J. Nucl. Med.* **2007**, *48*, 2046–2055. [CrossRef] [PubMed]
30. Yokoi, F.; Hara, T.; Iio, M.; Nonaka, I.; Satoyoshi, E. 1-^{11}Cpyruvate turnover in brain and muscle of patients with mitochondrial encephalomyopathy. A study with positron emission tomography (PET). *J. Neurol. Sci.* **1990**, *99*, 339–348. [CrossRef]
31. Koho, N.; Maijala, V.; Norberg, H.; Nieminen, M.; Pösö, A.R. Expression of MCT1, MCT2 and MCT4 in the rumen, small intestine and liver of reindeer (Rangifer tarandus tarandus L.). *Comp. Biochem. Physiol. Part A Mol. Integr. Physiol.* **2005**, *141*, 29–34. [CrossRef]
32. de Araujo, G.G.; Gobatto, C.A.; de Barros Manchado-Gobatto, F.; Teixeira, L.F.; Dos Reis, I.G.; Caperuto, L.C.; Papoti, M.; Bordin, S.; Cavaglieri, C.R.; Verlengia, R. MCT1 and MCT4 kinetic of mRNA expression in different tissues after aerobic exercise at maximal lactate steady state workload. *Physiol. Res.* **2015**, *64*, 513–522. [CrossRef]
33. Sepponen, K.; Ruusunen, M.; Pakkanen, J.A.; Pösö, A.R. Expression of CD147 and monocarboxylate transporters MCT1, MCT2 and MCT4 in porcine small intestine and colon. *Vet. J.* **2007**, *174*, 122–128. [CrossRef]
34. Becker, H.M.; Mohebbi, N.; Perna, A.; Ganapathy, V.; Capasso, G.; Wagner, C.A. Localization of members of

MCT monocarboxylate transporter family Slc16 in the kidney and regulation during metabolic acidosis. *Am. J. Physiol. Renal Physiol.* **2010**, *299*, F141–F154. [CrossRef] [PubMed]

35. Wang, Q.; Lu, Y.; Yuan, M.; Darling, I.M.; Repasky, E.A.; Morris, M.E. Characterization of monocarboxylate transport in human kidney HK-2 cells. *Mol. Pharm.* **2006**, *3*, 675–685. [CrossRef] [PubMed]
36. Deuticke, B. Monocarboxylate transport in erythrocytes. *J. Membr. Biol.* **1982**, *70*, 89–103. [CrossRef] [PubMed]
37. Poole, R.C.; Cranmer, S.L.; Halestrap, A.P.; Levi, A.J. Substrate and inhibitor specificity of monocarboxylate transport into heart cells and erythrocytes. Further evidence for the existence of two distinct carriers. *Biochem. J.* **1990**, *269*, 827–829. [CrossRef] [PubMed]
38. Sadeghzadeh, M.; Moldovan, R.-P.; Teodoro, R.; Brust, P.; Wenzel, B. One-step radiosynthesis of the MCTs imaging agent [^{18}F]FACH by aliphatic ^{18}F-labelling of a methylsulfonate precursor containing an unprotected carboxylic acid group. *Sci. Rep.* **2019**, *9*, 18890. [CrossRef] [PubMed]

Metabolic Brain Network Analysis of FDG-PET in Alzheimer's Disease Using Kernel-Based Persistent Features

Liqun Kuang [1,*], Deyu Zhao [1], Jiacheng Xing [2], Zhongyu Chen [3], Fengguang Xiong [1] and Xie Han [1,*]

[1] School of Data Science and Technology, North University of China, Taiyuan 030051, China; 1307084309@st.nuc.edu.cn (D.Z.); hopenxfg@nuc.edu.cn (F.X.)

[2] School of Software, Nanchang University, Nanchang 330047, China; xingjiacheng628@163.com

[3] School of Software, East China Jiaotong University, Nanchang 330013, China; 15079561913@139.com

* Correspondence: kuang@nuc.edu.cn (L.K.); hanxie@nuc.edu.cn (X.H.)

Academic Editor: Peter Brust

Abstract: Recent research of persistent homology in algebraic topology has shown that the altered network organization of human brain provides a promising indicator of many neuropsychiatric disorders and neurodegenerative diseases. However, the current slope-based approach may not accurately characterize changes of persistent features over graph filtration because such curves are not strictly linear. Moreover, our previous integrated persistent feature (IPF) works well on an rs-fMRI cohort while it has not yet been studied on metabolic brain networks. To address these issues, we propose a novel univariate network measurement, kernel-based IPF (KBI), based on the prior IPF, to quantify the difference between IPF curves. In our experiments, we apply the KBI index to study fluorodeoxyglucose positron emission tomography (FDG-PET) imaging data from 140 subjects with Alzheimer's disease (AD), 280 subjects with mild cognitive impairment (MCI), and 280 healthy normal controls (NC). The results show the disruption of network integration in the progress of AD. Compared to previous persistent homology-based measures, as well as other standard graph-based measures that characterize small-world organization and modular structure, our proposed network index KBI possesses more significant group difference and better classification performance, suggesting that it may be used as an effective preclinical AD imaging biomarker.

Keywords: Alzheimer's disease (AD); network measure; graph theory; brain network; positron emission tomography (PET); persistent homology

---

1. Introduction

Alzheimer's disease (AD) is one of the most common neurodegenerative neurological diseases and is the most common form of dementia in the elderly [1]. Its clinical manifestations include long-term memory loss, cognitive decline, language disorders, and other symptoms. AD seriously affects the normal life of the elderly. However, the pathology of AD is not yet clear [1]. Some existing imaging technologies are used to explore the mechanisms of human brain function. Compared to magnetic resonance imaging (MRI), fluorodeoxyglucose positron emission tomography (FDG-PET) has been demonstrated to be a more precise predictor of both AD and mild cognitive impairment (MCI), and is more suitable for monitoring disease progression [2]. It collects and measures changes in glucose metabolism values in brain regions or local brain cells. The signals are then converted into effective three-dimensional images and the connectivity between brain regions are analyzed.

The topological organization of metabolic brain networks have been successfully characterized in many cases using various measures based on graph theory [3–5], such as characteristic path length

(CPL) [6], global efficiency [7], modularity (Mod) [7,8], and network diameter (ND) [9], to name but a few. Specifically, in patients with AD and MCI, several research groups have reported topological alterations in the whole-brain connectome, including a loss of small-worldness [10], a redistribution of hubs [9,11], and a disrupted modular organization [12]. Traditionally, weighted networks usually require defining a set of thresholding values before quantifying network topology [13–15], which may result in inconsistent network features when the thresholding values vary. Generally, the choice of threshold is rather arbitrary and there are no widely accepted criteria [16,17].

Recently, persistent homology [18] in algebraic topology has been studied to detect persistent structures generated over all possible thresholds [19–23] in brain network analysis. There have been significant efforts to model evolution of brain networks and to link network topology to network dynamics. This method constructs multiscale network for all possible thresholds wherever the persistent topological features over the evolution of the network changes are identified. Its ability to handle noisy data and provide homological information has turned it into a successful tool for the analysis of brain network structures [24]. One typical application of persistent homology is in a Betti number plot (BNP) [18], which has been successfully applied to the brain network research on epilepsy [20], autism spectrum disorder, and attention-deficit hyperactivity disorder [19,23]. As BNP ignores the association between persistent features and forthcoming thresholding value changes, we proposed an integrated persistent feature (IPF) by integrating an additional feature of connected component aggregation cost with BNP, and applied it to measure an AD network using resting state functional MRI (rs-fMRI) in our prior study [25]. However, both BNP and IPF applied linear regression analysis for computing the slope of the plot over all thresholds as a univariate network index. Such a slope-based approach may not accurately characterize the changes of persistent features over graph filtration because the curves are not strictly linear. Moreover, our previous IPF works well on an rs-fMRI cohort though it has not been used to study metabolic brain networks yet.

In this paper, we borrow the idea of kernel methods [26,27] on persistent homology and propose a kernel-based IPF (KBI) index based on our prior work on IPF. We hypothesized that our KBI index may help to better reveal the difference between brain networks. With the cross-sectional FDG-PET imaging data of 140 AD, 280 MCI, and 280 normal control (NC) individuals, we set out to test this hypothesis by computing the KBI indices that measure the differences between AD, MCI, and NC groups. We further perform statistical inference and classification to validate the power of KBI.

2. Results

In this section, we use FDG-PET data to evaluate statistical power and classification performance of our proposed KBI index for the analysis of brain metabolic networks related to AD. We further compared it with prior persistent features, BNP [19,21,23] and SIP [25], as well as some other standard graph-based indices.

2.1. Metabolic Brain Networks

After data preprocessing, the summarized point cloud were extracted from PET 3D imaging using predefined automated anatomical labeling atlas with 90 (AAL-90) regions of interests (ROI) [28]. We obtained the SUV matrix for all 700 subjects in all 90 ROIs and plot three histograms, in Figure 1, to show the global distributions of FDG uptake in AD, MCI, and NC. As the number of AD is half of MCI and NC, we have normalized the SUV distribution of AD by doubling its statistics. We observed that the AD cohort has lower glucose metabolism than MCI and NC, but no significant differences were detected in the statistical inference of permutation test. We calculated the Pearson-based correlation distance of FDG uptake between each pair of brain regions using Equation (1) and constructed group-wise brain metabolic networks. The three multiscale networks of AD, MCI, and NC groups are shown in Figure 2, which visualizes the evolution of brain networks over different thresholds.

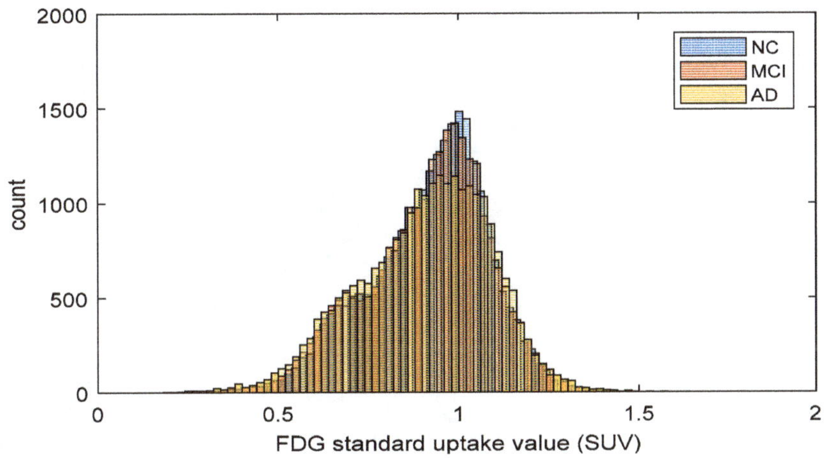

Figure 1. The fluorodeoxyglucose (FDG) uptake distribution of AD, MCI, and NC groups.

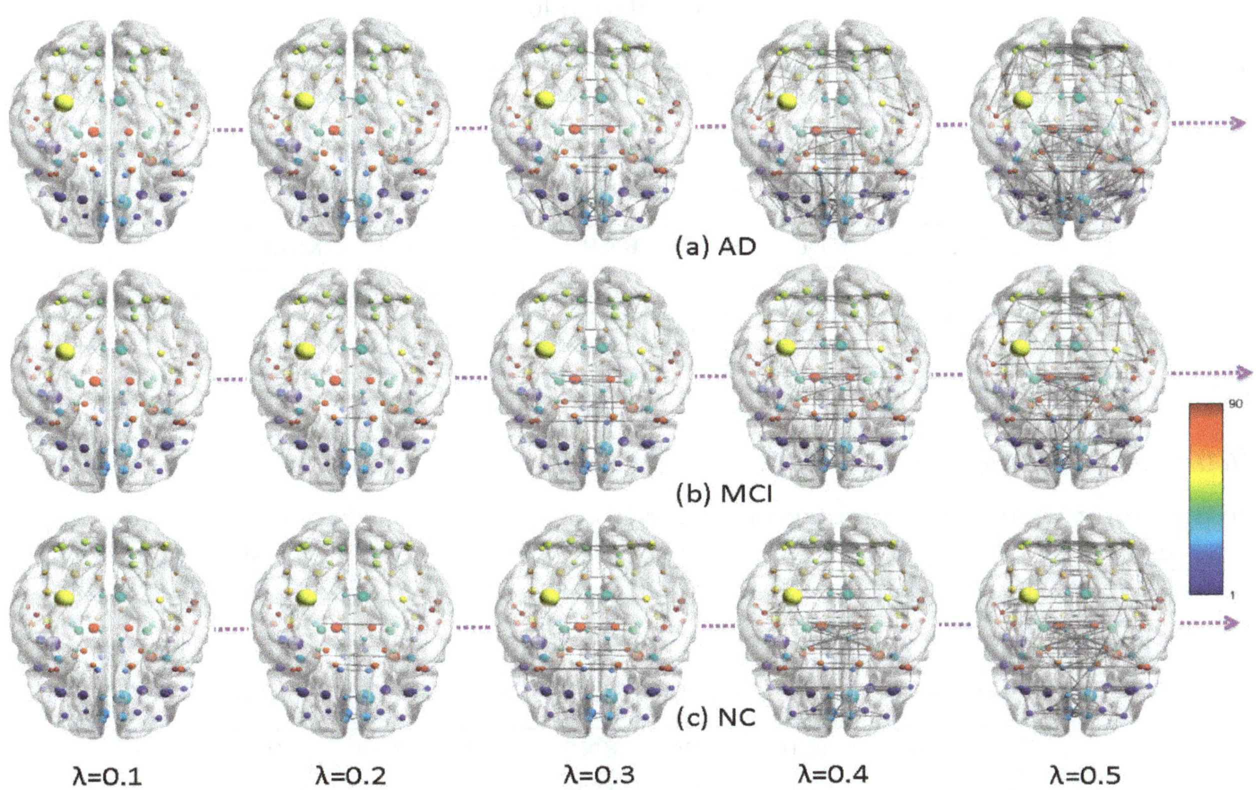

Figure 2. The constructed multiscale networks of AD, MCI, and NC by graph filtration λ, and the node color represents the ROI index predefined in AAL-90 atlas.

2.2. Brain Network Features

We computed the values of graph-based network indices (CPL, ND, and Mod) in three groups based on their weighted networks after filtering their edges, whose corresponding p-values passed a statistical threshold (Bonferroni corrected $p < 0.05$). We then obtained the multiscale network according to graph filtration and computed the BNP and IPF index (i.e., SIP), as well as KBI index. Figure 3 shows three separate IPF plots of AD, MCI, and NC. All brain network index values are shown in Table 1. The differences between groups need to be further verified by statistical inference and classification.

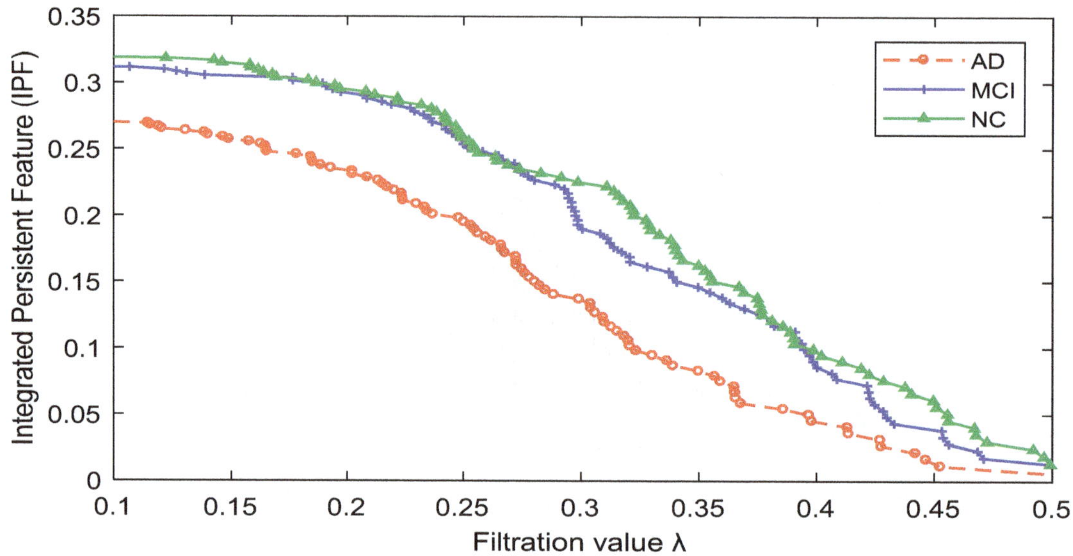

Figure 3. The proposed integrated persistent feature (IPF) plot for three group-wise networks of AD, MCI and NC, respectively.

Table 1. The network index values of three groups.

Cohort	KBI	SIP	BNP	CPL	ND	Mod
AD	0.577	0.790	268.7	1.20	1.601	1.289
MCI	0.826	0.842	265.2	1.17	1.457	0.770
NC	0.988	0.882	245.5	1.15	1.436	1.004

2.3. *Statistical Group Difference Performance*

In this study, we use the permutation test for 10,000 permutations between any two groups, and show the resulting p-value in Table 2. Only the proposed KBI index obtained a significant difference in any between-group at the significance level of 0.05.

Table 2. Statistical p-values for between-group differences by different graph indices on an AAL-90 atlas.

Cohort	KBI	SIP	BNP	CPL	ND	Mod
AD vs. MCI	**0.017**	0.036	0.048	0.058	0.397	0.074
AD vs. NC	**0.002**	0.042	0.054	0.285	0.266	0.063
MCI vs. NC	0.036	0.076	0.339	0.062	**0.031**	0.458

Only the proposed KBI index detected significant difference in any between-group (any p-value < 0.05).

2.4. *Classification Performance*

Furthermore, we resampled the networks 5000 times for each group with the resampling rate of 0.5, and obtained 5000 values of each network index for each group. We then performed leave-one-out crossvalidation to evaluate the classification powers of two-label (Figures 4 and 5) and three-label (Figure 6) by SVM. Our KBI shows better classification performance than prior persistent features, SIP and BNP, as well as other standard graph-based features, including CPL, ND, and Mod.

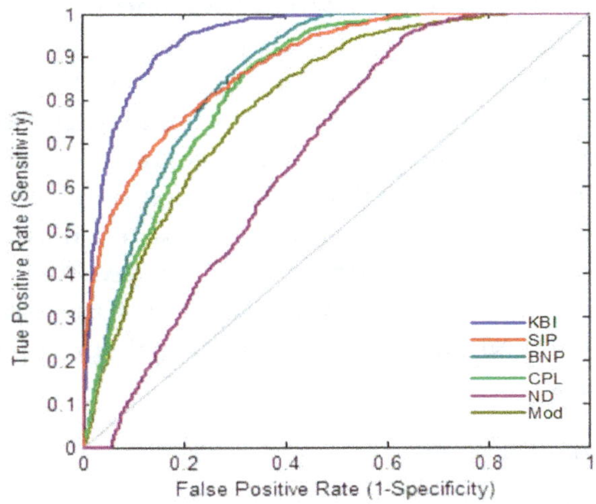

Figure 4. Comparison of ROC curves of different network indices for MCI vs. NC.

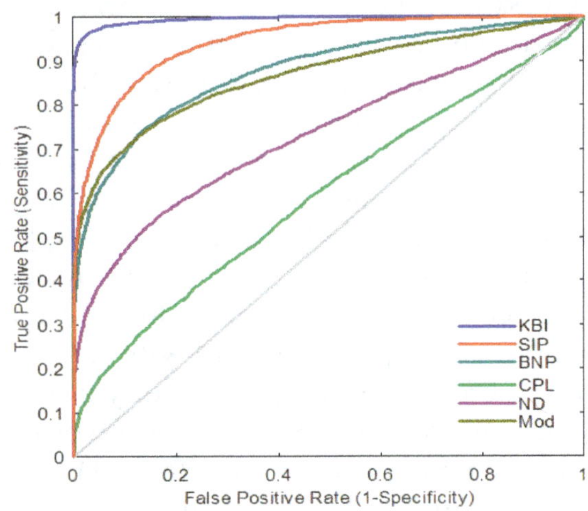

Figure 5. Comparisons of ROC curves of different network indices for AD vs. NC.

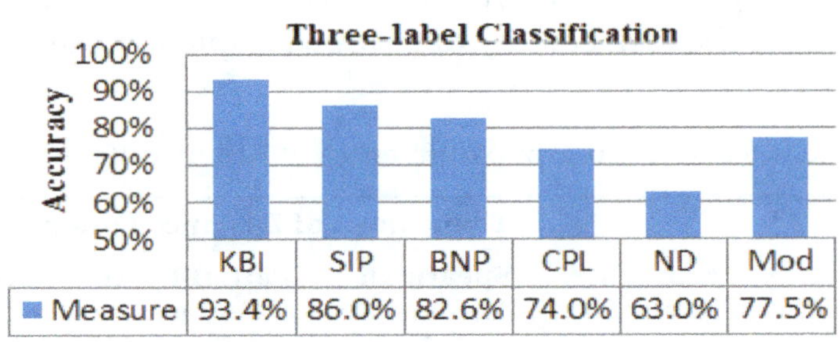

Figure 6. Three-label classification.

3. Discussion

3.1. Present Findings

This study has three main findings.

First, from Figure 1, we found that the AD cohort has lower glucose metabolism than MCI and NC. This may imply cognitive impairment in AD and MCI. Such an inference is further partly confirmed by graph theory analysis because a larger CPL is present in AD and MCI, while the network with smaller CPL is considered to be efficient.

Second, in our previous study [25], we had developed a univariate network index, SIP, based on homology to model graph dynamics over all possible scales and applied it to study the rs-fMRI data of

AD. We found the SIP values of AD were lower than MCI and much lower than NC. In the current PET data, we still find the SIP values show the same pattern AD < MCI < NC, suggesting a slower network integration rate in AD and MCI groups. Thus, the results from both independent cohorts provide consistent empirical evidence for decreased functional integration in AD dementia and MCI.

Finally, we propose a novel univariate network index KBI to enhance our previous study based on persistent homology. With our univariate KBI index, the difference of persistent features between cognitive dysfunction and NC brain network can be measured more accurately. Our preliminary experimental results demonstrate that the proposed KBI may greatly boost prior SIP and BNP power in both statistical inference and classification analyses. The KBI also outperforms other standard graph-based methods, such as CPL, ND, and Mod, suggesting that our method may serve as a valuable preclinical AD imaging biomarker.

3.2. Exploring Other Connectivity Definitions

There are many types of distance functions to construct weighted networks in brain network analysis [29], such as Pearson correlation, partial correlation, psycho–physiological interactions, ReHo, partial least squares, wavelet-based correlation, mutual information, synchronization likelihood, principal component analysis, independent component analysis, cluster analysis, dynamic causal modeling, Granger causality modeling, structural equation modeling, and multivariate autoregressive modeling, among others. At present, it is difficult to put forward the evaluation criteria of these methods, and few studies have compared them comprehensively. Although the Pearson correlation that we used in this study may be the most practical scheme to define the connectome in AD studies, there is still debate about the choice of connectivity definition [29,30]. Therefore, we performed four other connectivity definitions to explore more potentials in defining connectivity network. They were Kendall correlation [31], Spearman correlation [32], partial least squares [33], and Granger causality modeling [34]. The obtained p-values of our proposed KBI with these distance functions are shown in Table 3. There was no significant difference if Granger causality modeling was used, while the other three methods detected at least one significant difference. It should be noted that none of these methods performed significantly better than Pearson correlation (Table 1) in our current dataset. Moreover, when we checked all measures to discriminate AD, MCI, and NC by these methods, we found that the three-label classification accuracy of BNP (88.3%) was improved greatly if the partial least squares method was applied, while the performances in other cases have not been improved significantly. Such an empirical study may justify the connectivity definition adopted in our current work.

Table 3. Statistical p-values for between-group differences of KBI by different connectivity definitions.

Between-Group	Definitions of Distance Function			
	Kendall Correlation	Spearman Correlation	Partial Least Squares	Granger Causality Modeling
AD vs. MCI	**0.003**	0.007	0.159	0.399
AD vs. NC	0.005	**0.003**	0.047	0.375
MCI vs. NC	**0.109**	0.224	0.198	0.238

3.3. Ways of Network Construction

Graph-based brain connectome analyses are sensitive to the choice of parcellation schemes. To assess the effects of different parcellation strategies, we carried out the same set of analyses with another commonly employed atlas, the Harvard–Oxford atlas [35,36] with 110 ROIs (HOA-110). The detailed statistical significances of between-group difference on HOA-110 are presented in Table 4. Again, our proposed KBI achieved better statistical power.

Table 4. Statistical p-values for between-group difference of different network indices on HOA-110 atlas.

Between-Group	KBI	SIP	BNP	CPL	ND	Mod
AD vs. MCI	**0.022**	0.032	0.063	0.092	0.424	0.035
AD vs. NC	**0.013**	0.053	0.033	0.458	0.290	0.081
MCI vs. NC	**0.042**	0.051	0.242	0.088	0.076	0.404

Similarly, only the proposed KBI index detected significant difference in any between-group.

In the metabolic network construction, the common practice is building a group-wise brain network for each group as there is only one summarized value (average SUV) in each ROI. However, we notice that some studies [37] constructed subject-wise networks by dividing each ROI of a subject into blocks to obtain the correlation distance between any two ROI. Thus, subject-wise networks were constructed. We did not study this method in as it would require additional discussion that would exceed the scope of this paper.

In addition, we defined the connectivity between two brain regions as 1-Pearson correlation in Equation (1) in our study. Although some existing studies [19,23] also define such kinds of connectivity in analyzing brain network properties, the common practice in brain network analysis based on graph theory is to directly specify the Pearson correlation as the edge weight. To assess the effect of different connectivity definitions on other graph-based measures, we performed statistical inference on the brain networks whose edges were defined as directly based on Pearson correlation, and the statistical p-values of graph-based measures are shown in Table 5. We found the results were different from the previous results in Table 2, suggesting that graph-based measures could be affected by way of connectivity definition. We also found that none of the graph-based measures could detect all between-group differences significantly in either connectivity definition.

Table 5. Statistical p-values for between-group differences by specifying Pearson correlation as connectivity directly.

Between-Group	CPL	ND	Mod
AD vs. MCI	0.214	0.040	0.081
AD vs. NC	0.063	0.083	0.173
MCI vs. NC	0.004	0.281	0.005

3.4. Limitations and Future Work

Despite the promising results obtained by applying our proposed network index KBI based on persistent homology to PET, there are three important caveats. First, the current study only takes the zeroth persistent homology into account. Higher-order persistent features are also worth studying. In future, we will try to improve the performance of our method by considering higher dimensional persistent homology, such as the first Betti number, which is designed to calculate the number of holes in a graph and may boost the performance, especially in sparse networks that tend to have more holes. Then, although the subject-wise network is more convenient, efficient, and useful than group-wise network for brain network analysis, as we discussed in our prior study [25], we only measured the group-wise metabolic brain network according to regular practice in PET data analysis. In future, we will validate the KBI in a subject-wise metabolic network. Finally, this study was based on cross-sectional PET analysis, and we compared their network indices. With longitudinal PET analysis, we may further study the evolution between longitudinal brain networks by quantifying the difference of their persistent features.

4. Materials and Methods

Figure 7 shows the pipeline of our framework, where the data flow from FDG-PET brain images to some network indices. The details are described in following subsections.

4.1. Participants

Data used in the preparation of this article were obtained from the Alzheimer's Disease Neuroimaging Initiative (ADNI) database (adni.loni.usc.edu) [38,39]. ADNI was launched in 2003 as a public–private partnership led by Principal Investigator Michael W. Weiner, MD. The primary goal of ADNI has been to test whether serial magnetic resonance imaging (MRI), positron emission tomography (PET), other biological markers, and clinical and neuropsychological assessment can be combined to measure the progression of mild cognitive impairment (MCI) and early Alzheimer's disease (AD).

In this study, we chose 700 subjects with FDG-PET data from ADNI2. To match the three research cohorts of AD, MCI, and NC in gender and age, 140 AD, 280 MCI, and 280 NC subjects from 57 sites across North America were selected. The detailed cohort information is described in Table 6.

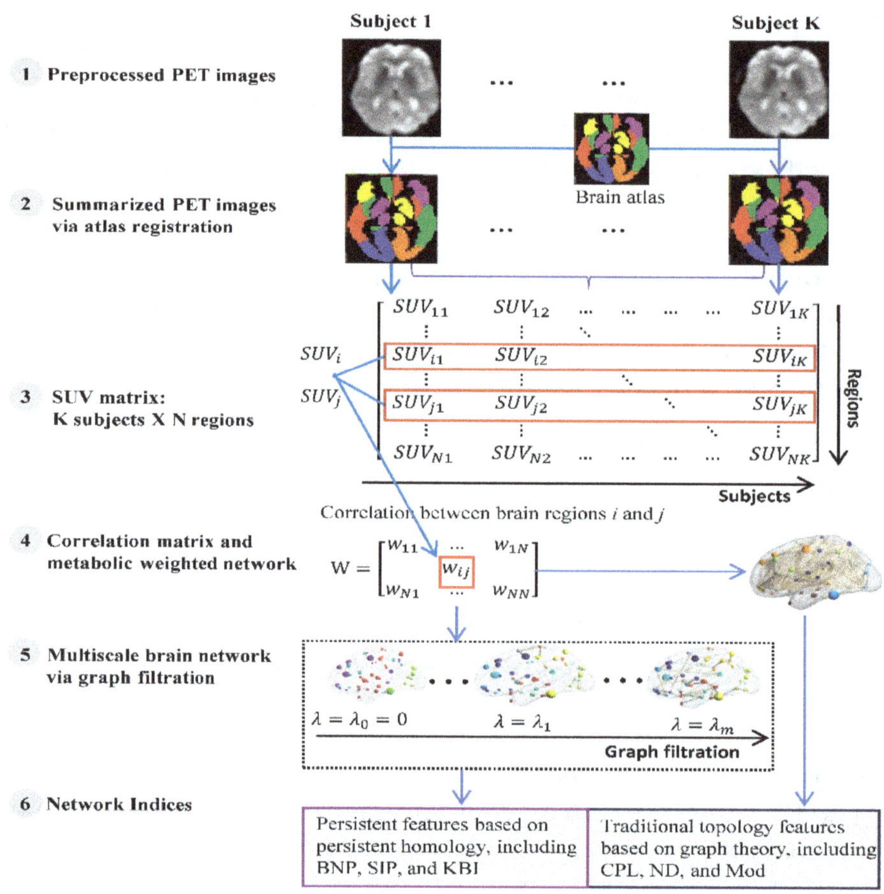

Figure 7. The pipeline of the brain network analysis based on a group of subjects. SUV, support vector machine; BNP, Betti number plot; SIP, slope of IPF plot; KBI, kernel-based IPF; CPL, characteristic path length; ND, network diameter; Mod, modularity.

Table 6. Demographic information of the subjects in this study.

	AD (n = 140)	**MCI (n = 280)**	**NC (n = 280)**	**p-value [c]**
Age [a]	74.2 ± 7.8	73.9 ± 8.0	75.0 ± 6.6	0.20
Gender [b]	70/70	140/140	140/140	1
CDR	≥ 1	0.5	0	–

Key: AD, Alzheimer's disease; MCI, mild cognitive impairment; NC, normal control; [a] mean ± SD; [b] male/female number; [c] statistical group significance using ANOVA test.

4.2. FDG-PET Data Acquisition and Preprocessing

All FDG-PET scans were obtained using Siemens, GE, and Philips PET scanners. Details of the PET data acquisition is described at http://adni.loni.usc.edu/methods/pet-analysis/pre-processing/. All FDG-PET scans used in this research are preprocessed (step 1 of Figure 7) as follows [40]. First, in order to eliminate the individual differences in brain morphology between subjects such that they can completely coincide and be subject to effective statistical analysis, we used the software toolkit Statistical Parametric Mapping (SPM8) [41] in MATLAB (Mathworks Inc, Natick, MA, USA) to linearly align the images into the Montreal Neurological Institute (MNI) space using the TPM.nii template file released with SPM. Second, we borrow a brain mask from SPM, exclude the brain stem and only keep the cerebral cortex (because the cerebral cortex is the object of this study), and then segmented all the images with this cerebral mask. Third, we conducted spatial smoothing with a Gaussian kernel of the full width at half maximum (FWHM) equal to (8,8,8) in three directions (x,y,z) to improve signal-to-noise.

4.3. Network Construction

A weighted graph is a natural and efficient way to represent metabolic brain network because it represents a discretized version of original PET images. In computer graphics, polygon meshes, as a class of graphs with particular connectivity restrictions, are extensively used to represent the topology of an object [42]; however, the mesh representation may not be the most suitable representation for analyzing PET images because of connectivity restrictions [43]. Here, we extend polygon meshes to general graphs by relaxing the connectivity restrictions. Such graphs are easier to construct and are flexible enough to capture metabolic information. We construct a weighted network by encoding the metabolic information through an adjacency matrix $W = \{w_{ij}\}$. The node corresponds to the brain regions, and the edge corresponds to the interregional correlation of brain metabolism. Specifically, the region parcellation in brain imaging is usually defined based on an anatomical atlas. In this study, we applied a predefined atlas, an automated anatomical labeling atlas with 90 (AAL-90) regions of interests (ROI) [28]. Once an ROI is specified, an overall summary measure within it can be calculated to assess the response as a whole, rather than on a voxel-by-voxel basis (step 2 of Figure 7). The most straightforward way to do so is by taking the average standard uptake values (SUV) of all voxels within the ROI. The SUV of a specific ROI is $\frac{1}{M}\sum_{p=1}^{M} v_p$, where M is the total voxel number in a given ROI and v_p is the FDG uptake value of voxel p. Given K subjects and N brain regions, let $SUV_i = \{SUV_{i1}, SUV_{i2}, \ldots, SUV_{iN},\}(1 \le i \le N)$ be the vector of average SUV in i-th ROI of all K subjects (step 3 of Figure 7), and the edge weight w_{ij} between two brain regions is defined as 1-Pearson correlation of SUV between them (step 4 of Figure 7), i.e.

$$w_{ij} = 1 - \frac{cov\left(SUV_i, SUV_j\right)}{\sigma_{SUV_i}\sigma_{SUV_j}}, \tag{1}$$

where SUV_i, SUV_j are the average SUV in i-th and j-th brain region respectively, cov is the covariance, σ is the standard deviation, and $\frac{cov(SUV_i, SUV_j)}{\sigma_{SUV_i}\sigma_{SUV_j}}$ is coefficient of Pearson correlation.

4.4. Network Indices

In clinical settings, doctors prefer single indices as biomarkers because a single neuroimaging index provides a practical reference for evaluating disease progression and for effective treatments. Generally, there are some available network indices based on graph theory that measure brain global attributes. In addition, we focus on some univariate indices that were developed from persistent homology in algebraic topology, and compare them with the network indices from traditional graph theory in our experiments.

4.4.1. Traditional Graph Theory Indices

Traditionally, graph theoretical analysis has been applied to measure brain network topological features. In this study, three global network indices based on graph theory are investigated, including characteristic path length (CPL) [6], network diameter (ND) [9], and modularity (Mod) [7].

Briefly, CPL can be understood as indicating a network with "easily" transferred information. It is the average shortest path length between all pairs of nodes in the graph, and is calculated as $CPL = \frac{1}{N(N-1)} \sum_{i \in V, j \in V, i \neq j} d_{i,j}$, where $d_{i,j}$ is the shortest path length between nodes i and j. Note that infinitely long paths (i.e., paths between disconnected nodes) are not included in computations. ND is the greatest distance between any pair of nodes, and is defined as $ND = \max_{i \in V} \max_{j \in V} d_{i,j}$. It enables understanding of the size of a network. A graph with a large ND and small CPL would therefore be considered an efficient network. Mod describes the extent to which a network has modules that differ from others, each of which is independent and functionally specialized [7]. Computationally, it is expressed as $Mod = \sum_{i \in M} \left[c_{ii} - \left(\sum_{j \in M} c_{ij} \right)^2 \right]$, where i and j are individual modules in the set of all modules M, and c is the proportion of existing connections between two modules.

In practice, we filtered the weighted network before computing these graph-based indices by only selecting the edges whose corresponding p-values passed through a statistical threshold (Bonferroni corrected $p < 0.05$) and then adopted the Brain Connectivity Toolbox (https://sites.google.com/site/bctnet/) [7] for their implementation (step 6 (right) of Figure 7).

4.4.2. Persistent Features Based on Persistent Homology

Persistent homology is an emerging mathematical concept for characterizing shapes in complex data, and the persistence features based on BNP are widely recognized as a useful feature descriptor. BNPs can distinguish robust and noisy topological properties over a wide range of graph filtrations based on the connectivity of k-dimensional simplicial complexes [18] (step 6 (left) of Figure 7). Graph filtration is an important tool [24] in persistent homology that constructs nesting subnetworks in a coherent manner and avoids thresholding selection (step 5 of Figure 7). BNPs have been successfully applied to measure brain networks based on FDG-PET and structural MRI data [23] in some neurodegenerative diseases. In our previous study [25], we proposed an integrated persistent feature (IPF) by integrating an additional feature of connected component aggregation cost with BNP to achieve holistic descriptions of graph evolutions. The IPF at filtration λ_i is defined as [25]

$$IPF_{\lambda_i} = \begin{cases} \frac{m-i}{m(m-1)} \sum_{k=i+1}^{m-1} \lambda_k, \ 0 \leq i \leq m-2 \\ 0, \ i = m-1 \end{cases}, \tag{2}$$

where the maximal graph filtration is $\lambda_0 = 0 < \lambda_1 < \lambda_2 < \cdots < \lambda_{m-1}$. As the IPF plot over all possible filtration values is a monotonically decreasing convergence function, the absolute value of the slope of IPF plot (SIP) was defined as a univariate network index and was successfully applied to quantify brain network dynamics on rs-fMRI data of AD. Both the BNP and SIP indices indicate the rate of connecting components converging over the filtration value, and can be thought as the information diffusion rate or the convergence speed with said network.

4.4.3. The Kernel-Based IPF (KBI) Index

Although the SIP has been developed as a univariate network index in our previous study, it may not be the most appropriate way to describe IPF plot as it is nonlinear, strictly speaking. Recently, some kernel methods [26,27] have been defined on persistent homology to measure the distance between persistence diagrams, which are not only provably stable but also discriminative. Therefore, we employ the framework of kernel embedding of the IPF plot into reproducing kernel Hilbert spaces [26]. Given a point set of IPF plot $X = \{x_1, x_2, \cdots x_N\}$ and a template $T = \{t_1, t_2, \cdots t_N\}$ that are obtained from an average metabolic network of all NC subjects, the kernel-based IPF (KBI) index is defined as

$$KBI(X) = \frac{1}{N} \sum_{x_i \in X,\, t_i \in T,\, i=1}^{N} tan^{-1}(C(\lambda_i^X)^p)\, tan^{-1}(C(\lambda_i^T)^p) e^{-\frac{x_i - t_i^{\ 2}}{2\sigma^2}}, \tag{3}$$

where $tan^{-1}(C(\lambda_i^X)^p)$ and $tan^{-1}(C(\lambda_i^T)^p)$ are both increasing functions with respect to maximal graph filtrations $\lambda^{(X)}$ of X and $\lambda^{(T)}$ of T, and are used for weighting the persistence (λ is a sequence of persistence of zeroth homology in fact). Hence, an essential persistence gives a large weight and a noisy persistence produces a small weight. By adjusting the parameters p, σ, and C, we can control the effect of the persistence. In our practice, we set $p = 5$,

$$\sigma = \underset{\forall X}{median}\{ \underset{x_i, x_j \in X,\, i<j}{median} ||x_i - x_j||\}, \tag{4}$$

$$C = (\underset{\forall \lambda^X}{median}\{\underset{\lambda_i^X \in \lambda^X}{median}(\lambda_i^X)\})^{-p}, \tag{5}$$

so that they take close values to many $||x_i - t_i||$ and λ_i^X, respectively.

4.5. Statistical Analysis

We applied a group-wise statistical analysis of permutation test to all network indices in the last section between AD, MCI, and NC groups. As there are no prior studies on the statistical distribution of any network index, it is difficult to construct a parametric test procedure. Moreover, as there is only one group-wise network for each group, it is necessary to empirically construct the null distribution and determine the p-value. The steps of our permutation test are described as follows. First, the actual network index difference in means between two groups is calculated according to the actual grouping of their subjects. Second, the subjects are randomly assigned to two groups, each of which is assigned the same group size. We then construct two group-wise networks based on such permutated groups and recalculate their indices, whose difference is recorded. This process is repeated 10,000 times and 10,000 permuted differences are obtained. Finally, the total number of permuted differences larger than the actual difference is counted and divided by 10,000. The obtained value is the probability of no difference between the groups, that is, the p-value.

4.6. Classification

We evaluate the power of our method by classification analysis. In this study, our proposed KBI index and other comparison network indices have only one univariate feature to discriminate the global brain network structure. Since the samples are limited, we apply resampling technology beforehand. For a specific group, half subjects are removed randomly at a time and the remaining subjects are used to construct a group-wise network. Resampling all subjects for n times repeatedly in each group until the results are stable, we can obtain n group-wise networks. Each group-wise network is an average of all involved subjects graphs. In our practice, the number of resampling times is set to 5000 ($n = 5000$) and we obtain 5000 resampled networks for each group. Each network can yield a KBI index and other comparable network indices. Then, we compute the values of proposed KBI index, as well as other network measures for all resampled networks, and run support vector machine (SVM) [44] on them. We conduct leave-one-out crossvalidation experiments to evaluate the classification performance. The classification accuracy, sensitivity (i.e., true positive rate), specificity (i.e., true negative rate), and area under the curve (AUC) of receiver operating characteristic (ROC) are severed as criterion of classification performance.

5. Conclusions

This work proposed a novel network index KBI based on our prior work of persistent feature IPF to measure the metabolic brain network of FDG-PET on cognitively impaired cohort. The proposed KBI encoded a great deal of dynamic information over all possible scales that may be inaccessible by standard graph-based measures. Compared to previous slope-based approaches of persistent homology, our kernel-based network index is more accurate regarding the characterization of differences between persistent features. Our current results show that the slope of IPF plot present a pattern AD < MCI < NC in a FDG-PET cohort, consistent with our prior finding in an rs-fMRI cohort, and indicate a slower network integration rate in AD dementia and MCI. Moreover, the enhanced measurement KBI greatly boosted the performance of prior persistent features and outperformed some standard graph-based network indices in both statistical inference and classification experiments, suggesting that our method may serve as a valuable preclinical AD imaging biomarker.

Author Contributions: Conceptualization and methodology, L.K., D.Z. and X.H.; validation: D.Z., J.X. and Z.C.; formal analysis: L.K., F.X., and X.H.; writing: L.K., D.Z., and X.H. visualization, F.X.; software, J.X. and Z.C.

Acknowledgments: Data collection and sharing for this project was funded by the Alzheimer's Disease Neuroimaging Initiative (ADNI) (National Institutes of Health Grant U01 AG024904) and DOD ADNI (Department of Defense award number W81XWH-12-2-0012). ADNI is funded by the National Institute on Aging, the National Institute of Biomedical Imaging and Bioengineering, and through generous contributions from the following: AbbVie, Alzheimer's Association; Alzheimer's Drug Discovery Foundation; Araclon Biotech; BioClinica, Inc.; Biogen; Bristol-Myers Squibb Company; CereSpir, Inc.; Cogstate; Eisai Inc.; Elan Pharmaceuticals, Inc.; Eli Lilly and Company; EuroImmun; F. Hoffmann-La Roche Ltd. and its affiliated company Genentech, Inc.; Fujirebio; GE Healthcare; IXICO Ltd.; Janssen Alzheimer Immunotherapy Research & Development, LLC.; Johnson & Johnson Pharmaceutical Research & Development LLC.; Lumosity; Lundbeck; Merck & Co., Inc.; Meso Scale Diagnostics, LLC.; NeuroRx Research; Neurotrack Technologies; Novartis Pharmaceuticals Corporation; Pfizer Inc.; Piramal Imaging; Servier; Takeda Pharmaceutical Company; and Transition Therapeutics. The Canadian Institutes of Health Research is providing funds to support ADNI clinical sites in Canada. Private sector contributions are facilitated by the Foundation for the National Institutes of Health (www.fnih.org). The grantee organization is the Northern California Institute for Research and Education, and the study is coordinated by the Alzheimer's Therapeutic Research Institute at the University of Southern California. ADNI data are disseminated by the Laboratory for Neuro Imaging at the University of Southern California.

References

1. Lane, C.A.; Hardy, J.; Schott, J.M. Alzheimer's disease. *Eur. J. Neurol.* **2018**, *25*, 59–70. [CrossRef] [PubMed]
2. Ito, K.; Fukuyama, H.; Senda, M.; Ishii, K.; Maeda, K.; Yamamoto, Y.; Ouchi, Y.; Ishii, K.; Okumura, A.; Fujiwara, K. Prediction of outcomes in mild cognitive impairment by using 18F-FDG-PET: A multicenter study. *J. Alzheimers Dis.* **2015**, *45*, 543–552. [CrossRef] [PubMed]
3. Sporns, O. Graph theory methods: Applications in brain networks. *Dialogues Clin. Neuro.* **2018**, *20*, 111–121.
4. Bullmore, E.; Sporns, O. Complex brain networks: Graph theoretical analysis of structural and functional systems. *Nat. Rev. Neurosci.* **2009**, *10*, 186–198. [CrossRef] [PubMed]
5. Sporns, O. The human connectome: A complex network. *Ann. N. Y. Acad. Sci.* **2011**, *1224*, 109–125. [CrossRef] [PubMed]
6. Brier, M.R.; Thomas, J.B.; Fagan, A.M.; Hassenstab, J.; Holtzman, D.M.; Benzinger, T.L.; Morris, J.C.; Ances, B.M. Functional connectivity and graph theory in preclinical alzheimer's disease. *Neurobiol. Aging* **2014**, *35*, 757–768. [CrossRef] [PubMed]
7. Rubinov, M.; Sporns, O. Complex network measures of brain connectivity: Uses and interpretations. *NeuroImage* **2010**, *52*, 1059–1069. [CrossRef]
8. Sporns, O.; Betzel, R.F. Modular brain networks. *Annu. Rev. Psychol.* **2016**, *67*, 613–640. [CrossRef]
9. Fagerholm, E.D.; Hellyer, P.J.; Scott, G.; Leech, R.; Sharp, D.J. Disconnection of network hubs and cognitive impairment after traumatic brain injury. *Brain* **2015**, *138*, 1696–1709. [CrossRef]

10. Stam, C.; Jones, B.; Nolte, G.; Breakspear, M.; Scheltens, P. Small-world networks and functional connectivity in alzheimer's disease. *Cereb. Cortex* **2006**, *17*, 92–99. [CrossRef]
11. Qiu, T.; Luo, X.; Shen, Z.; Huang, P.; Xu, X.; Zhou, J.; Zhang, M. Disrupted brain network in progressive mild cognitive impairment measured by eigenvector centrality mapping is linked to cognition and cerebrospinal fluid biomarkers. *J. Alzheimers Dis.* **2016**, *54*, 1483–1493. [CrossRef] [PubMed]
12. De Haan, W.; Van Der Flier, W.M.; Koene, T.; Smits, L.L.; Scheltens, P.; Stam, C.J. Disrupted modular brain dynamics reflect cognitive dysfunction in alzheimer's disease. *NeuroImage* **2012**, *59*, 3085–3093. [CrossRef] [PubMed]
13. Tong, T.; Aganj, I.; Ge, T.; Polimeni, J.R.; Fischl, B. Functional density and edge maps: Characterizing functional architecture in individuals and improving cross-subject registration. *NeuroImage* **2017**, *158*, 346–355. [CrossRef] [PubMed]
14. Daianu, M.; Jahanshad, N.; Nir, T.M.; Jack, C.R.; Weiner, M.W.; Bernstein, M.A.; Thompson, P.M. Rich club analysis in the alzheimer's disease connectome reveals a relatively undisturbed structural core network. *Hum. Brain Mapp.* **2015**, *36*, 3087–3103. [CrossRef] [PubMed]
15. McKenna, F.; Koo, B.B.; Killiany, R. Comparison of apoe-related brain connectivity differences in early mci and normal aging populations: An fmri study. *Brain Imaging Behav.* **2016**, *10*, 970–983. [CrossRef] [PubMed]
16. Woo, C.-W.; Krishnan, A.; Wager, T.D. Cluster-extent based thresholding in fmri analyses: Pitfalls and recommendations. *NeuroImage* **2014**, *91*, 412–419. [CrossRef]
17. Zalesky, A.; Cocchi, L.; Fornito, A.; Murray, M.M.; Bullmore, E. Connectivity differences in brain networks. *NeuroImage* **2012**, *60*, 1055–1062. [CrossRef] [PubMed]
18. Edelsbrunner, H.; Harer, J. *Computational Topology: An Introduction*; American Mathematical Society: Heidelberg, Germany, 2010.
19. Lee, H.; Kang, H.; Chung, M.K.; Kim, B.-N.; Lee, D.S. Persistent brain network homology from the perspective of dendrogram. *IEEE Trans. Med. Imaging* **2012**, *31*, 2267–2277.
20. Choi, H.; Kim, Y.K.; Kang, H.; Lee, H.; Im, H.-J.; Kim, E.E.; Chung, J.-K.; Lee, D.S. Abnormal metabolic connectivity in the pilocarpine-induced epilepsy rat model: A multiscale network analysis based on persistent homology. *NeuroImage* **2014**, *99*, 226–236. [CrossRef]
21. Chung, M.K.; Hanson, J.L.; Ye, J.; Davidson, R.J.; Pollak, S.D. Persistent homology in sparse regression and its application to brain morphometry. *IEEE Trans. Med. Imaging* **2015**, *34*, 1928–1939. [CrossRef]
22. Yoo, K.; Lee, P.; Chung, M.K.; Sohn, W.S.; Chung, S.J.; Na, D.L.; Ju, D.; Jeong, Y. Degree-based statistic and center persistency for brain connectivity analysis. *Hum. Brain Mapp.* **2017**, *38*, 165–181. [CrossRef] [PubMed]
23. Lee, H.; Kang, H.; Chung, M.K.; Lim, S.; Kim, B.N.; Lee, D.S. Integrated multimodal network approach to pet and mri based on multidimensional persistent homology. *Hum. Brain Mapp.* **2017**, *38*, 1387–1402. [CrossRef] [PubMed]
24. Giusti, C.; Ghrist, R.; Bassett, D.S. Two's company, three (or more) is a simplex: Algebraic-topological tools for understanding higher-order structure in neural data. *J. Comput. Neurosci.* **2016**, *41*, 1–14. [CrossRef] [PubMed]
25. Kuang, L.; Han, X.; Chen, K. A concise and persistent feature to study brain resting-state network dynamics: Findings from the alzheimer's disease neuroimaging initiative. *Hum. Brain Mapp.* **2019**, *40*, 1062–1081. [CrossRef] [PubMed]
26. Kusano, G.; Hiraoka, Y.; Fukumizu, K. *Persistence Weighted Gaussian Kernel for Topological Data Analysis*; International Conference on Machine Learning: New York, NY, USA, 2016; pp. 2004–2013.
27. Carrière, M.; Cuturi, M.; Oudot, S. Sliced wasserstein kernel for persistence diagrams. *Working Papers* **2017**.
28. Tzourio-Mazoyer, N.; Landeau, B.; Papathanassiou, D.; Crivello, F.; Etard, O.; Delcroix, N.; Mazoyer, B.; Joliot, M. Automated anatomical labeling of activations in spm using a macroscopic anatomical parcellation of the mni mri single-subject brain. *NeuroImage* **2002**, *15*, 273–289. [CrossRef] [PubMed]
29. Friston, K.J. Functional and effective connectivity: A review. *Brain Connect* **2011**, *1*, 13–36. [CrossRef]
30. Valdes-Sosa, P.A.; Roebroeck, A.; Daunizeau, J.; Friston, K. Effective connectivity: Influence, causality and biophysical modeling. *NeuroImage* **2011**, *58*, 339–361. [CrossRef]
31. Kendall, M.G. A new measure of rank correlation. *Biometrika* **1938**, *30*, 81–93. [CrossRef]
32. Best, D.; Roberts, D. Algorithm as 89: The upper tail probabilities of spearman's rho. *J. R. Stat. Soc. Ser. C (Appl. Stat.)* **1975**, *24*, 377–379. [CrossRef]

33. McIntosh, A.R.; Chau, W.K.; Protzner, A.B. Spatiotemporal analysis of event-related fmri data using partial least squares. *NeuroImage* **2004**, *23*, 764–775. [CrossRef] [PubMed]
34. Roebroeck, A.; Formisano, E.; Goebel, R. The identification of interacting networks in the brain using fmri: Model selection, causality and deconvolution. *NeuroImage* **2011**, *58*, 296–302. [CrossRef] [PubMed]
35. Kennedy, D.; Lange, N.; Makris, N.; Bates, J.; Meyer, J.; Caviness Jr, V. Gyri of the human neocortex: An mri-based analysis of volume and variance. *Cereb. Cortex* **1998**, *8*, 372–384. [CrossRef] [PubMed]
36. Makris, N.; Meyer, J.W.; Bates, J.F.; Yeterian, E.H.; Kennedy, D.N.; Caviness, V.S. Mri-based topographic parcellation of human cerebral white matter and nuclei: Ii. Rationale and applications with systematics of cerebral connectivity. *NeuroImage* **1999**, *9*, 18–45. [CrossRef] [PubMed]
37. Yu, Z.; Yao, Z.; Zheng, W.; Jing, Y.; Ding, Z.; Mi, L.; Lu, S. *Predicting mci Progression with Individual Metabolic Network Based on Longitudinal FDG-PET*; IEEE International Conference on Bioinformatics & Biomedicine: Kansas City, MO, USA, 2017.
38. Jagust, W.J.; Bandy, D.; Chen, K.; Foster, N.L.; Landau, S.M.; Mathis, C.A.; Price, J.C.; Reiman, E.M.; Skovronsky, D.; Koeppe, R.A. The alzheimer's disease neuroimaging initiative positron emission tomography core. *Alzheimer's Dement.* **2010**, *6*, 221–229. [CrossRef]
39. Jack, C.R.; Bernstein, M.A.; Fox, N.C.; Thompson, P.; Alexander, G.; Harvey, D.; Borowski, B.; Britson, P.J.L.; Whitwell, J.; Ward, C. The alzheimer's disease neuroimaging initiative (adni): Mri methods. *J. Magn. Reson. Imaging* **2008**, *27*, 685–691. [CrossRef] [PubMed]
40. Mi, L.; Zhang, W.; Zhang, J.; Fan, Y.; Goradia, D.; Chen, K.; Reiman, E.M.; Gu, X.; Wang, Y. An optimal transportation based univariate neuroimaging index. In Proceedings of the IEEE International Conference on Computer Vision, Venice, Italy, 2017; pp. 182–191.
41. Penny, W.D.; Friston, K.J.; Ashburner, J.T.; Kiebel, S.J.; Nichols, T.E. *Statistical Parametric Mapping: The Analysis of Functional Brain Images*; Academic press: Pittsburgh, PA, USA, 2011.
42. De Floriani, L.; Magillo, P. Multiresolution mesh representation: Models and data structures. In *Tutorials on Multiresolution in Geometric Modelling*; Springer: Berlin/Heidelberg, Germany, 2002; pp. 363–417.
43. Chen, S.; Tian, D.; Feng, C.; Vetro, A.; Kovačević, J. Fast resampling of 3d point clouds via graphs. *arXiv* **2017**, arXiv:1702.06397. [CrossRef]
44. Cortes, C.; Vapnik, V. Support-vector networks. *Mach. Learn.* **1995**, *20*, 273–297. [CrossRef]

11

The Rise of Synaptic Density PET Imaging

Guillaume Becker *,†, Sylvestre Dammicco †, Mohamed Ali Bahri † and Eric Salmon †

GIGA-Cyclotron Research Center-in vivo imaging, University of Liège, Allée du 6 Août, B30, 4000 Liege, Belgium; sdammicco@uliege.be (S.D.); m.bahri@uliege.be (M.A.B.); eric.salmon@uliege.be (E.S.)

* Correspondence: g.becker@uliege.be

† These authors have equally contributed.

Academic Editors: Anne Roivainen and Xiang-Guo Li

Abstract: Many neurological disorders are related to synaptic loss or pathologies. Before the boom of positrons emission tomography (PET) imaging of synapses, synaptic quantification could only be achieved in vitro on brain samples after autopsy or surgical resections. Until the mid-2010s, electron microscopy and immunohistochemical labelling of synaptic proteins were the gold-standard methods for such analyses. Over the last decade, several PET radiotracers for the synaptic vesicle 2A protein have been developed to achieve in vivo synapses visualization and quantification. Different strategies were used, namely radiolabelling with either ^{11}C or ^{18}F, preclinical development in rodent and non-human primates, and binding quantification with different kinetic modelling methods. This review provides an overview of these PET tracers and underlines their perspectives and limitations by focusing on radiochemical aspects, as well as preclinical proof-of-concept and the main clinical outcomes described so far.

Keywords: SV2A protein; PET radiotracers; synaptic loss; radiochemistry; preclinical development; clinical outcomes

---

1. Introduction

The synaptic vesicle glycoprotein 2A (SV2A) has been studied for three decades which were punctuated by important milestones. Among others, the discovery by Lynch et al. of SV2A being the binding site of the first-in-class antiepileptic drug levetiracetam is one of these significant steps [1]. The most recent milestone is undoubtedly the current possibility to study SV2A in vivo via PET imaging with specific radiopharmaceuticals. The protein is ubiquitously expressed throughout the brain and is known to be essential for proper brain development and functioning [2,3]. Numerous functions have been hypothesized for SV2A and were recently reviewed [4]. It is noteworthy that pharmacological modulation of SV2A protein may have an impact on Alzheimer's disease (AD) progression [5,6]. Besides the obvious importance of SV2A in epilepsy, AD is a perfect illustration of the clinical interest of synaptic density quantification [7,8]. Before the onset of synaptic density PET imaging, the quantification of synaptic density in brain tissue was performed using immunohistochemistry of key proteins located in the pre- or postsynaptic neurons, such as synaptophysin, or using electron microscopy. Terry et al. used the immunohistochemistry of synaptophysin and demonstrated a lower synaptic density in the midfrontal and inferior parietal cortices of AD patients. Moreover, they reported a positive correlation between the synaptophysin optical density (as an index of synaptic density) and the mini-mental state examination (MMSE) score of the patients [7]. More than a decade later, Scheff et al. counted the synapses in the hippocampus of AD patients using electron microscopy and found a decreased synaptic density in early AD compare to MCI and healthy controls. Consistently with previously mentioned results, Scheff et al. described a positive correlation between the number of synapses in the hippocampus and the MMSE score [8]. Another pertinent example consists in

Parkinson's disease of which the synaptopathy in mainly consists in dysfunction of dopaminergic nigrostriatal terminals and corticostriatal synapses, probably due to the toxic effect of misfolded α-Synuclein. In that case, the majority of genes implicated in PD have a critical role in presynaptic function and thus presumably lead to synaptic dysfunctions. With this in mind, the underlying concept is that PET imaging of synaptic density could be achieved by targeting proteins embedded in synaptic vesicles thanks to appropriate specific radiotracers. Strongly supported by the experience of UCB Pharma in the development of SV2A ligands, several PET research centres embarked on the development of SV2A PET radiotracers. In this review, we return to this "success story" with an emphasis on updated radiochemical considerations of available PET tracers for SV2A. In a second part, we summarize the preclinical developments that were made with these radiotracers, and finally, we report the major clinical outcomes achieved by the existing PET radiotracers.

2. Radiochemistry of SV2A PET Radiotracers

Over the last decades UCB has developed several effective antiepileptic drugs sharing the same mode of action for binding SV2A: levetiracetam (Keppra®) and brivaracetam (Briviact®) (Figure 1) [9–12].

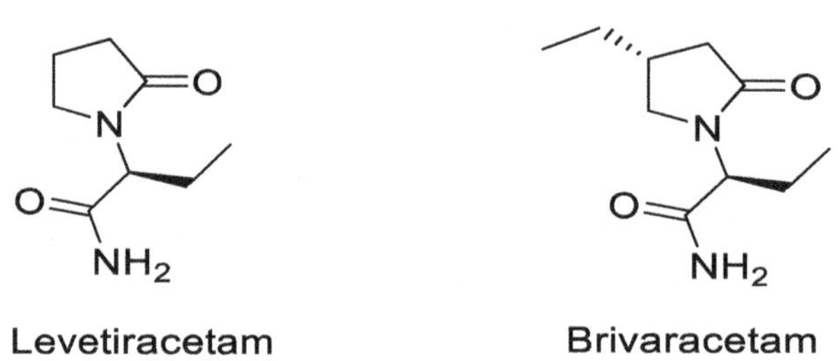

Figure 1. Two antiepileptic drugs: Levetiracetam and Brivaracetam.

After further exploration, the acetamide motif was replaced by different heteroaryl groups as imidazole and pyridine derivatives mimicking the acetamide motif [13]. The modification of the substitution of the alky group on the lactam function was also studied and revealed that (poly)-fluorinated aryls provided the best affinities at SV2A obtained so far.

Quantification of SV2A-PET signal aims to provide a measure of brain synaptic density. Specific requirements for designing CNS PET ligands have been recently reviewed extensively [14–17]. Several parameters are required to obtain a good PET tracer. The radioligand must have a high affinity for the target (nanomolar or subnanomolar) and a B_{max}/Kd ratio in a suitable range to measure a specific signal in vivo (above 10). It has to be able to cross the BBB to reach its target in the CNS. Typically, the LogP of the compound should be between 1 and 3. Since the target density is usually low, the molar activity of the tracer has to be as high as possible. Finally, the radiosynthesis of the tracer with a PET radionuclide as fluorine-18 or carbon-11 must be fast and easily implemented.

Initially, in 2014, the radiochemical synthesis of levetiracetam was performed with carbon-11 (Table 1, entry 1) by Cai et al. but the affinity for SV2A of levetiracetam (Ki = 2.5 μM) was too low for in vivo imaging application [18]. Several other candidates presenting good affinity for SVA were also developed by UCB and were labelled with fluorine-18 and carbon-11: [^{18}F]UCB-H, [^{11}C]UCB-A and [^{11}C]UCB-J (Table 1, entry 2–5). All these compounds were synthesized in partnership with PET centers, in the University of Liège for [^{18}F]UCB-H, in Uppsala University in Sweden for [^{11}C]UCB-A and finally, in Yale University in New Haven for [^{11}C]UCB-J. These compounds have two enantiomeric forms due to the chiral carbon on the lactam ring. In every case, the *R* form presents best affinity for the SV2A target.

The first published radiotracer was [^{18}F]UCBH. A multi-step synthesis was described in 2013 by Aerts et al. involving nucleophilic ^{18}F-labelling (entry 2) of a pyridine derivative precursor followed by reductive amination, reduction and ring closure reaction [19,20]. This approach afforded UCB-H with a no decay corrected radiochemical yield (ndc RCY) of 30%. The duration of the synthesis including the purification and formulation steps was of 150 min and the molar activity of 96.2 GBq.μmol^{-1}. This process was fully automated on a FASTlab synthesizer and was until recently used in the Liège laboratory for cGMP routine production of the radiopharmaceutical.

In 2014, an alternative at this time consuming multi step synthesis was proposed by the same laboratory and greatly simplified the automation process [21]. This late stage approach (entry 3) requires the labelling of a Pyridyl(4-methoxypehnyl)iodonium triflate salt precursor according to the Pike methodology [22]. In order to improve the yield of the labelling (< 1%), TEMPO was added as a radical scavenger to stabilize the diaryliodonium salt precursor. Indeed, these types of compounds are known to decompose into radical intermediates upon heating. Although TEMPO is known to be genotoxic, the QC study shows that the presence of traces of this radical in the final injectable solution was far below the specification (500–1000 times). This process, fully automated on an AIO from Trasis, proceeds at the Curie level with an RCY of 35% (dc). The duration of the synthesis is only of 50 min and the molar activity is very high (815 GBq·μmol^{-1}). However, even if the affinity of UCB-H is slightly lower compared to UCB-J, leading to more difficulties in detecting the variation of SV2A availability, this radiotracer has a more convenient half live of 110 min and its precursor is commercial available as the dedicated cassette for automated synthesis.

In 2016, [^{11}C]UCB-A was labelled with [^{11}C]methyl triflate reagent (entry 4) reacting with the triphenylmethyl UCB-A precursor [23]. After an acidic treatment and about 40 min of synthesis, the formulated radiotracer was obtained with a RCY of 14% (dc) and a molar activity of 62.9 GBq.μmol^{-1}. Unfortunately, [^{11}C]UCB-A showed slow kinetic and slow metabolism with a brain Tmax of 20 min with a maximum of 5 min for the two other radiotracers leading to quantification issue.

The same year, [^{11}C]UCB-J was produced by labelling the trifluoroborate precursor with [^{11}C]methyl iodide (entry 5) under Suzuki-Miyaura coupling conditions with a palladium catalyst [24]. In a first step, [^{11}C]methyl iodide was reacted with the palladium catalyst followed by in situ hydrolysis of the trifluorobrate precursor to activate it. This coupling reaction lead to a 35% decay corrected radiochemical yield and good molar activity (215 GBq·0μmol^{-1}). The authors noticed that the efficiency of the labelling by methylation depended from the purity of the precursor. The presence of traces amounts (a few percent) of the corresponding boronic acid was required to obtain good yield. Recently, Rokka et al. changed the solvent of the reaction (THF-H_2O instead of DMF-H_2O) and performed the reaction in a single step by mixing all the reagents before the addition of [^{11}C] methyl iodide [25]. The RCY of the coupling reaction between [^{11}C]methyl iodide and the precursor was 39 ± 5% decay corrected within 40 min with a molar activity of 390 GBq·μmol^{-1} at the end of synthesis. More recently, Sephton et al. proposed a completely automated radiosynthesis of [^{11}C]UCB-J with cGMP compliant conditions [26]. The precursor was preactivated with HCl to form the more reactive boronic acid derivative. The RCY of the coupling was 35 ± 4% dc and 11 ± 1 ndc with a molar activity around 30 GBq·μmol^{-1}. UCB-J presents the best in class SV2A radiotracer with fast kinetic, high brain uptake and rapid metabolization [24]. However, the low half-life of the carbone-11 (20.4 min) requires on-site cyclotron production resulting in some issue for commercial distribution to PET centers.

To circumvent this half-life issue, Li et al. from Yale University have investigated the feasibility of ^{18}F-labelling one of the three fluorine atoms presents on the aromatic ring of the UCB-J molecule [27]. First, the authors tried the traditional ^{18}F-fluorine nucleophilic substitution of a halogen leaving group and the isotopic exchange but none of these methods were successful. They managed to obtain [^{18}F]UCB-J by ^{18}F-labelling an iodonium salt and a iodonium ylide (entry 6). Both reactions generated a racemization of the compound due to the high temperature of the labelling reaction (above 170 °C) requiring a chiral HPLC purification. Those syntheses provided very low RCY (1–2%) and the molar activity was moderate (59 ± 36 GBq·μmol^{-1}). Other radiofluorination methods with arylstannanes, phenofluor derivatives and boronic ester were tested without further success. Although [^{18}F]UCB-J presented similar imaging properties (clearance, metabolism, kinetic) than [^{11}C]UCB-J due to equivalent chemical structure, the radiosynthesis issue led to a need for new SV2A tracers.

In 2018, and a few months apart, the Yale University group and Invicro published a new UCB-J analogue with two fluorine atoms instead of three on the aromatic cycle [28,29]. This compound was initially named [^{18}F]SDM-8 by the Yale University group and [^{18}F]MNI-1126 by Invicro. The two groups agreed to call it [^{18}F]SynVesT-1 (entry 7) for later publication and this name will be used in this paper. This tracer has an affinity comparable to UCB-J (8.4 vs 8.2 respectively) and offers the advantage of a fluorine-18 labelling. Different synthesis route for the preparation of desired tracer were investigated by Li et al. They tried iodonium ylide, boronic ester and arylstannane precursors. The ^{18}F-fluorination of the iodonium precursor afforded very low yield (< 1%) partially due to the chiral HPLC purification of the racemate resulting from the high temperature use for the labelling. Note that the authors did not tested the addition of a radical scavenger as TEMPO in the previous study [21]. The boronic ester derivative provided better yields (11% at 150 °C and 6% at 110 °C) but the stannic precursor is the most promising with a RCY of 19% (ndc) after 95min of radiosynthesis and a significant molar activity of 242 MBq·μmol^{-1}. The radiolabelling occurred at 110 °C which is lower than the critical racemization temperature of 120 °C. Only the synthesis of the R-enantiomer is reported in this publication. Constantinescu et al. (Invicro) worked also on the tin precursor but they synthesized all the enantiomeric forms of the compound (SynVesT-1 (R), MNI-1128 (S) and the racemate) and compared their PET imaging properties. They managed to obtain RCY between 10 and 20% decay corrected with high specific activities (100–370 GBq·μmol^{-1}).

The synthesis of another analogue of UCB-J was also published by the Yale University group. This compound ([^{18}F]SMD-2) with only one fluorine atom on the aromatic ring was renamed later in [^{18}F]SynVesT-2 [30,31]. Like SynVest-1, SynVesT-2 is also an interesting candidate for SV2A imaging probe. It has been synthesized via an iodonium ylide and an arylstannane precursor. The iodonium approach did not provide high radiochemical yield (1%) but radiosynthesis from the tin precursor provided higher RCY (7%, dc). An average molar activity of 141 Gb·μmol^{-1} was obtained after a 90 min synthesis including the purification and formation processes.

In 2019, a screening of a large panel of potential radioligands for SV2A imaging, was performed to identify compounds with similar binding affinities to UCB-J. From these in vitro homogenate binding, autoradiography and in vivo micro-PET studies [32], it appears that SynVesT-1 and SynVesT-2 are promising candidates for SV2A PET imaging, confirming the previous studies (19–22).

In 2019, the synthesis of a ^{18}F-difluoromethyl analogue of UCB-J was reported by Trump et al. [33]. As the substitution of the methyl group presents on the pyridine ring of UCB-J by a fluorine atom slightly reduced the affinity of the molecule for SV2A, these authors investigated the possibility to have a CHF^{18}F function instead of the methyl. The radiosynthesis of this difluoromethylated compound [^{18}F]**1** (entry 9) implied a late-stage ^{18}F-difluoromethylation step. This method proceeds by C-H activation and does not require the synthesis of a specific precursor. The catalyzed addition of the CHF^{18}F moiety is generated by UV from a previously synthesized [^{18}F]difluorobenzothiazole sulfone. The reaction is not regiospecific and several isomers can be obtained. Even if the RCY (dc) was of only 1.5%, the fully automated process affords sufficient amount of the labelled molecule, with relatively high molar activity (40–80 GBg·μmol^{-1}) for subsequent preliminary μPET animal studies [34]. This ^{18}F-fluoromethyl labelling approach of *N*-heteroaromatic compounds by C-H activation represents an interesting way to rapidly evaluate new SV2A PET tracers. However, for future PET clinical imaging applications, the radiochemical synthesis of the [^{18}F]difluorobenzothiazole sulfone should be improved.

Table 1. Affinity, molar activity and radiochemical yield (RCY) of published SV2A tracers.

Entry	Tracer	Ref	Synthesis of the Radiotracer	pIC_{50} for Human SV2A	Ki (nM) for Human SV2A	Molar Activity (GBq. μmol^{-1})	RCY (%)
1	[11C]Levetir-acetam	[18]	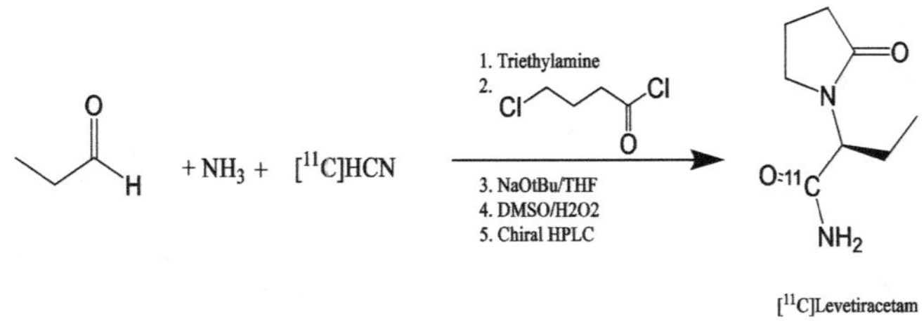	5.7 [24]	2500	17	8.3 (dc)
2	[18F]UCB-H	[19]	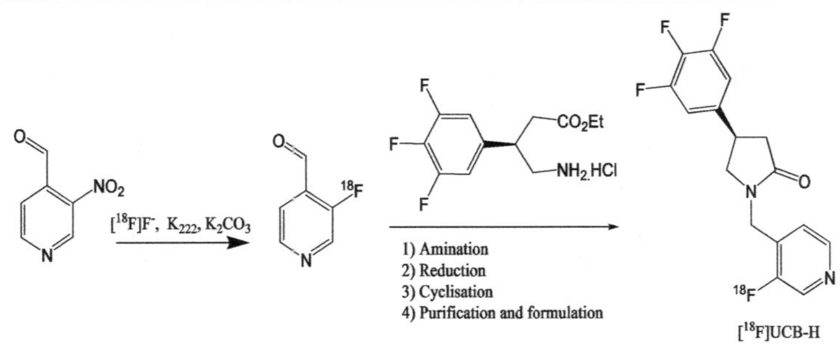	7.8	9.0	518	15 (ndc)
3		[21]	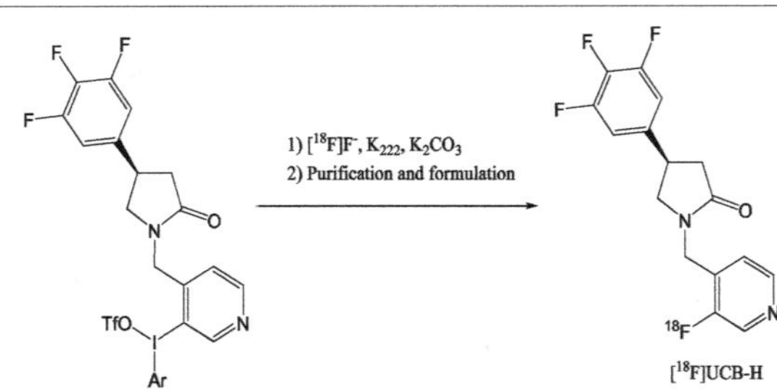			815 ± 185	35 (ndc)

Table 1. *Cont.*

Entry	Tracer	Ref	Synthesis of the Radiotracer	pIC_{50} for Human SV2A	Ki (nM) for Human SV2A	Molar Activity (GBq. μmol^{-1})	RCY (%)
4	[^{18}F]UCB-A	[23]	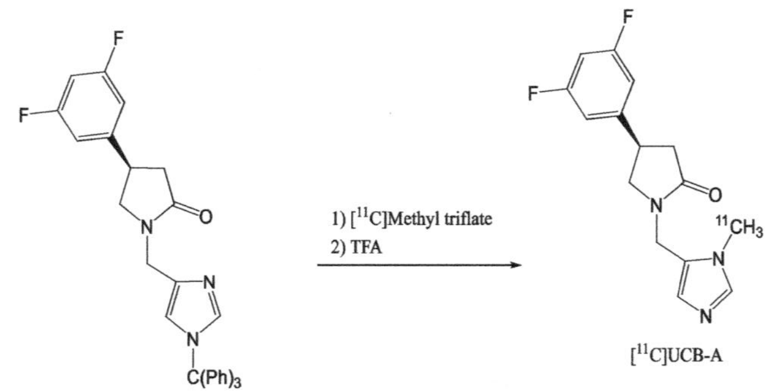	7.9 [24]	ND [a]	65	14 (dc)
5	[^{11}C]UCB-J	[24]	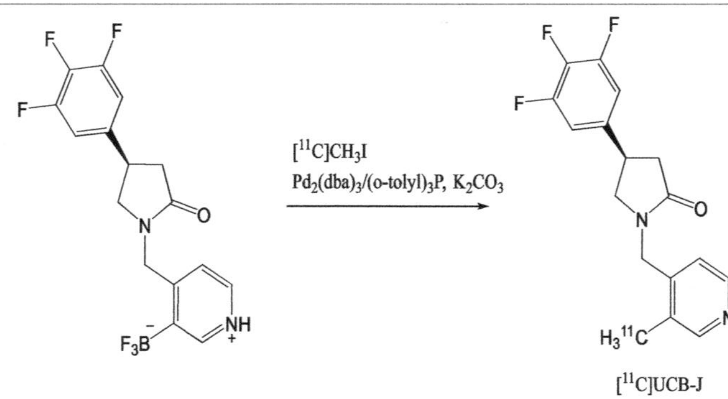	8.2	1.5	215	35 (dc)
6	$[^{18}F]$UCB-J	[27]	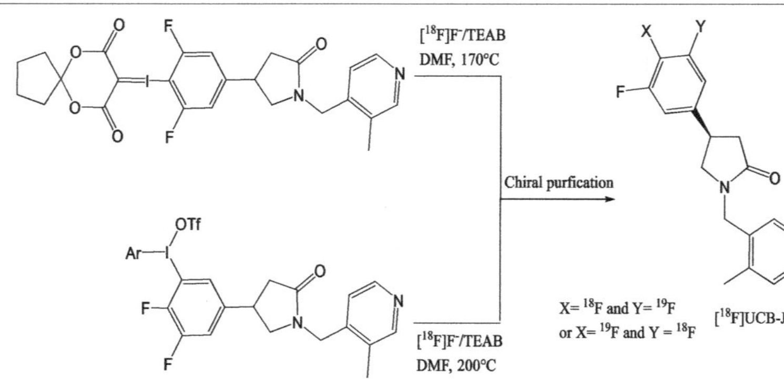	Similar to $[^{11}C]$UCB-J	Similar to $[^{11}C]$UCB-J	59 ± 36	1–2 (ndc)

Table 1. *Cont.*

Entry	Tracer	Ref	Synthesis of the Radiotracer	pIC_{50} for Human SV2A	Ki (nM) for Human SV2A	Molar Activity (GBq. µmol^{-1})	RCY (%)
7	[^{18}F]SynVesT-1	[28,29]	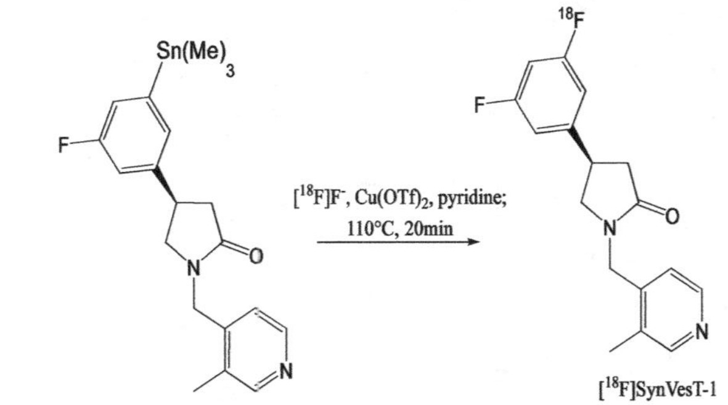	8.4	2.2–4.7 [b]	242	19 (ndc)
8	[^{18}F]SynVesT-2	[31]	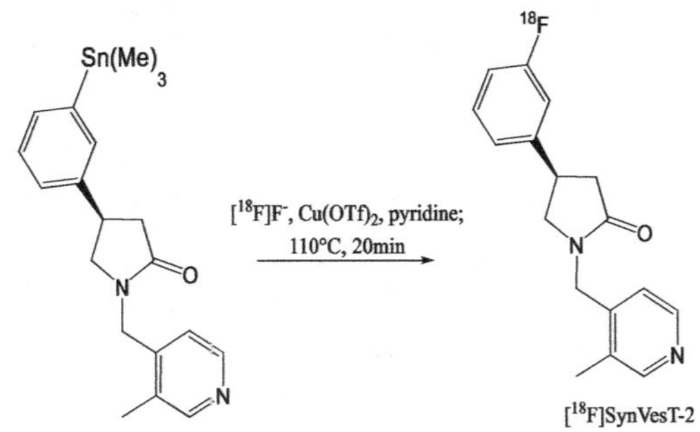	ND [a]	12	141	7(dc)
9	[^{18}F]1	[33]	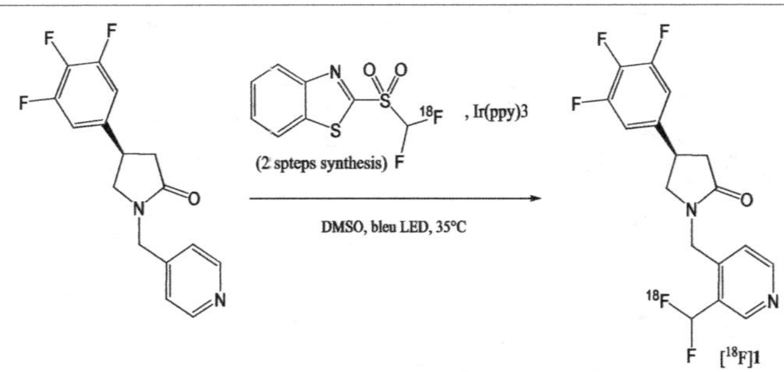	8.3	ND [a]	40–80	1.5 (dc)

[a] Unpublished information. [b] Respectively the value obtained by Invicro and Yale University.

[^{11}C]UCB-J and [^{18}F]UCB-H are currently the two most widely used radio tracers for SV2A imaging. [^{11}C]UCB-J has a higher affinity for the target but the half-life of ^{11}C drastically limits its use in PET centers without cyclotron. Conversely, the synthesis of [^{18}F]UCB-H is commercially available with good yield and high specific activity. However, due to the limited imaging properties of [^{18}F]UCB-H, a new generation of radiotracer has recently been released. [^{18}F]SynVesT-1 and [^{18}F]SynVesT-2 were produced via labelling of an arylstannane precursor. The disadvantage of this chemistry is the toxicity of organotin compounds as well as copper used as a catalyst which could lead to complications for GMP applications. Indeed, an ICP-MS analysis seems essential to quality control for injection to the patient. On the other hand, the iodonium precursors radiolabelling did not show as interesting yields as for the [^{18}F]UCB-H. The use of radical scavenger has not yet been considered, which has however proved its usefulness for the labelling of [^{18}F]UCB-H.

3. Preclinical Developments of SV2A PET Radiotracers

3.1. Drug Metabolism and Pharmacokinetic (DMPK)

The first generation of SV2A PET radiotracers, namely UCB-A, UCB-H and UCB-J shared the same chemical backbone and were profiled with DMPK studies in male Wistar rats (single intravenous injection at 0.1 mg·kg^{-1} for each compound) [13]. We report here the main DMPK features for these three radiotracers.

Among the three compounds, UCB-A displayed good affinity for SV2A protein (Table 1, entry 4) and a good logD value of 1.4 (measured from octanol/water partition coefficient at 25 °C and pH 7.4). The A > B apparent permeability (P_{app}) was measured on CACO-2 cells and the Efflux ratio (ER) was defined as the ratio of apparent permeabilities (B > A / A > B) with values of 383 nm·s^{-1} and 1.2 respectively. The intrinsic clearance (Clint) measured in human microsomes was 20 μL·min^{-1}·mg·protein^{-1}. Finally, the fraction unbound in rat brain tissue (Fu% brain) is 12% with a ratio of free brain concentration versus free plasma concentration at 20 min post-administration (Free B/P ratio) is 0.6.

As a comparison, UCB-H and UCB-J displayed a good affinity as well (Table 1, entry 2,3,5). The reported logD values were 2.3 for UCB-H and 2.5 for UCB-J. The P_{app}/ER were 707 nm·s^{-1} /0.7 for UCB-H and 323 nm·s^{-1} /0.8 for UCB-J. The Clint were 12 μL·min^{-1}·mg·protein^{-1} for UCB-H and 16 μL·min^{-1}·mg·protein^{-1} for UCB-J. Finally, the Fu% brain and the Free B/P ratio were 8 and 1.6, and 4.5 and 1.6 for UCB-H and UCB-J respectively.

Overall, these data (summarized in Table 2) highlighted that the UCB compounds family have a high permeability and suitable PKPD profile as PET radiotracers. The LogD, a key feature for brain PET radiotracers, is nearly equal for UCB-H and UCB-J, and even lower for UCB-A. In all cases, it is in the suitable range for blood brain barrier crossing. However, another important feature, the free B/P ratio clearly highlights that UCB-H and UCB-J possess the greatest potential (free B/P ratio higher than 1 for both, whereas this ratio is less than 1 for UCB-A).

Table 2. Main PK/PD characteristics of the first-generation of SV2A radiotracers derived from IUCB Pharma library. LogP measured from octanol/water partition coefficient at 258C and pH 7.4, Efflux ratio (ER) derived from apparent permeabilities, the intrinsic clearance (Cl*int*) measured in human microsomes, the fraction unbound in rat brain tissue (Fu% brain) and the ratio of free brain concentration versus free plasma concentration (Free B/P ratio).

Tracers	LogD	ER	Cl*int* μL·min^{-1}·mg·Protein^{-1}	Fu% Brain	Free B/P Ratio
[^{11}C]UCB-A	1.4	1.2	20	12	0.6
[^{18}F]UCB-H	2.3	0.7	12	8	1.6
[^{11}C]UCB-J	2.5	0.8	16	4.5	1.6

Concerning the pharmacological profile, UCB-J exhibited a greater than 10-fold and greater than 100-fold selectivity for SV2A over SV2C and SV2B protein, respectively [24]. Regarding UCB-H, the in vivo selectivity for SV2A over the two other isoforms (B and C) was assessed by microPET imaging with pharmacological blocking experiment [35]. The authors performed pharmacological competitions with either vehicle, SV2A competitor (levetiracetam at 10 $mg \cdot kg^{-1}$), SV2B competitor (UCB5203 at 3 $mg \cdot kg^{-1}$), and SV2C competitor (UCB0949 at 3 $mg \cdot kg^{-1}$). Statistical analysis revealed differences between levetiracetam pre-treated group and all the other groups of the study, thereby highlighting the in vivo selectivity of UCB-H for SV2A.

To summarized, all of the three radiotracers initially developed by UCB Pharma displayed very good features for central nervous system PET imaging, with excellent brain penetration and the important requirement that none of them is substrate of P-glycoprotein (P-gp) efflux.

As previously mentioned, the second generation of SV2A PET radiotracers includes mainly the two compounds SynVesT-1 and SynVesT-2. SynVesT-1 seems the most promising compound with an IC50 of 3.52 nM and a logP value measured at 2.32. Plasma free fraction of SynVesT-1 was high, at 43 ± 2% [28]. SynVesT-2 hold a high affinity toward SV2A assessed by Ki values of 7.6 and 12 nM for rat and human SV2A, respectively. Finally, SynVesT-2 possesses a Log D of 2.17 ± 0.02 and a plasma free fraction similar of 41% ± 2% [31].

3.2. Preclinical PET Imaging with SV2A Radiotracers

The first in vivo description of SV2A PET radiotracer has been achieved in mice with UCB-H for dosimetric analysis purpose [36]. This study revealed by ex vivo tissue distribution that the brain is one of the mice organs most exposed to radioactive doses, along with the urinary bladder wall and the liver, all the three organs receiving a resulting effective dose of $1.88 \cdot 10^{-2}$ $mSv \cdot MBq^{-1}$. This study concluded that UCB-H tracer met the standard criteria for radiation exposure in clinical studies with an estimated effective dose of 2.8 mSv for an injected dose of 150 MBq and a maximum injectable dose of approximately 325 MBq per participant. Moreover, this study highlighted the high brain penetration of the tracer in mice.

Afterward, preclinical investigations with UCB-H were conducted in rats (Sprague Dawley) considering that their size better suits microPET brain imaging, as well as images quantification with invasive protocols [19]. Warnock et al. proceeded to a full quantification using an arterial input function (AIF). The AIF was measured thanks to an arteriovenous shunt and a beta-probe. To compute the full kinetic model, they used AIF corrected for plasma-to-whole blood ratio and in vivo metabolism. The metabolism was highly reproducible and fitted a bi-exponential curve. This parent fraction curve revealed that 40% of the UCB-H was metabolized 5 min after the injection, while it remains 20% of the parent compound 30 min after injection. The authors showed that the Logan graphic analysis (start time ranged from 7.5 to 15 min.) afforded a highly reproducible distribution volume (V_T) measurement in a test-retest experimental design. Moreover, they validated the pharmacological blocking by increasing doses of levetiracetam, which ranged from 0.1 to 100 $mg \cdot kg^{-1}$ leading respectively to −9.0 ± 4.6% and −43.8 ± 4.7% decreases in the V_T value for the whole brain.

This in vivo evaluation of UCB-H as a PET tracer for SV2A protein was followed by several studies that aimed at simplifying the binding quantification, AIF in rats being highly invasive and time consuming. The first step for a non-invasive quantification of UCB-H in rat brain used a population-based input function (PBIF) [37]. The authors averaged 8 individuals AIF to compute the PBIF and validate the used of the PBIF on each individual rat. They reported a high correlation of the V_T measured either by individual AIF or by the PBIF ($R^2 = 0.99$ for all fits, the reported V_T values for both methods being almost equals for each rat). Beyond the quantification part, the authors used HPLC-MS/MS to identify the *N*-oxide as the main plasmatic metabolite of UCB-H (the UCB-H-*N*-oxide represented 90.2% of the formed metabolites). Then, they proceed to the radiolabelling of this UCB-H-*N*-oxide and performed PET imaging with [^{18}F]UCB-H-*N*-oxide thereby establishing the complete absence of UCB-H radiometabolite in the rat brain.

The second simplification step for preclinical studies with UCB-H was the validation of a static PET acquisition and standardized uptake value assessment [38]. The authors compared the two parameters: the V_T obtained from Logan graphical analysis using the previously developed PBIF, and the standardized uptake value (SUV). The authors used pharmacological competition design with 1 and 10 mg·kg^{-1} of levetiracetam in rats to study the impact of the length of the dynamic acquisition (90 versus 60 min) and the correlations between V_T and SUV over 20 min consecutive timeframes. They reported no bias between the V_T values obtained for both dynamic acquisition times, and a high correlation between the V_T derived from 90 min acquisition time and the SUV computed from 20 to 40 min static acquisition. The authors identified the 20–40 min timeframe as the best situation for a static PET acquisition with UCB-H in rat. This method of static acquisition and SUV assessment was further used to investigate the in vivo modification in SV2A protein expression in a preclinical rat model of temporal lobe epilepsy. Although pathophysiological findings are beyond the scope of this review, this study highlights the efficiency of static PET analysis with UCB-H to detect variations in SV2A expression in the brain of an epileptic rat model, as well as physiological modifications related to brain development and maturation [39].

The UCB-J was initially developed in rhesus monkey [24]. As it has been shown with UCB-H, UCB-J displayed a fast metabolism, the parent fraction in the plasma accounted for approximately 40% and about 25% of the radioactivity at 30 and 90 min after injection, respectively. PET images revealed a high brain uptake throughout the grey matter, consistent with the ubiquitous distribution of SV2A. The pre-injection of levetiracetam (10 mg·kg^{-1}) substantially blocked [^{11}C]UCB-J binding and co-injection of cold UCB-J (150 mg·kg^{-1}) drastically decreased specific UCB-J binding. [^{11}C]UCB-J displayed a high uptake and rapid kinetics, with an SUV peak of 5–8 in grey matter areas and peak uptake times ranging from 10 to 50 min. Nabulsi et al. tested several kinetic models to quantify UCB-J binding and chose the 1-Tissu compartmental model (1T model) as it produced reliable V_T estimates with low variability (compared to the other kinetic analyses tested, the multilinear analysis and the 2-tissues compartmental model). Then, using the 1T model, the author reported a significant reduction in regional V_T due to levetiracetam pre-injection (10 and 30 mg·kg^{-1}). The resulting receptor occupancy analysis revealed that 59% and 89% of SV2A in rhesus monkey brain were occupied by 10 and 30 mg·kg^{-1} of levetiracetam respectively. The blocking experiment using 17, 50, and 150 mg·kg^{-1} of UCB-J showed respectively an occupancy of occupancies of 46%, 68%, and 87%. Thanks to these results, the authors were able to compute the Kd value for UCB-J estimated 3.4 ± 0.2 nM and the B_{max} for several brain regions (highest value in cingulate cortex 350 nmol·L^{-1}, and lowest value in the pons and the brain stem 123 and 124 nmol·L^{-1} respectively).

Regarding the dosimetry, they performed a whole-body distribution studies showing that the liver was receiving the largest doses for males (0.0199 mGy·MBq^{-1}) whereas the brain received the largest dose for females (0.0181 mGy·MBq^{-1}). They estimated the effective dose equivalent value of approximately 4.5 mSv·MBq^{-1} and conclude that the maximum effective dose equivalent from a single 740 MBq (20 mCi) administration of [^{11}C]UCB-J is equivalent to 3.4 mSv, thus being fully compliant with regulation for human PET imaging.

The same group published in 2016 the only complete validation of SV2A PET as marker of synaptic density [40]. This well-designed study was realized in vivo with [^{11}C]UCB-J PET imaging in an olive baboon (Papio anubis), after which the animal was sacrificed, and the brain was dissected for post-mortem tissue studies. The post-mortem analyses (involving 12 brain regions) consisted in western blotting, SV2A homogenate binding assays and immunohistochemical staining for SV2A and synaptophysin protein as reference marker for synaptic density measures. To established that SV2A can be used as marker of synaptic density, they compared regional densities of SV2A and the "gold standard" synaptic marker synaptophysin using selective antibodies. SV2A and synaptophysin signals were strong and specific in all grey matter regions but absent or weak in the centrum semiovale (CS). There was an excellent linear correlation between SV2A and synaptophysin across all grey matter regions. They were able to establish that SV2A can be used as an alternative to Synaptophysin for accurate synapse quantification. In addition, the authors established a strong correlation between the in vitro regional distribution of SV2A and the [^{11}C]UCB-J V_T measured in vivo by PET. Afterward, to further evaluate the relationship between in vivo [^{11}C]UCB-J binding and SV2A density, homogenate binding studies were performed to determine affinity (*Kd*) and regional SV2A densities B_{max}. The authors reported a clear correlation between the in vitro B_{max} values measured in the 12 brain regions and the in vivo V_T values. As a cross validation, there was an excellent correlation between the *Kd* derived from homogenate binding and the regional SV2A Western blot measurements.

Recently, UCB-J was investigated in mice and more specifically in the amyloid precursor protein and presenilin 1 double-transgenic (APPswe/PS1DE9 [APP/PS1]) mouse model of Alzheimer disease [41]. The authors intended to perform a longitudinal [^{11}C]UCB-J PET on these AD mice to measure the treatment effects of saracatinib, an inhibitor of the tyrosine kinase Fyn which is believed to be useful in AD treatment. The experimental design consisted in the testing of two groups: the control group with wild type (WT) mice and the test group with APPswe/PS1DE9 mice. Both groups underwent three [^{11}C]UCB-J PET measurements: at baseline, after treatment, and during drug washout (more than 27 d after the end of treatment). The quantification was achieved with several parameters, the first to be used was the BP_{ND}, computed by the simplified reference tissue model with the brain stem as reference region. Then the authors compared this BP_{ND} with the SUVratio using the brain stem signal for normalization ($SUVR_{BS}$, static acquisition time of 30 min between 30 and 60 min post-injection). The authors also tested another SUVratio normalized by the whole brain ($SUVR_{WB}$). The authors found that BP_{ND} and $SUVR_{BS}$ demonstrate excellent agreement with correlation coefficient $R^2 = 0.85$ for the whole brain region. However, for treatment response assessment, the authors claimed that $SUVR_{WB}$ gave less variability mainly due to the small size of the used regions of interest. Then, Toyonaga et al. stated that [^{11}C]UCB-J PET allows to differentiate hippocampal $SUVR_{WB}$ in APP/PS1 mice and in WT mice at baseline and to detect a significant increase in hippocampal $SUVR_{WB}$ after AD treatment with saracatinib.

In 2016, UCB Pharma, in collaboration with Yale University, reported preclinical data on their newly developed antiepileptic drug named Brivaracetam (acting on SV2A, like its predecessor compound levetiracetam). They used PET imaging to prove a faster SV2A occupancy by brivaracetam compared with levetiracetam [42]. Displacement experiments using [^{11}C]UCB-J were performed in rhesus monkeys to estimate the time course of tracer exit from the brain after single IV dosing of brivaracetam (5 $mg \cdot kg^{-1}$) or levetiracetam (30 $mg \cdot kg^{-1}$). The estimated displacement half-times were 10 min for brivaracetam and 30 min for levetiracetam. Further, using kinetic modelling, they were able to predict drug entry half-times, which were 3 min for brivaracetam and 23 min for levetiracetam.

The third SV2A radiotracer belonging to the first generation is the UCB-A [23]. Unlike the two other UCB tracers, UCB-A displayed a relatively slow metabolism, with 93% and 42% intact tracer present at 5 and 40 min post-injection. Surprisingly, the [^{11}C]UCB-A showed a slow kinetic profile with an accumulation during the first 60 min, followed by a slow wash out from the brain. The time activity curves of the whole brain clearly demonstrated a successful blocking of [^{11}C]UCB-A binding by the pre-injection of an acetamide-based ligand of SV2A (named compound 4 in the study, 10 $mg \cdot kg^{-1}$). Further, the reversible binding of [^{11}C]UCB-A was demonstrated by the administration of brivaracetam (21 $mg \cdot kg^{-1}$), at 45 min post-injection, which fully and rapidly displaced [^{11}C]UCB-A. Afterward, the [^{11}C]UCB-A was further developed in pig where PET images were quantified by whole blood time-activity measures and metabolite-corrected arterial input curves for kinetic modelling. The authors used the Akaike criteria to determine that [^{11}C]UCB-A kinetics were best described by a 1T model. With this model, they could estimate both V_T and k_1 parameters. However, the 1T model was unable to properly estimate V_T in the blocking condition. The authors found that Logan graphical analysis could reliably fit baseline and blocking conditions and therefore decided to use it in the occupancy analysis of their blocking conditions. Regarding the dosimetry in rats, the organ receiving the highest absorbed dose was the liver, at 12.5 and 26.3 $\mu Gy \cdot MBq^{-1}$ in males and females, respectively. Effective doses were 2.9 $\mu Sv \cdot MBq^{-1}$ and 4.6 $\mu Sv \cdot MBq^{-1}$, for males and females, respectively. The authors claimed that given the effective doses observed in rats, an effective dose of no more than 1.8 mSv per typical administration of 400 MBq would be achievable.

Currently, UCB-J has been fluorinated and tested in vivo in non-human primates [27]. As the chemical structure is the same as UCB-J, all features of UCB-J radiotracer remain the same and the authors stated that the tracer possesses the same in vivo behavior has its parent compounds UCB-J.

The second generation of radiotracer is leaded by two tracers: SynVesT-1 and SynVesT-2. Both tracers display a very high affinity for SV2A (reported previously in this review). Both of them were evaluated in non-human primates [28,31]. SynVesT-1 and SynVesT-2 share a very similar metabolism rate in plasma. The first one displayed 42 ± 13% of parent radiotracer remaining at 30 min after injection, which further decreased to 27 ± 5% and 23 ± 5%, respectively, at 60 and 90 min. post-injection. For the second one, the authors reported that 34% ± 0.1% of intact parent radiotracer remains at 30 min post-injection, which further decreased to 24% ± 3% and 22% ± 4%, at 60 and 90 min, respectively. In rhesus monkeys, both tracer with high tracer uptake in gray matter and very low uptake in white matter (the lower value being found in the CS, as in the case of UCB-J PET imaging). SynVesT-1 has been drastically displaced by the administration of levetiracetam (30 $mg{\cdot}kg^{-1}$) at 90 min post-injection. The binding specificity was emphasized by blocking studies, either by pretreatment with levetiracetam (30 $mg{\cdot}kg^{-1}$) or UCB-J (0.15 $mg{\cdot}kg^{-1}$). Both competitors dramatically decreased regional uptake levels across all brain regions and resulted in earlier peak uptake. Regarding SynVesT-2 preblocking study with unlabelled UCB-J (150 $\mu g{\cdot}kg^{-1}$) completely reduced the specific binding of the tracer. Although both tracers look very similar, it is worth mentioning that their brain kinetics largely differ. Indeed, SynVesT-1 displayed an SUV peak within 30 min post-injection in all brain regions followed by a moderate rate of clearance over time, whereas SynVesT-2 showed a much faster brain kinetic with a SUV peak reached at 10 min post-injection. On the contrary, both tracers display a very similar uptake pattern with the highest tissue uptake levels found in the frontal cortex and putamen (SUV > 8 for both), and lowest in CS (SUV < 2 for both). Concerning the quantification of PET images, both tracers were analyzed with either the 1T model or the simplified reference tissue model (SRTM) using the CS as reference tissue. The 1T model allows to compute the V_T parameter which has proven to be more than two times higher for SynVesT-1 than for SynVesT-2 across all brain regions. In addition, the V_T values for SynVesT-1 are much closer to those obtained with UCB-J in rhesus monkeys. Similarly, with the BP_{ND} obtained with SRTM, values for SynVesT-1 were higher for all brain regions, but this time BP_{ND} values for SynVesT-2 are closer to those obtained with UCB-J.

In a nutshell, SynVesT-1 and SynVesT-2 share lots of common features in terms of metabolism and in vivo behavior, although SynVesT-1 seems the most promising one with close outcomes to UCB-J PET imaging.

4. Clinical Studies with SV2A PET Radiotracers

4.1. Quantification of SV2A PET Radiotracers Binding

4.1.1. UCB-H in Human Brain

The distribution of UCB-H in the human brain was studied using the full kinetic modelling approach [43,44]. Authors have motivated their orientation to the full kinetic modelling by the ubiquitous distribution of SV2A in the brain, which makes very unlikely the identification of a "reference region" with all its necessary characteristics for modelling the radiotracer distribution [45]. Moreover, the white matter usually used as reference region for several tracers and studies was also discarded because of the presence of white matter lesions in several elderly and AD participants [46]. In order to overcome the problem of patient discomfort during the arterial input function (AIF) sampling, an alternative method using carotid artery image-derived input function was developed for UCB-H quantification [43]. Even with this image-derived input function, blood sampling was not completely discarded, and authors collected venous blood samples in a group-representative number of subjects at six time-points post injection in order to determine the plasmatic parent fraction needed for image-derived input function correction.

The input function was derived from dynamic PET images [43]. Briefly, the method extracts time series of radiotracer activity in the carotid arteries [47]. The identification of voxels belonging to the carotids is based on the computation of the Pearson product-moment correlation coefficient between a "seeding region" and voxels in a mask containing the carotid. As, during the first 2min, radioactivity is mainly localized in the vessels, inducing a large spill-out effect [47], the signal was corrected for this spill-out effect using the geometric transfer matrix approach [48]. The extracted time-series signal was then corrected for the mean unchanged plasma fraction and used for kinetic modelling.

As image analysis and kinetic modelling, UCB-H PET dynamic data frames underwent a series of processing steps before voxel-wise parametric map extraction. Indeed, data frames were corrected for participant's motion during the acquisition and co-registered to the corresponding MRI structural image (the sum of frames between 2 and 30 min as source image), and then partial volume corrected. The PET scanner low resolutions as well the small structures of interest (e.g., hippocampus and the basal forebrain that are atrophied in early Alzheimer's disease are the main raisons for partial volume correction [49]. The iterative Yang (PETPVC toolbox, [50]) voxel-wise PVC method was used, with grey matter, white matter, CSF as ROI mask. Kinetic modelling using PVE-corrected dynamic PET data and image-derived input function was done with PMOD software (PMOD Technologies, Zurich, Switzerland). Logan graphical analysis method was used to calculate the V_T map of UCB-H in the brain with t* of 25 min. The obtained V_T map was then spatially normalized into the MNI space using the transformation parameters obtained during structural MRI spatial normalization. Spatial normalization is usually done through the structural MRI image as the last one has a higher resolution. Mean regional V_T values were then extracted from V_T map using the AAL atlas [51].

4.1.2. UCB-J in Human Brain

UCB-J in vivo quantification in human brain was presented in the publication of Finnema 2016 where the authors proposed the CS as a reference region for non-displaceable binding [40]. Regional non-displaceable binding potential (BP_{ND}) was calculated as the ratio between the distribution volume in region of interest and the distribution volume in the CS minus one ($V_{T,region}$ / $V_{T,centrum\_semiovale}$ −1). The volume of distribution was calculated using a full kinetic modelling through the 1T model with measured arterial input function and regional time activity curves (TACs). The extraction of the regional time activity curves was done on the subject PET space using AAL atlas. Briefly, the inverse transformation parameters obtained during the spatial normalization of the motion corrected UCB-J dynamic data were applied to the AAL atlas to bring it into the PET space. Then, regional TACs were extracted end expressed in SUV by normalization of the regional activity concentration by the ratio of injected dose to subject weight.

Parametric BPND maps were also generated with the simplified reference tissue model 2 using the CS as a reference region [52]. The author showed that CS has some degree of specific binding and further follow-up studies and analysis were still needed to justify its use as a reference region.

In a recent study aiming at the validation of the CS, Rossano et al. investigated the region of interest definition and the reconstruction parameters (number of iteration of the ordered subset expectation minimization "OS-EM" [53]. Indeed, optimization of the CS ROI definition aims to minimize the inclusion of grey matter and partial volume effects that would lead to erroneous CS V_T values. This was done using an improved ROI definition strategy based on the use of the CS AAL to mask the individual white matter and the definition of a group CS ROIs with increasing volume (2, 4, and 6 mL). Additionally, convergence using the OS-EM algorithm was investigated by increasing the iterations used to reconstruct the PET image, which would minimize any positive bias that may be observed in the low-intensity white matter, surrounded by the high-intensity grey matter. Moreover, baseline and blocking (levetiracetam and brivaracetam) UCB-J scans were used to estimate the V_{ND} of the grey matter, and the validity of using CS V_T to estimate V_{ND} in calculating BP_{ND} was evaluated. Even if the results showed a specific uptake in the white matter lower than 10% of that in the grey matter and the CS uptake was predominantly due to non-displaceable binding, the authors stressed the importance of assessing differences in white matter uptake when investigating differences across disease groups, especially in diseases with white matter pathology. Koole et al. also investigated CS as reference region for UCB-J quantification showing considerable agreement with Rossano conclusions [54]. Compared to a full kinetic analysis, with 1T compartment method with measured AIF, simplified reference tissue model approach using a 90 min acquisition interval and the CS as reference tissue provided a negligible bias of less than 6%. Moreover, the authors suggested shortening the dynamic acquisition time to 70 min instead of 120 min. Alternately to dynamic tracer uptake modelling, SUV ratio relative to the CS for 30 min acquisition starting 60 min after tracer injection was proposed as a quantitative approximation for UCB-J brain PET imaging. The use of CS white matter as reference region for [^{11}C]UCB-J quantification has been further supported by in vitro autoradiographic observations of low binding for [^{11}C]UCB-J in this region, in either human non-human primates [55].

4.2. Clinical Outcomes with SV2A PET Imaging

The first in-human study with SV2A specific PET tracer was published by Bretin et al. and concerned biodistribution description and radiation dosimetry assessment [56]. The authors reported the results of dynamic whole-body PET with UCB-H on five healthy males with an injected activity between 139.1–156.5 MBq. The radiation dosimetry was calculated using OLINDA/EXM. Regarding the brain, as main organ of interest, the absorbed dose was $1.89\times10^{-2} \pm 2.32 \times 10^{-3}$ mGy·MBq^{-1}. The methodological aspects of UCB-H brain images quantification have been described above in this review [43]. Thanks to the implementation of the image-derived blood input function, the same group reported the outcomes of UCB-H PET imaging in twenty-four patients with mild cognitive impairment or Alzheimer's disease (with positive [^{18}F]Flutemetamol amyloid-PET) compared to 19 healthy controls (Figure 2., [44]). Using voxel-wise analysis on V_T maps after partial volume effect correction (amyloid positive patients vs control group), the authors described a significant reduction of synaptic density in the right anterior hippocampus extending to the entorhinal cortex (26.9% decrease in right hippocampal [^{18}F]UCB-H V_T). A sub-analysis focusing only on mild AD patient (n = 14) showed reduced synaptic density in the right superior temporal gyrus. Finally, the authors computed Pearson correlations between [^{18}F]UCB-H values in selected ROIs and cognitive measures. When taking into account the correction for multiple comparisons, the authors showed correlations between awareness of memory problems and MMSE scores on the one hand and [^{18}F]UCB-H values in the hippocampus on the other hand (Pearson correlation coefficient of −0.75 and 0.57 respectively, at $p < 0.005$). Thus, Bastin et al. clearly confirmed that SV2A-PET imaging with [^{18}F]UCB-H, allows to image in vivo synaptic changes in Aβ-positive patients with neurocognitive disorder and to relate them to cognitive impairment with regional specificity according to the cognitive domain.

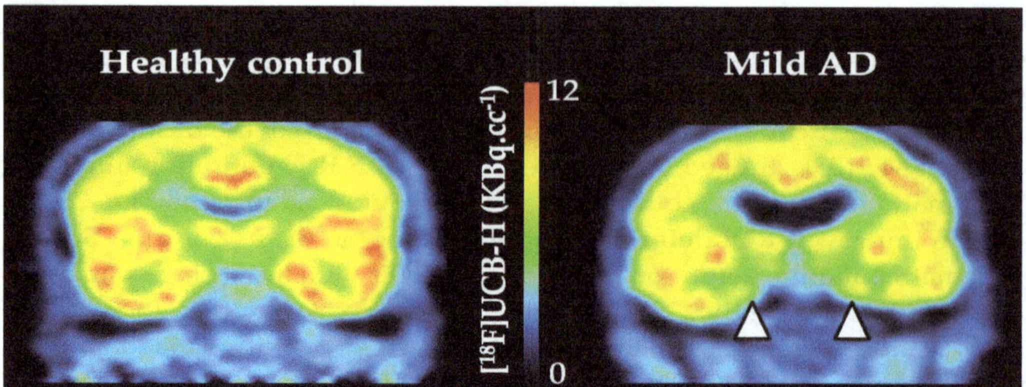

Figure 2. Individual example of [^{18}F]UCB-H in healthy control and in mild AD patient. The white arrow heads highlight the reduced [^{18}F]UCB-H uptake in temporal lobe areas of the mild AD patient.

The first study reporting SV2A PET assessment in AD was published by the University of Yale and used UCB-J [57]. The outcomes parameters used as imaging outcomes were the V_T, the delivery rate constant K_1 and the BP_{ND} (obtained with the 1T and the SRTM 2 models). The study included twenty-one participants, with 10 amnestic MCI due to AD or mild AD dementia participants and 11 healthy controls. The results were consistent with the hypothesis derived from AD Braak staging, showing that [^{11}C]UCB-J binding was significantly reduced in the hippocampus of participants with AD compared to the control group. In the hippocampus of AD participants, the V_T was 28% lower and the BP_{ND} was reduced by 44%. Parametric map of K1 value, reflecting the cerebral blood flow clearly highlighted that the pattern of regional k_1 reduction in the participant with AD was similar to that of hypometabolism observed with FDG-PET in AD. Finally, Chen et al. reported Pearson correlations between [^{11}C]UCB-J values in the hippocampus and cognitive measures. Notably, statistically significant correlations were found between SRTM2-derived hippocampus BP_{ND} and episodic memory on one hand (R = 0.56; p =0.01), and with clinical dementia rating–sum of boxes (CDR-SB) score on the other hand (R = −0.61; p =0.003). These results were later confirmed in a study conducted by the group of KU Leuven where prodromal AD patients (aMCI) were tested with both [^{11}C]UCB-J and [^{18}F]MK-6240 that allows the assessment of Tau protein deposition [58]. Within the median temporal lobe, there was a clear correlation between [^{11}C]UCB-J SUVR decrease and [^{18}F]MK-6240 SUVR increase (r = −0.076, p = 0.02). The authors corroborated previous results with SV2A PET imaging while highlighting the hippocampus as the most prominent region for synapse loss. Moreover, synaptic loss correlates with cognitive decline measured by MMSE score and episodic memory test (r = 0.77 and 0.7 respectively).

As a logical follow-up of the preclinical study that supported the development of the brivaracetam anti-epileptic drug, UCB Pharma and Yale University released a drug occupancy study in human for brivaracetam using [^{11}C]UCB-J PET [59]. Three cohorts with four, five, and four healthy subjects were tested for baseline and displacement, displacement and 4 h post-dose and steady state of oral dosing of brivaracetam respectively. The [^{11}C]UCB-J PET scanning procedure consisted of an intravenous bolus plus constant infusion. The regional V_T parameter was derived from 1T model and SV2A occupancy computed by regressing the change in V_T against the baseline V_T across regions. The main occupancy results were 66% and 70% for intravenous 100 mg of brivaracetam, 84% and 85% for intravenous 200 mg of brivaracetam, and 78–84% for intravenous 1500 mg of levetiracetam approximately 4 h post-dose. Moreover, the combined IC_{50} estimate across Cohorts 2 and 3 was 0.46 $\mu g{\cdot}mL^{-1}$ for brivaracetam and 4.02 $\mu g{\cdot}mL^{-1}$ for levetiracetam, leading the authors to state that brivaracetam has 8.7-fold higher affinity for SV2A than levetiracetam.

Recently, the group of Yale University published a PET imaging study with [^{11}C]UCB-J in a cohort of Parkinson's disease patients [60]. Based on current pathophysiological knowledge of PD, more precisely on the fact that synaptic changes are centrally involved in PD and characteristic of the disease pathogenesis, the authors seek to detect synaptic loss in vivo with [^{11}C]UCB-J PET in individuals with mild bilateral PD [61]. Twelve PD subjects, assessed according to the Movement Disorders Society Unified PD Rating Scale, were compared to 12 matched normal controls. As previously described, the PET data were processed using SRTM2 kinetic modelling with BP_{ND} as imaging outcome. Statistical lower SV2A-specific binding values were found in PD subjects in several brain regions, the substantia nigra (−45%; p <0.001), red nucleus (−31%; p =0.03), locus coeruleus (−17%; p =0.03), and parahippocampal gyrus (−12%; p <0.01). The lower SV2A binding in the substantia nigra was further confirmed by in vitro autoradiography (−17%; p <0.005). The authors concluded that their results were in line with the hypothesis claiming that clinical symptomatology of PD may begin in the synapses of brainstem nuclei and remain present throughout the course of the disease [61].

Concerning psychiatric disorders, a recent article reported the in vivo investigation of synaptic density in schizophrenia [62]. This study is in line with evidences implicating synaptic dysfunction in the pathophysiology of schizophrenia. The authors included 18 individuals with a DSM-5 diagnosis of schizophrenia and compared them to 18 healthy volunteers using [11C]UCB-J V_T, derived from the 1T model, as imaging outcome. Post-hoc analyses revealed that mean [^{11}C]UCB-J V_T (ml·cm^{-3}) was significantly reduced in schizophrenic patients relative to the control group in the frontal cortex (t = 2.51, df = 34.0, p =0.03), and in the anterior cingulate cortex (t = 2.83, df = 34.0, p =0.02) with large effect sizes (Cohen's d = 0.8 and 0.9 respectively). Interestingly, Onwordi et al. computed the distribution volume ratio (DVR, using the CS as reference region) in the selected ROIs and found a significant reduction in the hippocampus, in addition to the frontal cortex (FC) and the anterior cingulate cortex (ACC). This discrepancy was analyzed in the sense that DVR values show lower variability and so are likely to have greater sensitivity to detect group differences. Furthermore, the authors stated the absence of significant associations between [^{11}C]UCB-J V_T and corrected grey matter volume in any of the analyzed ROIs, as well as between [^{11}C]UCB-J V_T in the FC, ACC and the assessed clinical variables. The authors completed their clinical results by preclinical in vitro experiment that showed the absence of effect of chronic haloperidol administration on SV2A levels in the rat frontal cortex. This study raised the question whether these results rely on specific loss of SV2A protein or indicate lower synaptic terminal levels. So far, there is no evidence that antipsychotic drugs act on synaptic density, but it would be clinically relevant to compare longitudinally patients who do not respond to antipsychotic treatments and patients who do so.

In parallel, the group from Yale university investigated major depressive disorder (MDD) and post-traumatic stress disorder (PTSD) with the hypothesis that synaptic density, measured by [^{11}C]UCB-J PET, would be negatively associated with severity of depressive symptoms [63]. The study included twenty-six unmedicated clinical subjects and twenty-one age, sex, and smoking-matched healthy control subjects. The [^{11}C]UCB-J V_T derived from 1T model after partial volume correction used to correct for effects of tissue atrophy. Three regions of interest were considered: the hippocampus, the dorsolateral prefrontal cortex (dlPFC), and the anterior cingulate cortex (ACC). In each of these regions, a significant lower [^{11}C]UCB-J V_T in individuals with high severity depressive symptoms was detected in comparison to healthy controls. Strikingly, the authors reported significant negative correlations between the [^{11}C]UCB-J V_T and the severity of depressive symptoms (scored with the HAMD-17 scale) across all clinical subjects in dlPFC (r = −0.633, p = 0.001), ACC (r = −0.634, p = 0.001) and hippocampus (r = −0.487, p = 0.012). Finally, Holmes et al. looked at the functional connectivity in the study cohort and performed voxel-wise correlations to associate the seed connectivity data from the dlPFC to synaptic density. They found a significant negative correlation between dlPFC-posterior cingulate cortex (PCC) connectivity and SV2A density in the dlPFC in the clinical group (r = −0.60, p = 0.002). The authors concluded that their results prompt the discovery and evaluation of new treatments that should target synaptic density to increase synaptic connections.

Overall, the clinical outcomes of SV2A PET imaging suggest that this technic might bring new outcomes in clinical trials for disease monitoring and treatment response assessment, as well as in the refinement of the studies by providing new inclusion/exclusion criteria.

5. Conclusions

Currently, [^{11}C]UCB-J and [^{18}F]UCB-H are the two most widely used radiotracers for SV2A PET imaging in patients with neurological or psychiatric disorders, but they both present disadvantages. On one hand, the half-life of ^{11}C drastically limits the availability of [^{11}C]UCB-J, and [^{18}F]UCB-H provides a lower specific binding signal on the other hand. Notwithstanding, clinical outcomes obtained with both of them were very coherent with each other. The second generation of SV2A tracers is leaded by [^{18}F]SynVesT-1 and [^{18}F]SynVesT-2 which are both produced via labelling of an arylstannane precursor. The use of organotin compounds required ICP-MS analysis to ensure the injectability to the patients. Improvements of the radiochemical yield of iodonium precursors labelling could be an alternative to this stannic derivatives limitation. Alternatively, another radiotracer, a ^{18}F-difluoromethyl analogue of UCB-J that can be produced by C-H activation, does not require the synthesis of a specific precursor. However, for future PET clinical imaging applications, the radiochemical synthesis should also be improved. Nevertheless, and despite the quality of the newly designed fluorinated radiotracers, SV2A PET imaging still faces its biggest challenge, that is, in being included in a clinical routine for patient care and management.

Author Contributions: Conceptualization, G.B. and S.D.; writing—original draft preparation, G.B., S.D., M.A.B. and E.S.; writing—review and editing, G.B., S.D., M.A.B. and E.S. All authors have read and agreed to the published version of the manuscript.

Acknowledgments: In this section you can acknowledge any support given which is not covered by the author contribution or funding sections. This may include administrative and technical support, or donations in kind (e.g., materials used for experiments).

References

1. Lynch, B.A.; Lambeng, N.; Nocka, K.; Kensel-Hammes, P.; Bajjalieh, S.M.; Matagne, A.; Fuks, B. The Synaptic Vesicle Protein Sv2a Is the Binding Site for the Antiepileptic Drug Levetiracetam. *Proc. Natl. Acad. Sci. USA* **2004**, *101*, 9861–9866. [CrossRef] [PubMed]
2. Bajjalieh, S.M.; Frantz, G.D.; Weimann, J.M.; McConnell, S.K.; Scheller, R.H. Differential Expression of Synaptic Vesicle Protein 2 (Sv2) Isoforms. *J. Neurosci.* **1994**, *9*, 5223–5235. [CrossRef]
3. Crowder, K.M.; Gunther, J.M.; Jones, T.A.; Hale, B.D.; Zhang, H.Z.; Peterson, M.R.; Scheller, R.H.; Chavkin, C.; Bajjalieh, S.M. Abnormal Neurotransmission in Mice Lacking Synaptic Vesicle Protein 2a (Sv2a). *Proc. Natl. Acad. Sci. USA* **1999**, *26*, 15268–15273. [CrossRef] [PubMed]
4. Bartholome, O.; Van den Ackerveken, P.; Sánchez Gil, J.; de la Brassinne Bonardeaux, O.; Leprince, P.; Franzen, R.; Rogister, B. Puzzling out Synaptic Vesicle 2 Family Members Functions. *Front. Mol. Neurosci.* **2017**, 148. [CrossRef]
5. Bakker, A.; Krauss, G.L.; Albert, M.S.; Speck, C.L.; Jones, L.R.; Stark, C.E.; Yassa, M.A.; Bassett, S.S.; Shelton, A.L.; Gallagher, M. Reduction of Hippocampal Hyperactivity Improves Cognition in Amnestic Mild Cognitive Impairment. *Neuron* **2012**, *3*, 467–474. [CrossRef]
6. Pascal, E.S.; Zhu, L.; Verret, L.; Vossel, K.A.; Orr, A.G.; Cirrito, J.R.; Devidze, N.; Ho, K.; Yu, G.-Q.; Palop, J.J.; et al. Levetiracetam Suppresses Neuronal Network Dysfunction and Reverses Synaptic and Cognitive Deficits in an Alzheimer's Disease Model. *Proc. Natl. Acad. Sci. USA* **2012**, *109*, E2895–E2903.
7. Terry, R.D.; Masliah, E.; Salmon, D.P.; Butters, N.; DeTeresa, R.; Hill, R.; Hansen, L.A.; Katzman, R. Physical Basis of Cognitive Alterations in Alzheimer's Disease: Synapse Loss Is the Major Correlate of Cognitive Impairment. *Ann. Neurol.* **1991**, *4*, 572–580. [CrossRef]
8. Scheff, S.W.; Price, D.A.; Schmitt, F.A.; Mufson, E.J. Hippocampal Synaptic Loss in Early Alzheimer's Disease and Mild Cognitive Impairment. *Neurobiol. Aging* **2006**, *10*, 1372–1384. [CrossRef]
9. Klitgaard, H.; Verdu, P. Levetiracetam: The First Sv2a Ligand for the Treatment of Epilepsy. *Expert Opin. Drug Discov.* **2007**, *2*, 11. [CrossRef]
10. Gillard, M.; Fuks, B.; Michel, P.; Vertongen, P.; Massingham, R.; Chatelain, P. Binding Characteristics of [3h]Ucb 30889 to Levetiracetam Binding Sites in Rat Brain. *Eur. J. Pharmacol.* **2003**, *478*, 1–9. [CrossRef]
11. Klitgaard, H.; Matagne, A.; Gobert, J.; Wulfert, E. Evidence for a Unique Profile of Levetiracetam in Rodent Models of Seizures and Epilepsy. *Eur. J. Pharmacol.* **1998**, *353*, 191–206. [CrossRef]
12. Gillard, M.; Fuks, B.; Leclercq, K.; Matagne, A. Binding Characteristics of Brivaracetam, a Selective, High Affinity Sv2a Ligand in Rat, Mouse and Human Brain: Relationship to Anti-Convulsant Properties. *Eur. J. Pharmacol.* **2011**, *664*, 36–44. [CrossRef]
13. Mercier, J.; Archen, L.; Bollu, V.; Carré, S.; Evrard, Y.; Jnoff, E.; Kenda, B.; Lallemand, B.; Michel, P.; Montel, F.; et al. Discovery of Heterocyclic Nonacetamide Synaptic Vesicle Protein 2a (Sv2a) Ligands with Single-Digit Nanomolar Potency: Opening Avenues Towards the First Sv2a Positron Emission Tomography (Pet) Ligands. *Chem. Med. Chem.* **2014**, *9*, 693–698. [CrossRef]
14. Zhang, L.; Villalobos, A. Strategies to Facilitate the Discovery of Novel Cns Pet Ligands. *EJNMMI Radiopharm. Chem.* **2017**, 13. [CrossRef] [PubMed]

15. Need, A.; Kant, N.; Jesudason, C.; Barth, V. Approaches for the Discovery of Novel Positron Emission Tomography Radiotracers for Brain Imaging. *Clin. Transl. Imaging* **2017**, *5*, 265–274. [CrossRef]
16. Pike, V.W. Considerations in the Development of Reversibly Binding Pet Radioligands for Brain Imaging. *Curr. Med. Chem.* **2016**, *18*, 1818–1869. [CrossRef] [PubMed]
17. Zhang, L.; Villalobos, A.; Beck, E.M.; Bocan, T.; Chappie, T.A.; Chen, L.; Grimwood, S.; Heck, S.D.; Helal, C.J.; Hou, X.; et al. Design and Selection Parameters to Accelerate the Discovery of Novel Central Nervous System Positron Emission Tomography (Pet) Ligands and Their Application in the Development of a Novel Phosphodiesterase 2a Pet Ligand. *J. Med. Chem.* **2013**, *56*, 4568–4579. [CrossRef]
18. Hancheng, C.; Mangner, T.J.; Muzik, O.; Wang, M.-W.; Chugani, D.C.; Chugani, H.T. Radiosynthesis of (11)C-Levetiracetam: A Potential Marker for Pet Imaging of Sv2a Expression. *ACS Med. Chem. Lett.* **2014**, *10*, 1152–1155.
19. Warnock, G.I.; Aerts, J.; Bahri, M.A.; Bretin, F.; Lemaire, C.; Giacomelli, F.; Mievis, F.; Mestdagh, N.; Buchanan, T.; Valade, A.; et al. Evaluation of 18f-Ucb-H as a Novel Pet Tracer for Synaptic Vesicle Protein 2a in the Brain. *J. Nucl. Med.* **2014**, *8*, 1336–1341. [CrossRef]
20. Aerts, J.; Otabashi, M.; Giacomelli, F.; Warnock, G.; Bahri, M.; Bretin, F.; Sauvage, X.; Thielen, C.; Lemaire, C.; Salmon, E.; et al. Radiosynthesis and First Small Animal Micropet Imaging of [18f]Ucb-H, a New Fluorine-18 Labelled Tracer Targeting Synaptic Vesicle Protein 2a (Sv2a). *EANM Abstr.* **2013**, *40*, S158.
21. Warnier, C.; Lemaire, C.; Becker, G.; Zaragoza, G.; Giacomelli, F.; Aerts, J.; Otabashi, M.; Bahri, M.A.; Mercier, J.; Plenevaux, A.; et al. Enabling Efficient Positron Emission Tomography (Pet) Imaging of Synaptic Vesicle Glycoprotein 2a (Sv2a) with a Robust and One-Step Radiosynthesis of a Highly Potent 18f-Labeled Ligand ([18f]Ucb-H). *J. Med. Chem.* **2016**, *59*, 8955–8966. [CrossRef]
22. Pike, V.W.; Aigbirhio, F.I. Reactions of Cyclotron-Produced [18f] Fluoride with Diaryliodonium Salts—A Novel Single-Step Route to No-Carrier-Added [18] Fluoroarenes. *J. Chem. Soc. Chem. Commun.* **1995**, *21*, 2215–2216. [CrossRef]
23. Estrada, S.; Lubberink, M.; Thibblin, A.; Sprycha, M.; Buchanan, T.; Mestdagh, N.; Kenda, B.; Mercier, J.; Provins, L.; Gillard, M.; et al. [11c]Ucb-a, a Novel Pet Tracer for Synaptic Vesicle Protein 2a. *Nucl. Med. Biol.* **2016**, *43*, 325–332. [CrossRef] [PubMed]
24. Nabulsi, N.B.; Mercier, J.; Holden, D.; Carre, S.; Najafzadeh, S.; Vandergeten, M.C.; Lin, S.F.; Deo, A.; Price, N.; Wood, M.; et al. Synthesis and Preclinical Evaluation of 11c-Ucb-J as a Pet Tracer for Imaging the Synaptic Vesicle Glycoprotein 2a in the Brain. *J. Nucl. Med.* **2016**, *57*, 777–784. [CrossRef] [PubMed]
25. Rokka, J.; Schlein, E.; Eriksson, J. Improved synthesis of SV2A targeting radiotracer [11C]UCB-J. *EJNMMI Radiopharm. Chem.* **2019**, *4*. [CrossRef] [PubMed]
26. Sephton, S.M.; Miklovicz, T.; Russell, J.J.; Doke, A.; Li, L.; Boros, I.; Aigbirhio, F.I. Automated radiosynthesis of [11C]UCB-J for imaging synaptic density by positron emission tomography. *J. Label. Compd. Radiopharm.* **2020**, *63*, 151–158. [CrossRef]
27. Li, S.; Cai, Z.; Zhang, W.; Holden, D.; Lin, S.-F.; Finnema, S.J.; Shirali, A.; Ropchan, J.; Carre, S.; Mercier, J.; et al. Synthesis and in vivo evaluation of [18F]UCB-J for PET imaging of synaptic vesicle glycoprotein 2A (SV2A). *Eur. J. Nucl. Med. Mol. Imaging* **2019**, *46*, 1952–1965. [CrossRef]
28. Li, S.; Cai, Z.; Wu, X.; Holden, D.; Pracitto, R.; Kapinos, M.; Gao, H.; Labaree, D.C.; Nabulsi, N.; Carson, R.E.; et al. Synthesis and in Vivo Evaluation of a Novel PET Radiotracer for Imaging of Synaptic Vesicle Glycoprotein 2A (SV2A) in Nonhuman Primates. *ACS Chem. Neurosci.* **2018**, *10*, 1544–1554. [CrossRef]
29. Constantinescu, C.C.; Tresse, C.; Zheng, M.; Gouasmat, A.; Carroll, V.M.; Mistico, L.; Alagille, D.; Sandiego, C.M.; Papin, C.; Marek, K.; et al. Development and In Vivo Preclinical Imaging of Fluorine-18-Labeled Synaptic Vesicle Protein 2A (SV2A) PET Tracers. *Mol. Imaging Boil.* **2018**, *21*, 509–518. [CrossRef]
30. Cai, Z.; Li, S.; Finnema, S.; Lin, S.; Zhang, W.; Holden, D.; Carson, R.; Huang, Y. Imaging Synaptic Density with Novel 18f-Labeled Radioligands for Synaptic Vesicle Protein-2a (Sv2a): Synthesis and Evaluation in Nonhuman Primates. *J. Nucl. Med.* **2017**, *58* (Suppl. S1), 547.
31. Cai, Z.; Li, S.; Zhang, W.; Pracitto, R.; Wu, X.; Baum, E.; Finnema, S.J.; Holden, D.; Toyonaga, T.; Lin, S.-F.; et al. Synthesis and Preclinical Evaluation of an 18F-Labeled Synaptic Vesicle Glycoprotein 2A PET Imaging Probe: [18F]SynVesT-2. *ACS Chem. Neurosci.* **2020**, *11*, 592–603. [CrossRef] [PubMed]

32. Patel, S.; Knight, A.; Krause, S.; Teceno, T.; Tresse, C.; Li, S.; Cai, Z.; Gouasmat, A.; Carroll, V.M.; Barret, O.; et al. Preclinical In Vitro and In Vivo Characterization of Synaptic Vesicle 2A-Targeting Compounds Amenable to F-18 Labeling as Potential PET Radioligands for Imaging of Synapse Integrity. *Mol. Imaging Biol.* **2019**, 1–10. [CrossRef] [PubMed]
33. Trump, L.; Lemos, A.; Lallemand, B.; Pasau, P.; Mercier, J.; Lemaire, C.; Luxen, A.; Genicot, C. Late-Stage 18f-Difluoromethyl Labeling of N-Heteroaromatics with High Molar Activity for Pet Imaging. *Angew. Chem. Int. Ed.* **2019**, *131*, 13283–13288. [CrossRef]
34. Trump, L.; Lemos, A.; Jacq, J.; Pasau, P.; Lallemand, B.; Mercier, J.; Genicot, C.; Luxen, A.; Lemaire, C. Development of a General Automated Flow Photoredox 18F-Difluoromethylation of N-Heteroaromatics in an AllinOne Synthesizer. *Org. Process. Res. Dev.* **2020**. [CrossRef]
35. Serrano, M.E.; Becker, G.; Bahri, M.A.; Seret, A.; Mestdagh, N.; Mercier, J.; Mievis, F.; Giacomelli, F.; Lemaire, C.; Salmon, E.; et al. Evaluating the In Vivo Specificity of [18F]UCB-H for the SV2A Protein, Compared with SV2B and SV2C in Rats Using microPET. *Molecules* **2019**, *24*, 1705. [CrossRef]
36. Bretin, F.; Warnock, G.; Bahri, M.A.; Aerts, J.; Mestdagh, N.; Buchanan, T.; Valade, A.; Mievis, F.; Giacomelli, F.; Lemaire, C.; et al. Preclinical radiation dosimetry for the novel SV2A radiotracer [18F]UCB-H. *EJNMMI Res.* **2013**, *3*, 35. [CrossRef]
37. Becker, G.; Warnier, C.; Serrano, M.E.; Bahri, M.A.; Mercier, J.; Lemaire, C.; Salmon, E.; Luxen, A.; Plenevaux, A. Pharmacokinetic Characterization of [18F]UCB-H PET Radiopharmaceutical in the Rat Brain. *Mol. Pharm.* **2017**, *14*, 2719–2725. [CrossRef]
38. Serrano, M.E.; Bahri, M.A.; Becker, G.; Seret, A.; Mievis, F.; Giacomelli, F.; Lemaire, C.; Salmon, E.; Luxen, A.; Plenevaux, A. Quantification of [18F]UCB-H Binding in the Rat Brain: From Kinetic Modelling to Standardised Uptake Value. *Mol. Imaging Boil.* **2018**, *21*, 888–897. [CrossRef]
39. Serrano, M.E.; Bahri, M.A.; Becker, G.; Seret, A.; Germonpré, C.; Lemaire, C.; Giacomelli, F.; Mievis, F.; Luxen, A.; Salmon, E.; et al. Exploring with [18F]UCB-H the in vivo Variations in SV2A Expression through the Kainic Acid Rat Model of Temporal Lobe Epilepsy. *Mol. Imaging Boil.* **2020**, 1–11. [CrossRef]
40. Finnema, S.J.; Nabulsi, N.B.; Eid, T.; Detyniecki, K.; Lin, S.-F.; Chen, M.-K.; Dhaher, R.; Matuskey, D.; Baum, E.; Holden, D.; et al. Imaging synaptic density in the living human brain. *Sci. Transl. Med.* **2016**, *8*, 348ra96. [CrossRef]
41. Toyonaga, T.; Smith, L.M.; Finnema, S.J.; Gallezot, J.-D.; Naganawa, M.; Bini, J.; Mulnix, T.; Cai, Z.; Ropchan, J.; Huang, Y.; et al. In Vivo Synaptic Density Imaging with 11C-UCB-J Detects Treatment Effects of Saracatinib in a Mouse Model of Alzheimer Disease. *J. Nucl. Med.* **2019**, *60*, 1780–1786. [CrossRef] [PubMed]
42. Nicolas, J.-M.; Hannestad, J.; Holden, D.; Kervyn, S.; Nabulsi, N.; Tytgat, D.; Huang, Y.; Chanteux, H.; Staelens, L.; Matagne, A.; et al. Brivaracetam, a selective high-affinity synaptic vesicle protein 2A (SV2A) ligand with preclinical evidence of high brain permeability and fast onset of action. *Epilepsia* **2015**, *57*, 201–209. [CrossRef] [PubMed]
43. Bahri, M.A.; Plenevaux, A.; Aerts, J.; Bastin, C.; Becker, G.; Mercier, J.; Valade, A.; Buchanan, T.; Mestdagh, N.; LeDoux, D.; et al. Measuring brain synaptic vesicle protein 2A with positron emission tomography and [18 F]UCB-H. *Alzheimer's Dementia: Transl. Res. Clin. Interv.* **2017**, *3*, 481–486. [CrossRef] [PubMed]
44. Bastin, C.; Bahri, M.A.; Meyer, F.; Manard, M.; Delhaye, E.; Plenevaux, A.; Becker, G.; Seret, A.; Mella, C.; Giacomelli, F.; et al. In vivo imaging of synaptic loss in Alzheimer's disease with [18F]UCB-H positron emission tomography. *Eur. J. Nucl. Med. Mol. Imaging* **2019**, *47*, 390–402. [CrossRef]
45. Salinas, C.A.; Searle, G.E.; Gunn, R.N. The simplified reference tissue model: Model assumption violations and their impact on binding potential. *Br. J. Pharmacol.* **2014**, *35*, 304–311. [CrossRef]
46. Wahlund, L.O.; Barkhof, F.; Fazekas, F.; Bronge, L.; Augustin, M.; Sjögren, M.; Wallin, A.; Ader, H.; Leys, D.; Pantoni, L.; et al. A New Rating Scale for Age-Related White Matter Changes Applicable to MRI and CT. *Stroke* **2001**, *32*, 1318–1322. [CrossRef]
47. Schain, M.; Benjaminsson, S.; Varnäs, K.; Forsberg, A.; Halldin, C.; Lansner, A.; Farde, L.; Varrone, A. Arterial input function derived from pairwise correlations between PET-image voxels. *Br. J. Pharmacol.* **2013**, *33*, 1058–1065. [CrossRef]
48. Rousset, O.G.; Ma, Y.; Evans, A.C. Correction for partial volume effects in PET: Principle and validation. *J. Nucl. Med.* **1998**, *39*, 904–911.

49. Erlandsson, K.; Buvat, I.; Pretorius, P.H.; Thomas, B.A.; Hutton, B.F. A review of partial volume correction techniques for emission tomography and their applications in neurology, cardiology and oncology. *Phys. Med. Boil.* **2012**, *57*, R119–R159. [CrossRef]
50. Thomas, B.A.; Cuplov, V.; Bousse, A.; Mendes, A.; Thielemans, K.; Hutton, B.F.; Erlandsson, K. PETPVC: A toolbox for performing partial volume correction techniques in positron emission tomography. *Phys. Med. Boil.* **2016**, *61*, 7975–7993. [CrossRef]
51. Tzourio-Mazoyer, N.; Landeau, B.; Papathanassiou, D.; Crivello, F.; Etard, O.; Delcroix, N.; Mazoyer, B.; Joliot, M. Automated Anatomical Labeling of Activations in SPM Using a Macroscopic Anatomical Parcellation of the MNI MRI Single-Subject Brain. *NeuroImage* **2002**, *15*, 273–289. [CrossRef] [PubMed]
52. Wu, Y.; Carson, R.E. Noise Reduction in the Simplified Reference Tissue Model for Neuroreceptor Functional Imaging. *J. Cereb. Blood. Flow Metab.* **2002**, *22*, 1440–1452. [CrossRef] [PubMed]
53. Rossano, S.; Toyonaga, T.; Finnema, S.J.; Naganawa, M.; Lu, Y.; Nabulsi, N.; Ropchan, J.; De Bruyn, S.; Otoul, C.; Stockis, A.; et al. Assessment of a white matter reference region for 11C-UCB-J PET quantification. *Br. J. Pharmacol.* **2019**, 271678 19879230. [CrossRef]
54. Koole, M.; Van Aalst, J.; Devrome, M.; Mertens, N.; Serdons, K.; Lacroix, B.; Mercier, J.; Sciberras, D.; Maguire, R.P.; Van Laere, K. Quantifying SV2A density and drug occupancy in the human brain using [11C]UCB-J PET imaging and subcortical white matter as reference tissue. *Eur. J. Nucl. Med. Mol. Imaging* **2018**, *46*, 396–406. [CrossRef] [PubMed]
55. Varnäs, K.; Stepanov, V.; Halldin, C. Autoradiographic mapping of synaptic vesicle glycoprotein 2A in non-human primate and human brain. *Synapse* **2020**. [CrossRef]
56. Bretin, F.; Bahri, M.A.; Bernard, C.; Warnock, G.; Aerts, J.; Mestdagh, N.; Buchanan, T.; Otoul, C.; Koestler, F.; Mievis, F.; et al. Biodistribution and Radiation Dosimetry for the Novel SV2A Radiotracer [18F]UCB-H: First-in-Human Study. *Mol. Imaging Boil.* **2015**, *17*, 557–564. [CrossRef]
57. Chen, M.-K.; Mecca, A.P.; Naganawa, M.; Finnema, S.J.; Toyonaga, T.; Lin, S.-F.; Najafzadeh, S.; Ropchan, J.; Lu, Y.; McDonald, J.W.; et al. Assessing Synaptic Density in Alzheimer Disease With Synaptic Vesicle Glycoprotein 2A Positron Emission Tomographic Imaging. *JAMA Neurol.* **2018**, *75*, 1215–1224. [CrossRef]
58. Vanhaute, C.H.R.J.; Ceccarini, J.; Michiels, L.; Sunaert, S.; Lemmens, R.; Emsell, L.; Vandenbulcke, M.; Van Laere, K. Changes in Synaptic Density in Relation to Tau Deposition in Prodromal Alzheimer's Disease: A Dual Protocol Pet-Mr Study. In Proceedings of the European Association of Nuclear Medicine 2019, EANM, Barcelona, Spain, 12–16 October 2019; Volume 46, pp. S177–S178.
59. Finnema, S.J.; Rossano, S.; Naganawa, M.; Henry, S.; Gao, H.; Pracitto, R.; Maguire, R.P.; Mercier, J.; Kervyn, S.; Nicolas, J.; et al. A single-center, open-label positron emission tomography study to evaluate brivaracetam and levetiracetam synaptic vesicle glycoprotein 2A binding in healthy volunteers. *Epilepsia* **2019**, *60*, 958–967. [CrossRef]
60. Matuskey, D.; Tinaz, S.; Wilcox, K.C.; Naganawa, M.; Toyonaga, T.; Dias, M.; Henry, S.; Pittman, B.; Ropchan, J.; Nabulsi, N.; et al. Synaptic Changes in Parkinson Disease Assessed with in vivo Imaging. *Ann. Neurol.* **2020**, *87*, 329–338. [CrossRef]
61. Bellucci, A.; Mercuri, N.B.; Venneri, A.; Faustini, G.; Longhena, F.; Pizzi, M.; Missale, C.; Spano, P. Review: Parkinson's disease: From synaptic loss to connectome dysfunction. *Neuropathol. Appl. Neurobiol.* **2016**, *42*, 77–94. [CrossRef]
62. Onwordi, E.C.; Halff, E.F.; Whitehurst, T.; Mansur, A.; Cotel, M.C.; Wells, L.; Creeney, H.; Bonsall, D.; Rogdaki, M.; Shatalina, E.; et al. Synaptic Density Marker Sv2a Is Reduced in Schizophrenia Patients and Unaffected by Antipsychotics in Rats. *Nat Commun.* **2020**, *11*, 246. [CrossRef] [PubMed]
63. Holmes, S.E.; Scheinost, D.; Finnema, S.J.; Naganawa, M.; Davis, M.T.; DellaGioia, N.; Nabulsi, N.; Matuskey, D.; Angarita, G.A.; Pietrzak, R.H.; et al. Lower Synaptic Density Is Associated with Depression Severity and Network Alterations. *Nat. Commun.* **2019**, *10*, 1529. [CrossRef] [PubMed]

12

Thiol-Reactive PODS-Bearing Bifunctional Chelators for the Development of EGFR-Targeting [^{18}F]AlF-Affibody Conjugates

Chiara Da Pieve [1,*], Ata Makarem [2], Stephen Turnock [3], Justyna Maczynska [3], Graham Smith [1] and Gabriela Kramer-Marek [3,*]

1 PET Radiochemistry, Division of Radiotherapy and Imaging, the Institute of Cancer Research, 123 Old Brompton Road, London SW7 3RP, UK; Graham.Smith@icr.ac.uk
2 Division of Radiopharmaceutical Chemistry, German Cancer Research Center (DKFZ), Im Neuenheimer Feld 280, 69120 Heidelberg, Germany; a.makarem@dkfz-heidelberg.de
3 Preclinical Molecular Imaging, Division of Radiotherapy and Imaging, the Institute of Cancer Research, 123 Old Brompton Road, London SW7 3RP, UK; Stephen.Turnock@icr.ac.uk (S.T.); justyna.maczynska@icr.ac.uk (J.M.)
* Correspondence: chiara.daPieve@icr.ac.uk (C.D.P.); Gabriela.Kramer-Marek@icr.ac.uk (G.K.-M.)

Academic Editors: Anne Roivainen and Xiang-Guo Li

Abstract: Site-selective bioconjugation of cysteine-containing peptides and proteins is currently achieved via a maleimide–thiol reaction (Michael addition). When maleimide-functionalized chelators are used and the resulting bioconjugates are subsequently radiolabeled, instability has been observed both during radiosynthesis and post-injection in vivo, reducing radiochemical yield and negatively impacting performance. Recently, a phenyloxadiazolyl methylsulfone derivative (PODS) was proposed as an alternative to maleimide for the site-selective conjugation and radiolabeling of proteins, demonstrating improved in vitro stability and in vivo performance. Therefore, we have synthesized two novel PODS-bearing bifunctional chelators (NOTA-PODS and NODAGA-PODS) and attached them to the EGFR-targeting affibody molecule $Z_{EGFR:03115}$. After radiolabeling with the aluminum fluoride complex ([^{18}F]AlF), both conjugates showed good stability in murine serum. When injected in high EGFR-expressing tumor-bearing mice, [^{18}F]AlF-NOTA-PODS-$Z_{EGFR:03115}$ and [^{18}F]AlF-NODAGA-PODS-$Z_{EGFR:03115}$ showed similar pharmacokinetics and a specific tumor uptake of 14.1 ± 5.3% and 16.7 ± 4.5% ID/g at 1 h post-injection, respectively. The current results are encouraging for using PODS as an alternative to maleimide-based thiol-selective bioconjugation reactions.

Keywords: [^{18}F]AlF; NOTA; NODAGA; PODS; thiol-reactive; linker; affibody molecule; bioconjugation; EGFR; tumor imaging

1. Introduction

Reactive sulfhydryl groups of cysteine residues are attractive sites for the chemical attachment of dyes, chelators, or drugs to biomolecules. Targeting cysteine residues on biomolecules has several key benefits. Firstly, the presence of the thiol group, a highly reactive nucleophile, allows for a fast and selective reaction at physiological pH. The natural low abundance of accessible and reduced cysteine residues prevents the formation of heterogeneous mixtures of the bioconjugates. Moreover, a customized site-specific incorporation of cysteine residues into a biomolecule can be easily achieved [1]. Different classes of thiol-targeting electrophilic compounds have been used, with maleimides being the most common choice [2–4]. However, maleimide conjugates have shown instability mostly as a consequence of thiol exchange reactions in vivo (e.g., retro-Michael addition) [5,6]. When maleimide-based bioconjugates are used as imaging agents, the above mentioned succinimidyl thioether linkage instability can lead to reduced accumulation in target tissues due to the release of the radioactive payload from the conjugate. Additionally, the thiol exchange reaction with endogenous thiol-containing biomolecules (e.g., albumin, cysteine and glutathione) can result in a higher background-to-noise ratio and a consequently reduced imaging contrast [7]. Thiol-reactive reagents have been investigated aiming at the formation of selective, fast, high-yielding and, most importantly, stable linkages with biomolecules [2,8–10]. Among the promising molecules, oxadiazolyl methyl sulfone-based compounds showed not only rapid and selective reaction with thiols in proteins but also the capacity of forming conjugates (via an oxadiazole–protein thiolate bond) which were more stable than those derived from maleimides [11,12]. The preparation of thiol-reactive bifunctional chelators and prosthetic groups containing the oxadiazolyl methylsulfone moiety (e.g., phenyloxadiazolyl methylsulfone or PODS) and their attachment to proteins and peptides have been examined [13–15]. Once radiolabeled, the conjugates were found to be more stable in vitro than the maleimide-derived counterparts. Moreover, when used in vivo, the oxadiazolyl methylsulfone linker-derived agents demonstrated reduced uptake in non-targeted tissues than the maleimide equivalents [13–15]. Based on these promising reports, we have prepared two novel phenyloxadiazolyl methylsulfone-containing (PODS) bifunctional chelators (NOTA-PODS and NODAGA-PODS) for the conjugation and aluminum fluoride ([^{18}F]AlF) radiolabeling of a cysteine-containing biomolecule. For our study, an EGFR-targeting affibody molecule ($Z_{EGFR:03115}$) was used as a thiol-bearing protein representative. The effect of the chelator structure on the synthesis and radiolabeling of the two conjugates ([^{18}F]AlF-NOTA-PODS-$Z_{EGFR:03115}$ and [^{18}F]AlF-NODAGA-PODS-$Z_{EGFR:03115}$) was studied together with their in vitro and in vivo profile. Additionally, a comparison was carried out with the maleimide-bearing [^{18}F]AlF-NOTA-$Z_{EGFR:03115}$ to benchmark in vitro and in vivo performance.

2. Results and Discussion

2.1. *Preparation of Bifunctional Chelators NOTA-PODS and NODAGA-PODS*

The aluminum fluoride-18 ([^{18}F]AlF) radiolabeling procedure has generated significant interest by combining the convenient and straightforward metal-based radiochemistry (e.g., one-pot reaction, minimal purification steps, aqueous solution compatibility) and the excellent decay characteristics of fluorine-18 (97% positron emission, low positron energy, half-life of 109.8 min). This method was used to directly radiolabel small molecules, peptides and proteins containing macrocyclic chelators such as NOTA or NODA [16,17]. Accordingly, in this work, the NOTA and NODAGA chelators were selected for the [^{18}F]AlF radiolabeling of affibody molecule $Z_{EGFR:03115}$. However, instead of the conventional maleimide, thiol-reactive bifunctional chelators for the conjugation to the cysteine-containing small protein were developed by functionalizing the macrocycles with PODS. The reaction between PODS and the NHS ester of either NOTA or NODAGA was performed in DMF in the presence of base (Scheme 1). The products were obtained in a quantitative yield (Figure S1); NOTA-PODS and NODAGA-PODS were used for the subsequent conjugation reaction without further purification. Alternatively, pure bifunctional chelators could be isolated by semi-preparative RP–HPLC using formic acid instead of TFA in the mobile phase (Figures S2–S4). Of note, when NOTA-PODS solutions in DMF were stored at −20 °C, noticeable signs of degradation were detected already after 2 months. Conversely, NODAGA-PODS in DMF showed good stability for at least 10 months (Figure S5).

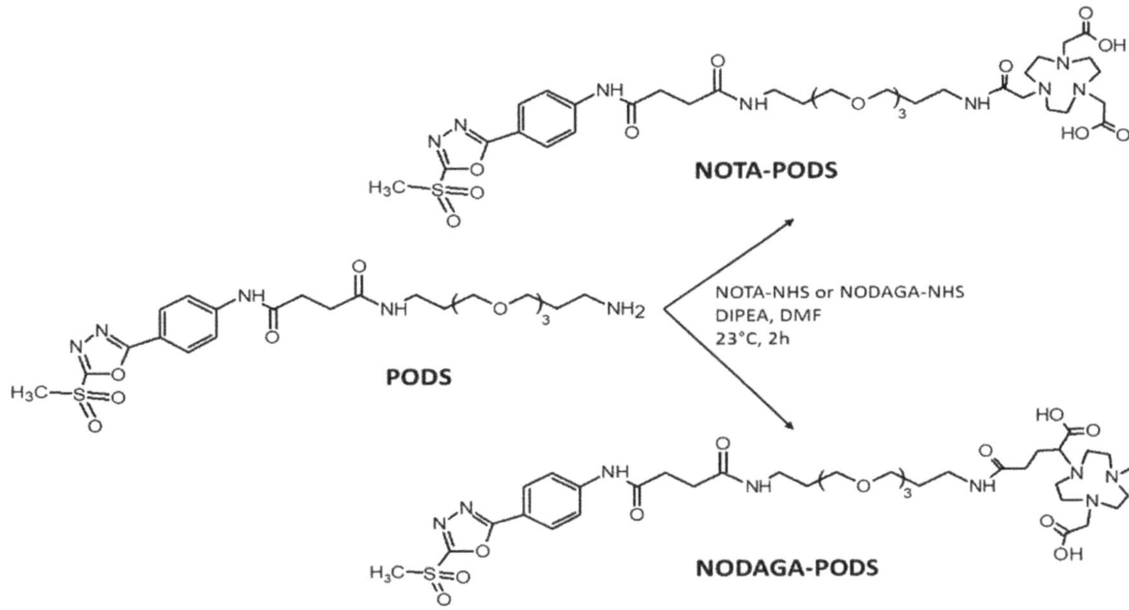

Scheme 1. Synthesis of NOTA-PODS and NODAGA-PODS.

2.2. *Preparation of NOTA-PODS-$Z_{EGFR:03115}$ and NODAGA-PODS-$Z_{EGFR:03115}$*

The bifunctional chelators were conjugated to $Z_{EGFR:03115}$ in a one-pot reaction using TCEP-HCl as the reducing agent (Scheme 2, Figure S6). A quantitative yield was achieved using a lower molar excess of PODS-bifunctional chelator to protein compared to a conventional maleimide-based chelator (15 vs. 35 equivalents). Being the great molar excess necessary as a consequence of the inhibition of the reactivity of maleimide-based compounds by TCEP, this result suggests that PODS is not as susceptible to TCEP as maleimides [18]. To obtain extremely pure products for the subsequent radiolabeling reaction, a single final purification of the conjugates by semi-preparative HPLC was performed (Figure 1). The pure compounds were isolated in a ca. 38% and ca. 24% yield for NOTA-PODS-$Z_{EGFR:03115}$ and NODAGA-PODS-$Z_{EGFR:03115}$, respectively. All products were characterized by ESI mass spectrometry (Figure S7).

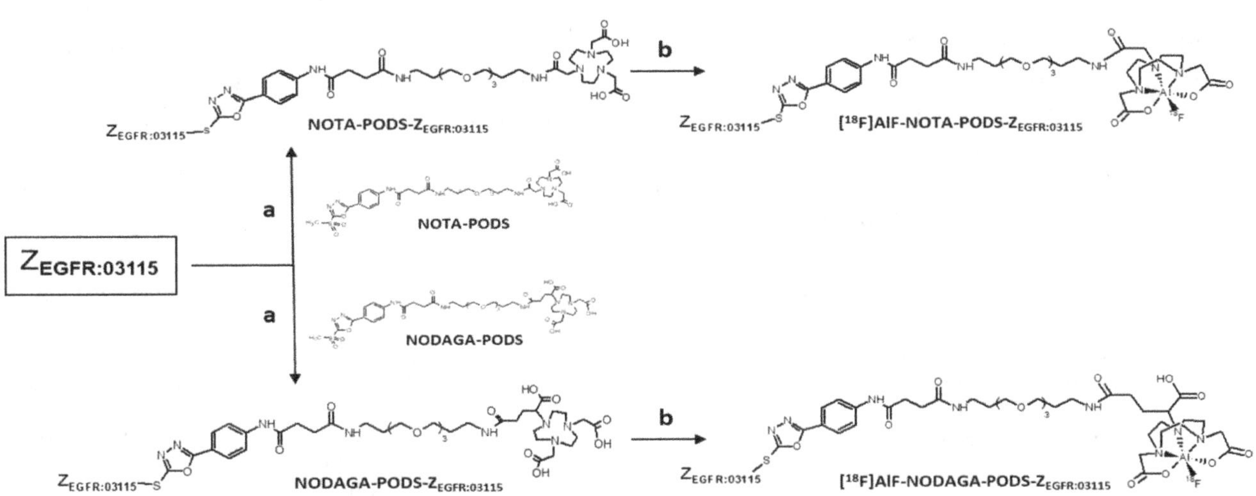

Scheme 2. Preparation of [^{18}F]AlF-NOTA-PODS-$Z_{EGFR:03115}$ and [^{18}F]AlF-NODAGA-PODS-$Z_{EGFR:03115}$. Reaction conditions: (a) TCEP-HCl, 1 M phosphate buffer pH 7; (b) $AlCl_3$ in sodium acetate pH 4, [^{18}F]F$^-$ aq./ethanol 1:1 (*v*/*v*), for 15 min, and at 100 °C.

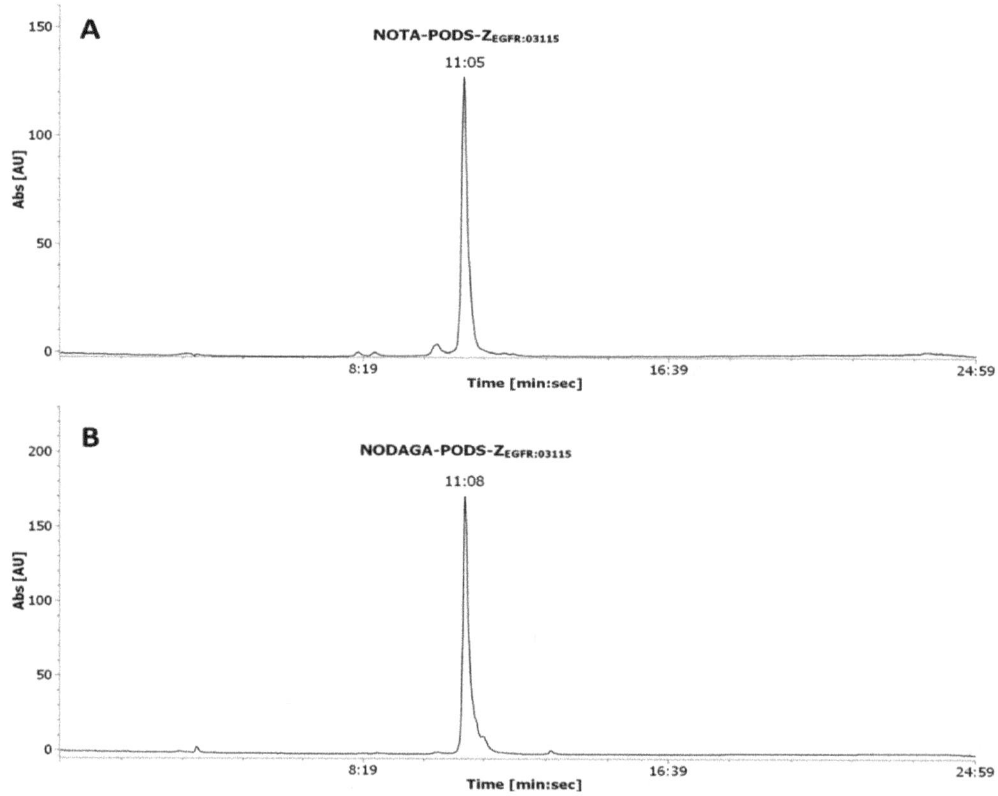

Figure 1. RP–HPLC analysis of NOTA-PODS-$Z_{EGFR:03115}$ (**A**), and NODAGA-PODS-$Z_{EGFR:03115}$ (**B**). The absorbance was recorded at the wavelength of 280 nm. The retention time (Rt) is indicated as min:sec.

2.3. [^{18}F]AlF Radiolabeling and In Vitro Stability

The affibody conjugates were radiolabeled with [^{18}F]AlF in a one-pot reaction at pH 4, 100 °C for 15 min using ethanol as organic co-solvent (50% *v/v*) (Scheme 2). Consistent with previously reported results for maleimide-derived affibody conjugates, some thermal degradation products were formed during the reaction (Figures S8,S9) [17]. Therefore, a RP–HPLC purification procedure, followed by HLB-SPE, was required to produce [^{18}F]AlF-NOTA-PODS-$Z_{EGFR:03115}$ and [^{18}F]AlF-NODAGA-PODS-$Z_{EGFR:03115}$ with a RCP > 98%, verified by RP–HPLC (Figure 2). As shown in Table 1, the radiochemical yields and the apparent specific/molar activities (SA/MA) achieved for [^{18}F]AlF-NODAGA-PODS-$Z_{EGFR:03115}$ were lower than for [^{18}F]AlF-NOTA-PODS-$Z_{EGFR:03115}$. Similar findings have been described by other research groups and attributed to the chelator structure and chelation capacity towards the [^{18}F]AlF complex [19,20].

Table 1. Summary of radiolabeling reactions. Radiochemical yields (RCY) and apparent specific (SA) and molar activities (MA) are decay corrected.

Radioconjugate	RCY	SA/MA	Protein Recovery
[^{18}F]AlF-NOTA-PODS-$Z_{EGFR:03115}$	11.0%–12.7%	0.40–0.59 MBq/μg 3.0–4.4 MBq/nmol	37.1%–38.0%
[^{18}F]AlF-NODAGA-PODS-$Z_{EGFR:03115}$	4.3%–8.1%	0.11–0.23 MBq/μg 0.8–1.7 MBq/nmol	23.9%–26.0%
[^{18}F]AlF-NOTA-$Z_{EGFR:03115}$	10.7%–38.0%	0.57–1.09 MBq/μg 4.1–7.8 MBq/nmol	10.6%–34.5%

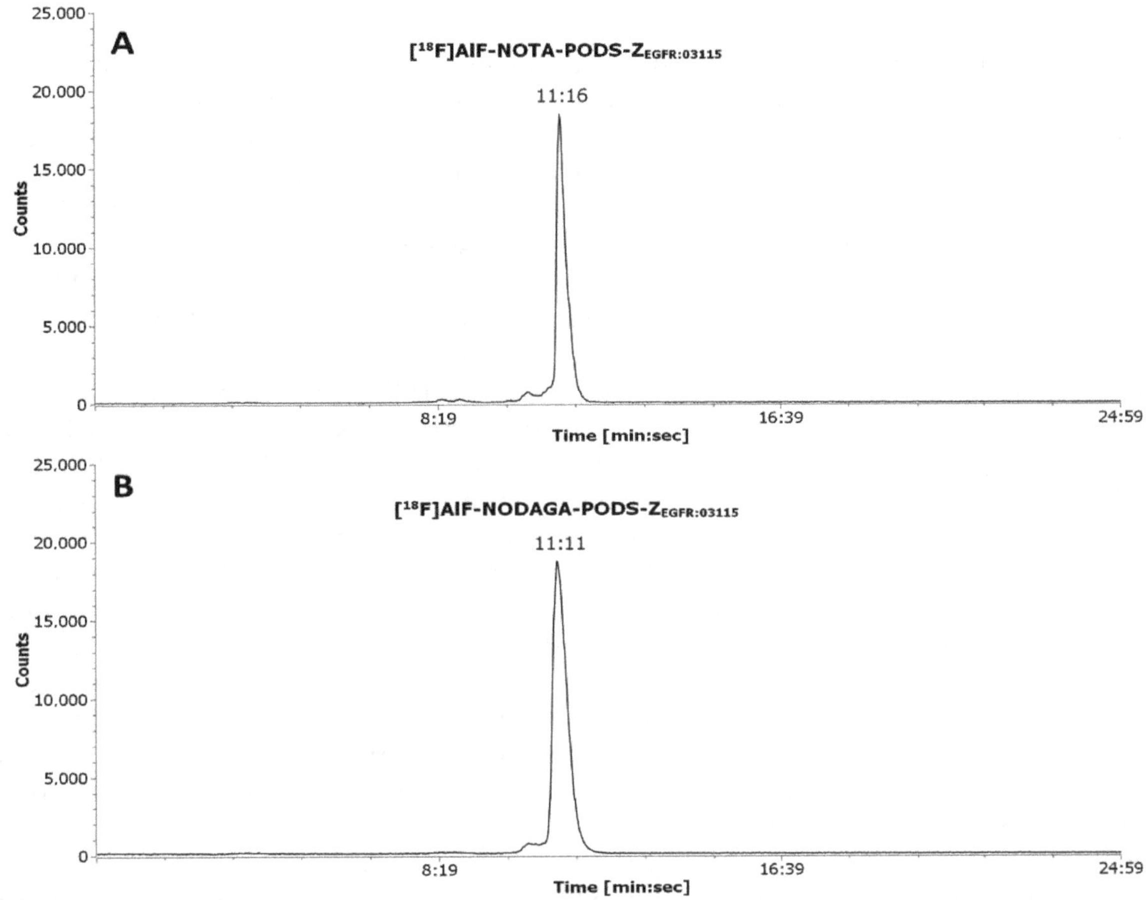

Figure 2. Radiochromatograms of pure [^{18}F]AlF-NOTA-PODS-$Z_{EGFR:03115}$ (**A**), and [^{18}F]AlF-NODAGA-PODS-$Z_{EGFR:03115}$ (**B**). The retention time (Rt) is indicated as min:sec.

To investigate the impact of the PODS linker on the radioconjugate properties, the distribution coefficient ($logD_{7.4}$) values of the two products were determined (Table S1). The $logD_{7.4}$ for [^{18}F]AlF-NOTA-PODS-$Z_{EGFR:03115}$ and [^{18}F]AlF-NODAGA-PODS-$Z_{EGFR:03115}$ was found to be hydrophilic, with values of -1.73 ± 0.07 and -3.62 ± 0.06, respectively. Including the maleimide-bearing product [^{18}F]AlF-NOTA-$Z_{EGFR:03115}$ $logD_{7.4}$ value of -1.13 ± 0.1, the NODAGA-radioconjugate proved to be the most hydrophilic of the tested compounds.

The stability of the PODS-bearing radioconjugates, with respect to change in radiochemical purity (RCP) and loss of radioactivity from the affibody molecule, was determined in mouse serum at 37 °C for 1 h (Table S2). As affibody molecules have short blood half-life, and the in vivo studies (imaging and biodistribution) are typically performed 1 h post-injection, a longer incubation time was not investigated [21]. According to RP–HPLC analysis, both conjugates exhibited good stability as 92.7 ± 2.6% of [^{18}F]AlF-NOTA-PODS-$Z_{EGFR:03115}$ and 97.2 ± 1.2% of [^{18}F]AlF-NODAGA-PODS-$Z_{EGFR:03115}$ remained intact after 1 h (Figure S10, Table S2). As previously observed for [^{18}F]AlF-NOTA-$Z_{EGFR:03115}$, a residual activity associated with the pelleted protein indicates some non-specific affinity of the radioconjugates towards the serum proteins (Table S2). However, amongst the tested compounds, the maleimide-bearing [^{18}F]AlF-NOTA-$Z_{EGFR:03115}$ demonstrated significantly higher protein-associated radioactivity than [^{18}F]AlF-NOTA-PODS-$Z_{EGFR:03115}$ and [^{18}F]AlF-NODAGA-PODS-$Z_{EGFR:03115}$ (30.5 ± 2.1% vs. 24.2 ± 3.4% and 20.4 ± 0.7%, respectively). Studies to determine whether this effect is connected to the maleimide linker are under investigation.

2.4. In Vivo Studies

To investigate the chelator effect on the pharmacokinetics and targeting properties of the conjugates, the two PODS-bearing radioactive agents were assessed in vivo in high EGFR-expressing U87MGvIII tumor-bearing mice. To determine the influence of PODS, a comparison to the maleimide derivative [^{18}F]AlF-NOTA-$Z_{EGFR:03115}$ was performed. Previous studies found that 12 μg of radiolabeled EGFR-targeting affibody conjugate with an apparent specific activity of 0.09–0.15 MBq/μg was able to partially saturate the endogenous EGFR expression (e.g., liver) and allowed for clear visualization of the tumors 1 h post-injection [22]; therefore, a dose of 12 μg (1.1–1.8 MBq) of each radioconjugate was injected. The biodistribution data indicate that the nature of the linker (i.e., PODS or maleimide) minimally influenced the radioconjugate pharmacokinetics, since similar distribution profiles were observed by both the NOTA-based products [^{18}F]AlF-NOTA-PODS-$Z_{EGFR:03115}$ and [^{18}F]AlF-NOTA-$Z_{EGFR:03115}$ (Figure 3, Table S3). However, compared to the NOTA-bearing products, [^{18}F]AlF-NODAGA-PODS-$Z_{EGFR:03115}$ showed an inconsistent radioactivity accumulation in the liver. This result suggests that the chelator can influence the radioconjugate pharmacokinetics and that chelator-customized injected protein doses and specific activities should be investigated further by dose-escalation studies. Among the non-targeted organs, the highest uptake of all three conjugates was found in the kidneys, which is due to renal excretion of the affibody molecule, and the reabsorption of the radioactive metabolites followed by their retention in the proximal tubular cells [23]. Based on this effect, the kidney uptake value for [^{18}F]AlF-NODAGA-PODS-$Z_{EGFR:03115}$ suggests a possible higher renal clearance of the NODAGA conjugate compared to [^{18}F]AlF-NOTA-PODS-$Z_{EGFR:03115}$. Moreover, both PODS-bearing radioconjugates show significantly lower kidney uptakes than the maleimide analogue, indicating a possible effect of the PODS linker on the renal retention (Figure 3 and Table S3). More experiments will be needed to confirm this observation. High accumulation of the conjugates was found in the tumors, with uptakes of 14.1 ± 5.3 and 16.7 ± 4.5 %ID/g for [^{18}F]AlF-NOTA-PODS-$Z_{EGFR:03115}$ and [^{18}F]AlF-NODAGA-PODS-$Z_{EGFR:03115}$, respectively (Figure 4, Table S3). The favorable tumor-to-muscle ratios for the two PODS-bearing radioconjugates resulted in high-contrast PET images already 1 h post-injection (Table 2). In contrast to Adumeau et al., there was no difference in both the biodistribution profile and the tumor-to-tissue ratios between the [^{18}F]AlF PODS-bearing conjugates and the malemide-based product (Table 2, Table S3) [15].

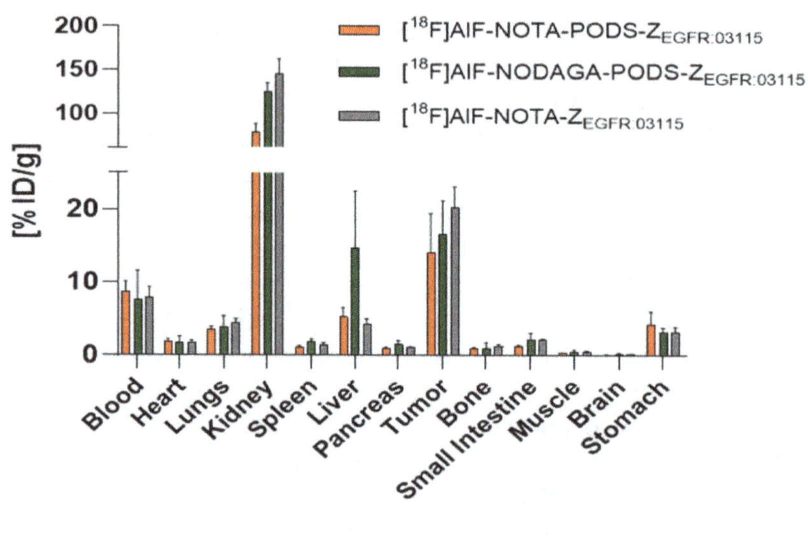

Figure 3. Biodistribution results for [^{18}F]AlF-NOTA-PODS-$Z_{EGFR:03115}$ and [^{18}F]AlF-NODAGA-PODS -$Z_{EGFR:03115}$ at 1 h p.i. [^{18}F]AlF-NOTA-$Z_{EGFR:03115}$ was used as a control. The data are reported as the mean percentage of the injected dose per gram of tissue (%ID/g) ± SD (for each group, n = 3).

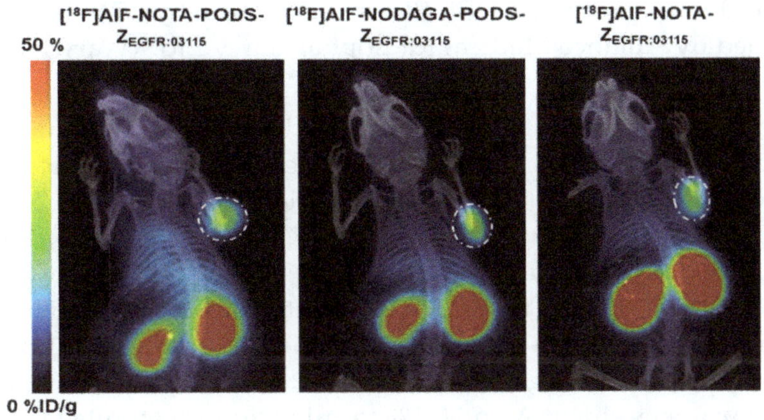

Figure 4. PET/CT images of U87MGvIII tumor-bearing mice using [^{18}F]AlF-NOTA-PODS-$Z_{EGFR:03115}$ and [^{18}F]AlF-NODAGA-PODS-$Z_{EGFR:03115}$. [^{18}F]AlF-NOTA-$Z_{EGFR:03115}$ was used as control. High-contrast images were acquired as early as 1 h p.i. The tumors are indicated by a white circle.

Table 2. Tumor-to-organ ratios at 1 h p.i. of the three examined [^{18}F]AlF conjugates. No differences were identified.

	Tumor-to-Organ Ratio			
	Blood	**Kidney**	**Liver**	**Muscle**
[^{18}F]AlF-NOTA-PODS-$Z_{EGFR:03115}$	1.6 ± 0.6	0.2 ± 0.1	2.7 ± 1.2	37.2 ± 12.4
[^{18}F]AlF-NODAGA-PODS-$Z_{EGFR:03115}$	2.6 ± 1.2	0.1 ± 0.0	1.3 ± 0.6	31.3 ± 8.2
[^{18}F]AlF-NOTA-$Z_{EGFR:03115}$	2.8 ± 0.9	0.1 ± 0.0	4.7 ± 0.8	34.9 ± 3.4

3. Materials and Methods

3.1. General Materials and Methods

Chemicals and solvents were purchased and used without further purification unless otherwise stated. The 2,2′-(7-{2-[(2,5-dioxopyrrolidin-1-yl)oxy]-2-oxoethyl}-1,4,7-triazonane-1,4-diyl)diacetic acid (NOTA-NHS) and 2,2′-(7-{1-carboxy-4-[(2,5-dioxopyrrolidin-1-yl)oxy)-4-oxobutyl]-1,4,7-triazonane-1,4-diyl}diacetic acid (NODAGA-NHS) were purchased from Chematech (Dijon, France). Tris(2-carboxyethyl)-phosphine hydrochloride (TCEP-HCl) was purchased from Thermo Fisher Scientific (Loughborough, UK). Ethanol (EtOH) and HPLC grade acetonitrile, trifluoroacetic acid (TFA) and formic acid were purchased from Thermo Fisher Scientific (Loughborough, UK). Phosphate-buffered saline (PBS) was purchased from Gibco (Life Technologies, Paisley, UK). Ethylenediaminetetraacetic acid (EDTA), *N*,*N*-diisopropylethylamine (DIPEA), mouse serum, dimethylformamide (DMF), *n*-octanol and Iso-Disc PVDF syringe filters (13 mm, 0.2 µm) were purchased from Sigma-Aldrich (Gillingham, UK). Aluminum chloride hexahydrate ($AlCl_3$, 99.9995%) was purchased from Alfa Aesar (Heysham, UK). Sodium acetate (AnalR Normapur) was purchased from VWR International (Lutterworth, UK). The $Z_{EGFR:03115}$-Cys affibody molecule was provided by Affibody AB (Solna, Sweden http://www.affibody.com) as a solution in 0.2 M sodium acetate. Phenyloxadiazolyl methylsulfone (PODS) was synthesized as described in the literature [15]. The maleimide-bearing affibody analogue NOTA-$Z_{EGFR:03115}$ was prepared and radiolabeled as previously reported [22]. Low-protein-binding microcentrifuge tubes (1.5 mL) were purchased from Eppendorf (Stevenage, UK). Dry bifunctional chelators and affibody conjugates were achieved using a Concentrator Plus (Eppendorf, Stevenage, UK). Incubation of the reaction mixtures was performed using a Grant Bio thermo shaker (Camlab, Stevenage, UK). Protein conjugate concentration was determined by measuring the UV absorbance at 280 nm on a NanoDrop 2000 spectrophotometer (Thermo Scientific, Loughborough, UK) using a molar extinction coefficient (ε_{280}) of 36345 cm^{-1} M^{-1}. Oasis HLB (1 mL, 30 mg sorbent) SPE cartridges were purchased from Waters

(Elstree, UK). [^{18}F]Fluoride was produced a GE PETrace cyclotron by 16 MeV irradiation of an enriched [^{18}O]H_2O target, supplied by Alliance Medical Radiopharmarcy Ltd. (Warwick, UK) and used without further purification.

Analytical and semi-preparative HPLC were carried out on an Agilent Infinity 1260 quaternary pump system equipped with a 1260 Diode array (Agilent Technologies, Didcot, UK). Elution profiles were recorded using Laura 4 software (Lablogic, Sheffield, UK, 2013). NOTA-PODS and NODAGA-PODS were analyzed on an Eclipse XDB C18 column, 4.6 × 150 mm, 5 μm (Agilent Technologies, Didcot, UK) using Gradient 1: 0–20 min 3%–60% B, at flow rate of 1 mL/min with 0.1% TFA in water as eluent A and 0.1% TFA in acetonitrile as eluent B. The bifunctional chelators were purified by semi-preparative RP–HPLC on a Ultracarb ODS C18 column, 10 × 250 mm, 7 μm (Phenomenex, Macclesfield, UK), using Gradient 1a: 0–20 min 3%–60% B, at a flow rate of 3mL/min with 0.1% formic acid in water as eluent A and 0.1% formic acid in acetonitrile as eluent B and. Affibody conjugates and radioconjugates were analyzed on a Zorbax 300SB C18 column, 4.6 × 250 mm, 5 μm (Agilent Technologies, Didcot, UK) using Gradient 2: 0–20 min. 30%–65% B, with 0.1% TFA in water as eluent A and 0.1% TFA in acetonitrile as eluent B at a flow rate of 1 mL/min. Affibody conjugates were purified by semi-preparative RP–HPLC on a Jupiter C18 column, 10 × 250 mm, 10 μm, 300 Å (Phenomenex, Macclesfield, UK), using Gradient 2 at a 3 mL/min flow rate. The radioactivity of the eluate was monitored using an IN/US Systems Gamma-ram Model 4 NaI radiodetector (Lablogic, Sheffield, UK). Retention times (Rt) are expressed as minutes:seconds (min:sec). Electro spray ionization high-resolution mass spectrometry (ESI–HRMS) was performed using an Agilent 1200 series LC pump with a 6210 time-of-flight (TOF) mass analyzer. Protein MS was performed on 6520 a Series qToF mass spectrometer fitted with a dual ESI ionization source (Agilent, Santa Clara, CA, USA).

3.2. *Preparation of NOTA-PODS and NODAGA-PODS*

The macrocyclic chelator NHS ester (10.32 μmol), was added solid to a solution of PODS (6.88 μmol) in DMF (400 μL) and DIPEA (7.2 μL, 41.3 μmol). The clear solution was incubated in a thermo shaker at 23 °C for 2 h (900 rpm). The product was analyzed by RP–HPLC and either purified by RP–HPLC (Gradient 1a) or used for the next reaction without further purification.

NOTA-PODS = Analytical RP–HPLC (Gradient 1): Rt: 12:15 min:sec; ESI–HRMS: $[M + H]^+$ (*m/z*) calcd: 827.9, found 827.3633.

NODAGA-PODS = Analytical RP–HPLC (Gradient 1): Rt: 12:13 min:sec; ESI–HRMS: $[M + H]^+$ (*m/z*) calcd: 899.9, found 899.3895.

3.3. *Preparation of NOTA-PODS-$Z_{EGFR:03115}$ and NODA-PODS-$Z_{EGFR:03115}$*

In a 1.5 mL low-protein-binding centrifuge tube, a freshly prepared solution of TCEP-HCl in 1 M phosphate buffer pH 7 (0.025 mg/μL, 9.8 μL, 1.71 μmol) was added to a solution of $Z_{EGFR:03115}$-Cys (200 μL, 2.3 mg/mL, 68.4 nmol). The mixture was incubated in a thermo shaker at 85 °C for 5 min (900 rpm) followed by 25 min at room temperature. Either NOTA-PODS or NODAGA-PODS solution in DMF was then added (1.03 μmol) and the solution was incubated in a thermo shaker at 37 °C for 1 h (900 rpm). The reaction mixture was analyzed by RP–HPLC. The product was purified by semi-preparative RP–HPLC. The collected fractions containing the product were dried and quantified by measuring the UV absorbance at 280 nm.

NOTA-PODS-$Z_{EGFR:03115}$ = yield 38.5%. Analytical RP–HPLC (Gradient 2): Rt: 11:06 min:sec; ESI–HRMS (*m/z*): $[M + H]^+$ expected: 7470, found: 7470.91.

NODAGA-PODS-$Z_{EGFR:03115}$ = yield 39.9%. Analytical RP–HPLC (Gradient 2): Rt: 11:08 min:sec; ESI–HRMS (*m/z*): $[M + H]^+$ expected: 7543, found: 7543.07.

3.4. *Radiosynthesis of [^{18}F]AlF-NOTA-PODS-$Z_{EGFR:03115}$ and [^{18}F]AlF-NODAGA-PODS-$Z_{EGFR:03115}$*

To a 1.5 mL low-protein-binding plastic tube containing either NOTA-PODS-$Z_{EGFR:03115}$ or NODAGA-PODS-$Z_{EGFR:03115}$ (lyophilized, 10–20 nmol), 2 mM $AlCl_3$ (4.0–6.5 μL, 7–13 nmol) in 0.5 M sodium acetate buffer pH 4, 50 mM ascorbic acid in 25 mM sodium acetate pH 4.5 (to a final concentration of 1 mM), and aqueous non-purified [^{18}F]fluoride (180–200 MBq) were added. A volume of ethanol was then added to achieve a final 1:1 *v*/*v* aqueous to organic solvent ratio. The mixture was heated at 100 °C for 15 min. After cooling to ambient temperature, the solution was purified by RP–HPLC using Gradient 2. The collected fraction containing the product was diluted with 0.1% aq TFA (3 mL) and loaded on an HLB-SPE cartridge (1 mL, 30 mg sorbent). The trapped radioactivity was washed with 0.1% aq TFA (4 mL) and then eluted with 60% ethanol/water (*v*/*v*, 120 μL). The product was quantified by measuring the UV absorbance at 280 nm. Synthesis time (from the beginning of the reaction) = ca. 45 min.

[^{18}F]AlF-NOTA-PODS-$Z_{EGFR:03115}$ = Analytical RP–HPLC (Gradient 2): Rt: 11:16 min:sec; RCY (decay corrected at the beginning of reaction): 11%–12.7%; apparent specific activity: 0.40–0.59 MBq/μg (apparent molar activity: 3.0–4.4 MBq/nmol).

[^{18}F]AlF-NODAGA-PODS-$Z_{EGFR:03115}$ = Analytical RP–HPLC (Gradient 2): Rt: 11:11 min:sec; RCY (decay corrected at the beginning of reaction): 4.3%–8.1%; apparent specific activity: 0.11–0.23 MBq/μg (apparent molar activity: 0.8–1.7 MBq/nmol).

3.5. Determination of Distribution Coefficient (LogD) at pH 7.4

To 0.5 mL of PBS (pH 7.4), either [^{18}F]AlF-NOTA-PODS-$Z_{EGFR:03115}$ or [^{18}F]AlF-NODAGA-PODS -$Z_{EGFR:03115}$ (0.08 MBq) was added followed by 0.5 mL of *n*-octanol. The mixture was vortexed for 10 min followed by centrifugation at 100× *g* for 10 min. The experiments were performed in triplicate. Three 100 μL samples were taken from each layer and the amount of activity was measured in a 2480 WIZARD^2 Automatic Gamma Counter (Perkin Elmer, Beaconsfield, UK) as counts per minutes (cpm). The distribution coefficient at pH 7.4 ($logD_{7.4}$) was expressed as the mean ± standard deviation (SD) and calculated using the following formula (Equation 1):

$$\text{LogD} = \log[(\text{counts}_{\text{octanol}})/(\text{counts}_{\text{PBS}})] \quad (1)$$

3.6. In Vitro Serum Stability Assay

The stability of [^{18}F]AlF-NOTA-PODS-$Z_{EGFR:03115}$ and [^{18}F]AlF-NODAGA-PODS-$Z_{EGFR:03115}$ was assessed as previously described by incubating the purified [^{18}F]AlF-radioconjugates (3.5–4 MBq) in mouse serum (500 μL) in a thermo shaker at 37 °C for 1 h (850 rpm) [17,24]. Each experiment was performed in triplicate. The data are expressed as the average of n = 3 measurements ± SD.

3.7. In Vivo Evaluation

All experiments were performed in compliance with license issued under the UK Animals (Scientific Procedures) Act 1986 and following local ethical review (project license PCC916B22, Animals in Science Regulation Unit, Home Office Science, London, UK). The studies followed the United Kingdom National Cancer Research Institute Guidelines for Animal Welfare in Cancer Research [25]. Female NCr athymic mice (6–8 weeks old) were subcutaneously injected on the right shoulder with U87MGvIII cells (0.5 × 10^6/mouse) suspended in 30% Matrigel. Tumors were allowed to grow to 100 mm^3. PET/CT studies were conducted on an Albira PET/SPECT/CT imaging system (Bruker, Coventry, UK). Mice were administered the radioconjugate (12 μg in 100 μL of 0.9% sterile saline, 1.1–1.8 MBq/mouse) by intravenous tail vein injection and were anesthetized using an isoflurane/O_2 mixture (1.5%–2.0% *v*/*v*) approximately 5 min prior to imaging. Whole-body static PET images were acquired 1 h post-radioconjugate injection for the duration of 10 min, with a 358 to 664 keV energy window, followed by CT acquisition as previously described [26]. The image data were processed and reconstructed as previously reported [26].

Immediately after image data acquisition, the mice were euthanized by cervical dislocation for the biodistribution studies. The major organs/tissues were dissected and weighed, and the radioactivity was measured in 2480 WIZARD^2 Automatic Gamma Counter (Perkin Elmer, Beaconsfield, UK).

The percentage of the injected dose per gram of tissue (%ID/g) was determined for each organ/tissue. The data are expressed as the average of $n = 3$ mice ± SD.

4. Conclusions

This study describes the preparation and attachment of two novel thiol-reactive PODS-bearing bifunctional chelators (NOTA-PODS and NODAGA-PODS) to the EGFR-targeting affibody molecule $Z_{EGFR:03115}$. When radiolabeled with [^{18}F]AlF, a RP–HPLC purification procedure followed by HLB-SPE was required to produce radioconjugates with a RCP > 98%. Overall, the radiolabeling efficiency for [^{18}F]AlF-NODAGA-PODS-$Z_{EGFR:03115}$ was found to be lower than for [^{18}F]AlF- NOTA-PODS-$Z_{EGFR:03115}$, a factor attributable to the chelator structure. Once purified, both radioconjugates showed a good serum stability. When injected in high EGFR-expressing tumor-bearing mice, [^{18}F]AlF-NOTA-PODS-$Z_{EGFR:03115}$ and [^{18}F]AlF-NODAGA-PODS-$Z_{EGFR:03115}$ showed similar pharmacokinetics and allowed for clear visualization of the tumors already 1 h post-injection. Additionally, the radiolabeling procedure, purification requirements, in vitro stability and in vivo behavior (at 1 h) of both PODS- and maleimide-bearing radioconjugates were found to be comparable. However, based on reports in the literature, it is possible that the benefits from the superior stability of PODS in vivo would be more noticeable at later time points. In conclusion, this investigation showed that PODS-based reagents are a viable alternative to maleimide for thiol-selective conjugation to cysteine-bearing proteins.

Supplementary Materials: The following are available online, Figure S1: RP–HPLC analysis (Gradient 1) of PODS (**A**), and the NODA-PODS (**B**) and NODAGA-PODS (**C**) reaction mixtures. NOTA-NHS and NODAGA-NHS elute with the mobile phase front, together with DMF (ca 3 min). The absorbance was recorded at the wavelength of 254 nm. The retention time (Rt) is indicated as min:sec. Figure S2: When the bifunctional chelators were purified by semi-preparative RPHPLC and subsequently dried using a speed-vacuum concentrator, the products showed clear signs of degradation RP–HPLC analysis (Gradient 1) of isolated NOTAPODS (**A**) and NODAGA-PODS (**B**). Each chromatogram shows the presence of one major degradation product (ca 10:40 min:sec). The absorbance was recorded at the wavelength of 254 nm. ESI–MS analysis of NOTA-PODS and the degradation product shows the expected mass of *m/z* 827 and a peak having a smaller mass (*m/z* 765) which could be associated to the hydrolysis derivative at the sulfone group (**C**). The prolonged presence of TFA in solution together with the type of drying process were possibly the cause. Figure S3: RP–HPLC analysis (Gradient 1) of pure NOTA-PODS (**A**) and NODAGAPODS (**B**) isolated by semi-preparative RP–HPLC using formic acid in the mobile phase instead of TFA. The absorbance was recorded at the wavelength of 254 nm. Figure S4: ESI–HRMS of NOTA-PODS (top) and NODAGA-PODS (bottom). Figure S5: RP–HPLC analysis of solutions of NOTA-PODS and NODAGA-PODS in DMF after being stored at −20 °C. Signs of degradation (peak at 10:36 min:sec) were detected already after 2 months for NOTA-PODS (**A**). Conversely, NODAGA-PODS showed good stability for at least 10 months (**B**). Figure S6: RP–HPLC analysis (Gradient 2) of NOTA-PODS-$Z_{EGFR:03115}$ (A), and NODAGA-PODS-$Z_{EGFR:03115}$ (**B**) reaction mixtures. NOTA-PODS and NODAGA-PODS elute with the mobile phase front, together with DMF (ca 3 min). The absorbance was recorded at the wavelength of 280 nm. The retention time (Rt) is indicated as min:sec. Figure S7: ESI–MS of purified NOTA-PODS-$Z_{EGFR:03115}$ (top) and NODAGA-PODS-$Z_{EGFR:03115}$ (bottom). Figure S8: Radiochromatograms (Gradient 2) of [^{18}F]AlF-NOTA-PODS-$Z_{EGFR:03115}$ (**A**), and [^{18}F]AlF-NODAGA-PODS-$Z_{EGFR:03115}$ (**B**) reaction mixtures. Free fluorine-18 elutes at ca 3 min. Labels on each peak on the chromatograms indicate the retention time (top) and the %ROI (bottom). Figure S9: Radiochromatograms (Gradient 2) of [^{18}F]AlF-NOTA-PODS-$Z_{EGFR:03115}$ (**A**), and [^{18}F]AlF-NODAGA-PODS-$Z_{EGFR:03115}$ (**B**) after purification by just HLB-SPE. As for [^{18}F]AlF-NOTA-$Z_{EGFR:03115}$ (**C**), the HLB-SPE-only purification step successfully removed the free fluorine-18 leaving the radioconjugate and the thermolysis products which elute at ca 3 min. The retention times (Rt) are expressed as min:sec. Figure S10: Representative radiochromatograms (Gradient 2) of [^{18}F]AlF-NOTA-PODS-$Z_{EGFR:03115}$ (**A**) and [^{18}F]AlF-NODAGA-PODS-$Z_{EGFR:03115}$ (**B**) after incubation in mouse serum for 1 h. The intact radioconjugates elute at ca 11 min. Activity non-associated with the conjugate elutes at ca 3 min. Labels on each peak on the chromatograms indicate the retention time (top) and the %ROI (bottom). Table S1: Summary of $LogD_{7.4}$ values measured for the three radioconjugates. Table S2: Summary of serum stability determined by RP–HPLC. The three radioconjugates were incubated in mouse serum at 37 °C for 1 h. The data are shown as the mean values of $n = 3$ experiments ± SD. Statistical analysis was performed using one-way ANOVA with Tukey correction using GraphPad Prism v8. Table S3: Summary of serum stability determined by RP–HPLC. The three radioconjugates were incubated in mouse serum at 37 °C for 1 h. The data are shown as the mean values of $n = 3$ experiments ± SD. Statistical analysis was performed using one-way ANOVA with Tukey correction using GraphPad Prism v8.

Author Contributions: Conceptualization, C.D.P., G.K.-M. and G.S.; methodology, C.D.P, A.M. J.M. and S.T.; formal analysis, C.D.P., S.T. and G.K.-M.; investigation, C.D.P., A.M., J.M., S.T., G.K.-M.; resources, G.S. and G.K.-M.; data curation, C.D.P., S.T. and G.K.-M.; writing—original draft preparation, C.D.P.; writing—review and editing, A.M., S.T., G.S. and G.K.-M.; visualization, C.D.P., S.T. and G.K.-M.; supervision, C.D.P. and G.K.-M.; project administration, G.S. and G.K.-M.; funding acquisition, A.M., G.S. and G.K.-M. All authors have read and agreed to the published version of the manuscript.

Acknowledgments: The authors gratefully thank Affibody AB for supplying the affibody molecule and the Structural Chemistry Facility (Cancer Therapeutics) for the provision of technical MS services.

References

1. Gunnoo, S.B.; Madder, A. Chemical protein modification through cysteine. *ChemBioChem* **2016**, *17*, 529–553. [CrossRef]
2. Koniev, O.; Wagner, A. Developments and recent advancements in the field of endogenous amino acid selective bond forming reactions for bioconjugation. *Chem. Soc. Rev.* **2015**, *44*, 5495–5551. [CrossRef] [PubMed]
3. Ravasco, J.M.J.M.; Faustino, H.; Trindade, A.; Gois, P.M.P. Bioconjugation with maleimides: A useful tool for chemical biology. *Chem. Eur. J.* **2019**, *25*, 43–59. [CrossRef] [PubMed]
4. Sabot, C.; Renard, P.-Y.; Renault, K.; Fredy, J.W. Covalent modification of biomolecules through maleimide-based labeling strategies. *Bioconjugate Chem.* **2018**, *29*, 2497–2513.
5. Alley, S.C.; Benjamin, D.R.; Jeffrey, S.C.; Okeley, N.M.; Meyer, D.L.; Sanderson, R.J.; Senter, P.D. Contribution of linker stability to the activities of anticancer immunoconjugates. *Bioconjugate Chem.* **2008**, *19*, 759–765. [CrossRef] [PubMed]
6. Baldwin, A.D.; Kiick, K.L. Tunable degradation of maleimide–thiol adducts in reducing environments. *Bioconjugate Chem.* **2011**, *22*, 1946–1953. [CrossRef] [PubMed]
7. Ponte, J.F.; Sun, X.; Yoder, N.C.; Fishkin, N.; Laleau, R.; Coccia, J.; Lanieri, L.; Bogalhas, M.; Wang, L.; Wilhelm, S.; et al. Understanding how the stability of the thiol-maleimide linkage impacts the pharmacokinetics of lysine-linked antibody-maytansinoid conjugates. *Bioconjugate Chem.* **2016**, *27*, 1588–1598. [CrossRef]
8. Szijj, P.A.; Bahou, C.; Chudasama, V. Minireview: Addressing the retro-Michael instability of maleimide bioconjugates. *Drug Discov. Today Technol.* **2018**, *30*, 27–34. [CrossRef]
9. Bernardim, B.; Cal, P.M.S.D.; Matos, M.J.; Oliveira, B.L.; Martínez-Sáez, N.; AlbuquerqueInês, S.; Perkins, E.; Corzana, F.; Burtoloso, A.C.B.; Jiménez-Osés, G.; et al. Stoichiometric and irreversible cysteine-selective protein modification using carbonylacrylic reagents. *Nat. Commun.* **2016**, *7*, 13128–13137. [CrossRef]
10. Kalia, D.; Malekar, P.V.; Parthasarathy, M. Exocyclic olefinic maleimides: Synthesis and application for stable and thiol-selective bioconjugation. *Angew. Chem. Int. Ed. Engl.* **2016**, *55*, 1432–1435. [CrossRef]
11. Toda, N.; Asano, S.; Barbas, C.F.I. Rapid, stable, chemoselective labeling of thiols with Julia-Kocieński-like reagents: A serum-stable alternative to maleimide-based protein conjugation. *Angew. Chem. Int. Ed. Engl.* **2013**, *52*, 12592–12596. [CrossRef] [PubMed]
12. Patterson, J.T.; Asano, S.; Li, X.; Rader, C.; Barbas, C.F.I. Improving the serum stability of site-specific antibody conjugates with sulfone linkers. *Bioconjugate Chem.* **2014**, *25*, 1402–1407. [CrossRef] [PubMed]
13. Zhang, Q.; Dall'Angelo, S.; Fleming, I.N.; Schweiger, L.F.; Zanda, M.; O'Hagan, D. Last-step enzymatic [^{18}F]-fluorination of cysteine-tethered RGD peptides using modified Barbas linkers. *Chem. Eur. J.* **2016**, *22*, 10998–11004. [CrossRef] [PubMed]
14. Chiotellis, A.; Sladojevich, F.; Mu, L.; Müller Herde, A.; Valverde, I.E.; Tolmachev, V.; Schibli, R.; Ametamey, S.M.; Mindt, T.L. Novel chemoselective ^{18}F-radiolabeling of thiol-containing biomolecules under mild aqueous conditions. *Chem. Commun.* **2016**, *52*, 6083–6086. [CrossRef] [PubMed]
15. Adumeau, P.; Davydova, M.; Zeglis, B.M. Thiol-reactive bifunctional chelators for the creation of site-selectively modified radioimmunoconjugates with improved stability. *Bioconjug. Chem.* **2018**, *29*, 1364–1372. [CrossRef]
16. McBride, W.J.; Sharkey, R.M.; Karacay, H.; D'Souza, C.A.; Rossi, E.A.; Laverman, P.; Chang, C.H.; Boerman, O.C.; Goldenberg, D.M. A novel method of 18F radiolabeling for PET. *J. Nucl. Med.* **2009**, *50*, 991–998. [CrossRef]

17. Da Pieve, C.; Allott, L.; Martins, C.D.; Vardon, A.; Ciobota, D.M.; Kramer-Marek, G.; Smith, G. Efficient [^{18}F]AlF radiolabeling of $Z_{HER3:8698}$ affibody molecule for imaging of HER3 positive tumors. *Bioconjug. Chem.* **2016**, *27*, 1839–1849. [CrossRef]
18. Kim, Y.; Ho, S.O.; Gassman, N.R.; Korlann, Y.; Landorf, E.V.; Collart, F.R.; Weiss, S. Efficient site-specific labeling of proteins via cysteines. *Bioconjug. Chem.* **2008**, *19*, 786–791. [CrossRef]
19. Liu, Y.; Hu, X.; Liu, H.; Bu, L.; Ma, X.; Cheng, K.; Li, J.; Tian, M.; Zhang, H.; Cheng, Z. A comparative study of radiolabeled bombesin analogs for the PET imaging of prostate cancer. *J. Nucl. Med.* **2013**, *54*, 2132–2138. [CrossRef]
20. D'Souza, C.A.; McBride, W.J.; Sharkey, R.M.; Todaro, L.J.; Goldenberg, D.M. High-yielding aqueous ^{18}F-labeling of peptides via Al^{18}F chelation. *Bioconjug. Chem.* **2011**, *22*, 1793–1803. [CrossRef]
21. Löfblom, J.; Feldwisch, J.; Tolmachev, V.; Carlsson, J.; Ståhl, S.; Frejd, F.Y. Affibody molecules: Engineered proteins for therapeutic, diagnostic and biotechnological applications. *Febs Lett.* **2010**, *584*, 2670–2680. [CrossRef] [PubMed]
22. Burley, T.A.; Da Pieve, C.; Martins, C.D.; Ciobota, D.M.; Allott, L.; Oyen, W.J.G.; Harrington, K.J.; Smith, G.; Kramer-Marek, G. Affibody-Based PET Imaging to Guide EGFR-Targeted Cancer Therapy in Head and Neck Squamous Cell Cancer Models. *J. Nucl. Med.* **2019**, *60*, 353–361. [CrossRef] [PubMed]
23. Behr, T.M.; Goldenberg, D.M.; Becker, W. Reducing the renal uptake of radiolabeled antibody fragments and peptides for diagnosis and therapy: Present status, future prospects and limitations. *Eur. J. Nucl. Med.* **1998**, *25*, 201–212. [CrossRef]
24. Su, X.; Cheng, K.; Jeon, J.; Shen, B.; Venturin, G.T.; Hu, X.; Rao, J.; Chin, F.T.; Wu, H.; Cheng, Z. Comparison of two site-specifically ^{18}F-labeled affibodies for PET imaging of EGFR positive tumors. *Mol. Pharm.* **2014**, *11*, 3947–3956. [CrossRef] [PubMed]
25. Workman, P.; Aboagye, E.O.; Balkwill, F.; Balmain, A.; Bruder, G.; Chaplin, D.J.; Double, J.A.; Everitt, J.; Farningham, D.A.H.; Glennie, M.J.; et al. Guidelines for the welfare and use of animals in cancer research. *Br. J. Cancer* **2010**, *102*, 1555–1577. [CrossRef]
26. Martins, C.D.; Da Pieve, C.; Burley, T.A.; Smith, R.; Ciobota, D.M.; Allott, L.; Harrington, K.J.; Oyen, W.J.G.; Smith, G.; Kramer-Marek, G. HER3-mediated resistance to Hsp90 inhibition detected in breast cancer xenografts by affibody-based PET imaging. *Clin. Cancer Res.* **2018**, *24*, 1853–1865. [CrossRef]

13

In Vitro and In Vivo Characterization of Dibenzothiophene Derivatives [^{125}I]Iodo-ASEM and [^{18}F]ASEM as Radiotracers of Homo- and Heteromeric α7 Nicotinic Acetylcholine Receptors

Cornelius K. Donat [1,2,*], Henrik H. Hansen [1], Hanne D. Hansen [1], Ronnie C. Mease [3], Andrew G. Horti [3], Martin G. Pomper [3], Elina T. L'Estrade [1,4,5], Matthias M. Herth [4,5], Dan Peters [6], Gitte M. Knudsen [1] and Jens D. Mikkelsen [1,*]

1 Neurobiology Research Unit, Copenhagen University Hospital, Rigshospitalet, DK-2100 Copenhagen, Denmark; hbh@gubra.dk (H.H.H.); Hanne.D.Hansen@nru.dk (H.D.H.); elina.nyberg@sund.ku.dk (E.T.L.); Gitte.Knudsen@nru.dk (G.M.K.)

2 Department of Brain Sciences, Imperial College London, London W12 0 LS, UK

3 Russell H. Morgan Department of Radiology and Radiological Science, The Johns Hopkins University School of Medicine, Baltimore, MD 21287, USA; rmease1@jhmi.edu (R.C.M.); ahorti1@jhmi.edu (A.G.H.); mpomper@jhmi.edu (M.G.P.)

4 Department of Drug Design and Pharmacology, University of Copenhagen, Jagtvej 162, 2100 Copenhagen, Denmark; matthias.herth@nru.dk

5 Department of Clinical Physiology, Nuclear Medicine & PET, Rigshospitalet, Blegdamsvej 9, 2100 Copenhagen, Denmark

6 DanPET AB, 216 19 Malmö, Sweden; info@danpet.eu

* Correspondence: cdonat@imperial.ac.uk (C.K.D.); jens_mikkelsen@dadlnet.dk (J.D.M.)

Academic Editor: Peter Brust

Abstract: The α7 nicotinic acetylcholine receptor (α7 nAChR) is involved in several cognitive and physiologic processes; its expression levels and patterns change in neurologic and psychiatric diseases, such as schizophrenia and Alzheimer's disease, which makes it a relevant drug target. Development of selective radioligands is important for defining binding properties and occupancy of novel molecules targeting the receptor. We tested the in vitro binding properties of [^{125}I]Iodo-ASEM [(3-(1,4-diazabycyclo[3.2.2]nonan-4-yl)-6-(^{125}I-iododibenzo[b,d]thiopentene 5,5-dioxide)] in the mouse, rat and pig brain using autoradiography. The in vivo binding properties of [^{18}F]ASEM were investigated using positron emission tomography (PET) in the pig brain. [^{125}I]Iodo-ASEM showed specific and displaceable high affinity (~1 nM) binding in mouse, rat, and pig brain. Binding pattern overlapped with [^{125}I]α-bungarotoxin, specific binding was absent in α7 nAChR gene-deficient mice and binding was blocked by a range of α7 nAChR orthosteric modulators in an affinity-dependent order in the pig brain. Interestingly, relative to the wild-type, binding in β2 nAChR gene-deficient mice was lower for [^{125}I]Iodo-ASEM (58% ± 2.7%) than [^{125}I]α-bungarotoxin (23% ± 0.2%), potentially indicating different binding properties to heteromeric α7β2 nAChR. [^{18}F]ASEM PET in the pig showed high brain uptake and reversible tracer kinetics with a similar spatial distribution as previously reported for α7 nAChR. Blocking with SSR-180,711 resulted in a significant decrease in [^{18}F]ASEM binding. Our findings indicate that [^{125}I]Iodo-ASEM allows sensitive and selective imaging of α7 nAChR in vitro, with better signal-to-noise ratio than previous tracers. Preliminary data of [^{18}F]ASEM in the pig brain demonstrated principal suitable kinetic properties for in vivo quantification of α7 nAChR, comparable to previously published data.

Keywords: alpha 7; nicotinic acetylcholine receptors; PET; nAChR; autoradiography

1. Introduction

The $\alpha7$ nicotinic acetylcholine receptor ($\alpha7$ nAChR) belongs to the superfamily of ligand-gated ion channels and is expressed across all mammalian species [1–4]. The receptor plays an important role in cognition [5], mood [6] and consistent with this, $\alpha7$ nAChR are particularly abundant in hippocampus and prefrontal cortex [7,8]. Furthermore, $\alpha7$ nAChR are implied in neuro-immune [9] and immune functions [10] under homeostatic conditions.

Changes in protein and mRNA levels of $\alpha7$ nAChR have been reported in a number of neuropsychiatric and neurodegenerative diseases [1,11–15]. Notably, certain polymorphisms in the promoter region of the $\alpha7$ nAChR gene (*CHRNA7*) [16] are probable risk factors for neuropsychiatric diseases, such as major depression [17] and schizophrenia [18] and are associated with developmental disorders and cognitive impairments [19]. Additionally, $\alpha7$ nAChRs are expressed by several central and peripheral immune cells and activation via agonists and positive allosteric modulators showed neuroprotective and immunomodulatory efficacy in different preclinical disease models [20–24].

Changes of $\alpha7$ nAChR in the healthy and diseased brain can only be detected in vivo by molecular imaging, such as positron emission tomography (PET) using specific radiotracers. A clinically usable radiotracer requires sufficient selectivity, specificity and suitable affinity, depending on the target [25]. Most of the previously described $\alpha7$ nAChR PET tracers, among those [^{18}F]NS14490, [^{11}C]NS14492, [^{11}C]CHIBA-1001 and [^{11}C]A-582941 (Table 1), studied in mice, pigs and non-human primates exhibited some shortcomings, such as poor specific and/or high nonspecific binding or radiometabolites crossing the blood–brain barrier [26–32]. Furthermore, the specificity of novel $\alpha7$ nAChR tracers has not always been tested in respective gene-deficient mice, e.g., using in vitro autoradiography.

While development of novel tracers from different lead structures is still ongoing [33–37], tilorone [38] provided a lead-structure for a number of derivatives subsequently developed into $\alpha7$ nAChR PET tracers. From those, [^{18}F]ASEM (JHU82132) [39] and the structurally related [^{18}F]DBT-10 (JHU82108) [40] have been most widely investigated. Initial studies have shown that ASEM is a potent antagonist [39] with subnanomolar affinity and high selectivity [39,41], further substantiated by the radiolabelled compounds [^{18}F]ASEM [26] and [^{125}I]Iodo-ASEM [42] as tested in human and rat recombinant $\alpha7$ nAChR. [^{18}F]ASEM and [^{125}I]Iodo-ASEM readily enter the mouse brain, are displaceable, and accumulate in regions with highest $\alpha7$ nAChR density [26,39,42,43].

More recent studies using [^{18}F]ASEM and [^{18}F]DBT-10 further supported the suitability of the tracers, showing high and reversible brain uptake with a regional binding pattern consistent with the distribution of $\alpha7$ nAChR receptors in the non-human primate brain [39,44,45]. Favourable brain pharmacokinetics, excellent test-retest reproducibility and regional uptake [^{18}F]ASEM pattern consistent with post-mortem $\alpha7$ nAChR distribution have been reported in human PET studies [43,46]. Several recent studies extended the available data in human subjects, showing good agreement with previous distribution volumes (V_T) and test-retest values in nonhuman primates and healthy volunteers [44]. A study in ageing subjects showed a significant positive correlation between age and [^{18}F]ASEM V_T in striatum and several cortical regions [47], however without any correlation between V_T and cognitive measures. A small sample of individuals with schizophrenia on stable antipsychotic medication showed lower [^{18}F]ASEM V_T in cingulate cortex and hippocampus [46] and individuals with recent onset of psychosis were also reported to show lower [^{18}F]ASEM V_T in hippocampus, after controlling for age [48]. Interestingly, patients with mild cognitive impairment showed higher [^{18}F]ASEM V_T when adjusted for age as compared to the control group [49], consistent with post-mortem findings from patients and animal models. Additionally, [^{18}F]ASEM has been employed in a rat 6-OHDA lesion model of Parkinson's disease, showing an initial increase of [^{18}F]ASEM SUVr in the ipsilateral striatum and substantia nigra between 3 and 7 days, which coincided with several histology markers of glia activation [50].

While this data shows the general applicability of [^{18}F]ASEM, binding properties and interpretation of novel α7 nAChR tracers might be complicated by the fact that α7 subunits can form heteromeric receptors together with other subunits, specifically β2 [51]. These receptors can be heterologously expressed in oocytes and are found in the rodent and human basal forebrain and cortex [52,53]. While these heteromeric receptors display different pharmacological properties [52,54], it is not clear how this translates to radiotracer binding. In vitro binding studies of [^{18}F]ASEM or [^{125}I]ASEM in gene-deficient mice could answer the question, and would also reveal the suitability of [^{125}I]ASEM for in vitro autoradiographic studies. The latter would offer a better comparability to in vivo PET data over the current gold-standard tracer [^{125}I]α-bungarotoxin. We therefore investigated the potential of [^{125}I]ASEM for in vitro studies of the α7 nAChR, by comparing binding of [^{125}I]Iodo-ASEM in rat, mouse and pig brain sections. Furthermore, [^{18}F]ASEM was characterized for in vivo brain uptake and target selectivity in a PET study conducted in the pig.

Table 1. Common α7 nAChR ligands and their structure, previously evaluated as radiotracers.

Tracer	Structure
[^{11}C]CHIBA-1001	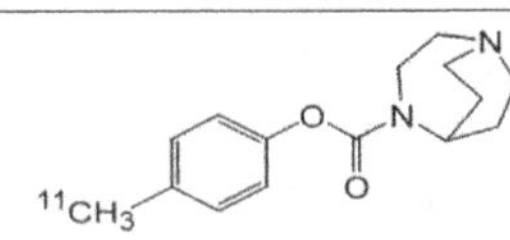
[^{11}C]A-582941	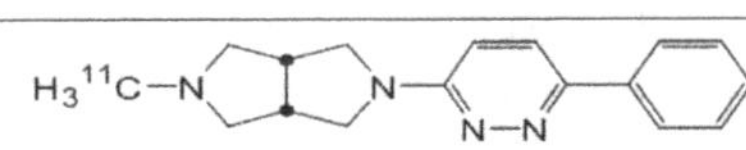
[^{18}F]NS14490	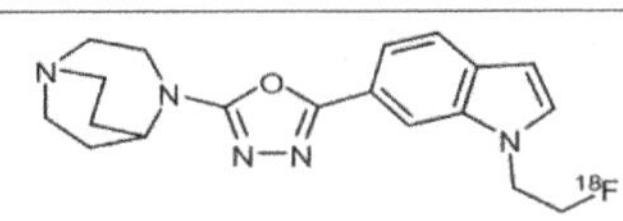
[^{11}C]NS14492	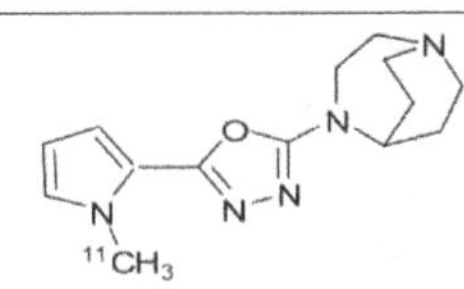
[^{18}F]ASEM	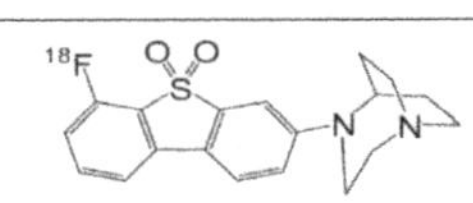
[^{18}F]DBT-10	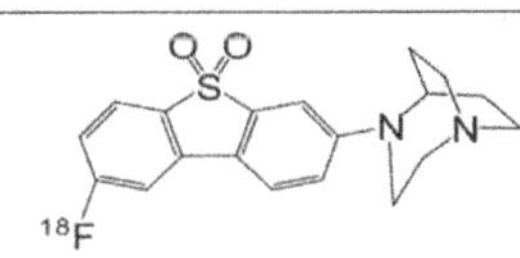
[^{125}I]ASEM	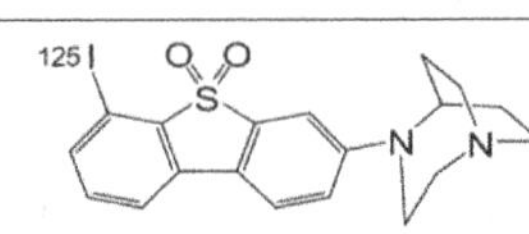

2. Results

2.1. In Vitro Autoradiography

Cerebral binding of [^{125}I]Iodo-ASEM was investigated across several mammalian species, i.e., rat (Figure 1A, upper row), mouse (Figure 2A) and pig brain (Figure 1A, lower row) and compared to [^{125}I]α-bungarotoxin (Figure 1B/2B). Total cortical [^{125}I]Iodo-ASEM binding was highest in the pig, and lower in the rat and mouse (Figures 1C and 2C), as compared to [^{125}I]α-bungarotoxin. [^{125}I]Iodo-ASEM binding was displaceable with (-)-nicotine (1 mMol/L, data not shown) and SSR-180,711 (10 μMol/L, Figures 1A and 2A, nonspecific binding) in all species.

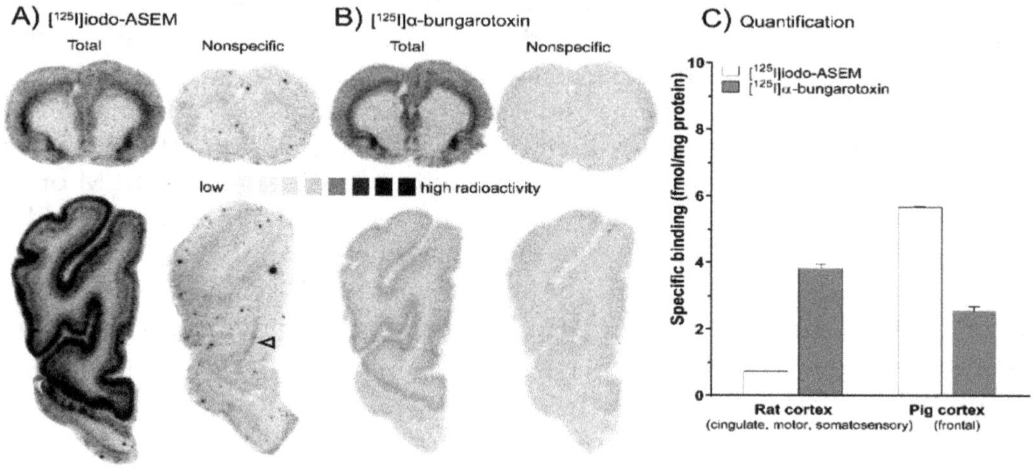

Figure 1. (**A,B**) Representative autoradiographs showing [^{125}I]Iodo-ASEM and [^{125}I]α-bungarotoxin total and non-specific binding (determined with 1 mMol/L (-)-nicotine for [^{125}I]α-bungarotoxin and 10 μMol/L SSR-180,711 for [^{125}I]Iodo-ASEM) in 12 μm sections of the rat (upper row) and pig brain (lower row). Arrowheads indicate residual white matter binding. (**C**) Comparative quantitative analysis of specific binding (± S.E.M.) of [^{125}I]Iodo-ASEM and [^{125}I]α-bungarotoxin from autoradiography in the rat (n = 1) and pig cortex (*n* = 2). All autoradiographic experiments and quantifications are carried out in 3-4 sections per animal.

A non-specific binding component remained detectable under the described experimental conditions at low levels in white matter structures (arrowheads, Figures 1A and 2A). The distribution pattern of [^{125}I]Iodo-ASEM binding in the rat, mouse and pig brain was comparable to that of [^{125}I]α-bungarotoxin (Figures 1B and 2B). In the pig, [^{125}I]Iodo-ASEM showed a laminar binding pattern in the frontal cortex, with highest density in cortical layers (1–3) (Figure 1A, lower row), while in the rat, binding in motor, cingulate and somatosensory cortex was more prominent in layers 5–6. However, this species difference was also observed for [^{125}I]α-bungarotoxin (Figure 1B).

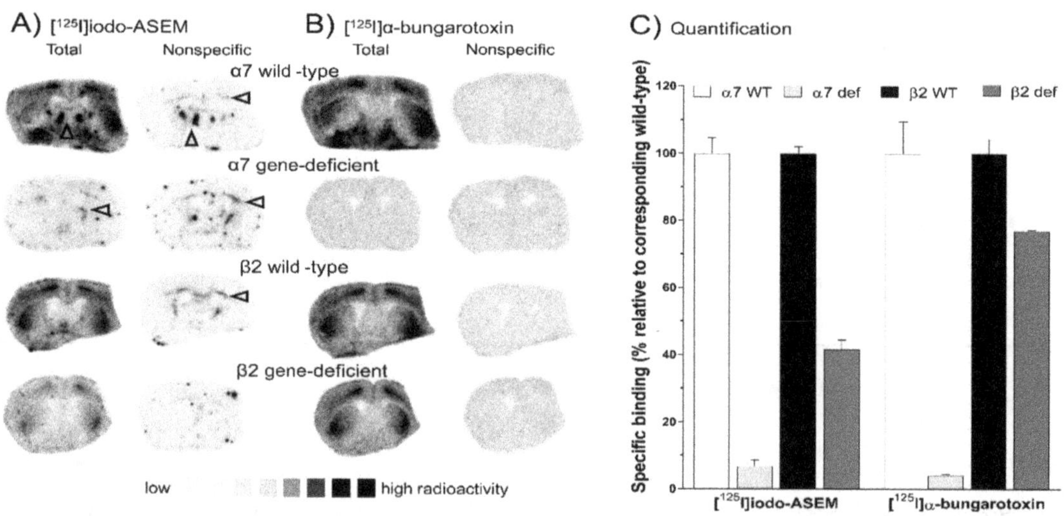

Figure 2. (**A,B**) Representative autoradiographs showing total [^{125}I]Iodo-ASEM (**A**) and [^{125}I]a-bungarotoxin (**B**) and non-specific (determined with 1 mMol/L (-)-nicotine for [^{125}I]α-bungarotoxin and 10 μMol/L SSR-180,711 for [^{125}I]Iodo-ASEM) binding in 12 μm brain sections of *α*7 and β2 nAChR wild-type vs. corresponding gene-deficient (def) mice (*n* = 1 each). Arrowheads indicate residual white matter binding. (**C**) Comparative quantitative analysis of specific binding (± S.E.M.) of [^{125}I]Iodo-ASEM and [^{125}I]a-bungarotoxin in *α*7 and β2 nAChR wild-type vs. corresponding gene-deficient mice (*n* = 1). All autoradiographic experiments and quantifications are carried out in 3-6 sections per animal.

The specificity of [^{125}I]Iodo-ASEM to α7 nAChR is further substantiated by tracer binding experiments in α7 nAChR gene-deficient mice. Specific [^{125}I]Iodo-ASEM binding was lacking in α7 nAChR gene-deficient mice (Figure 2A), as indicated by the overall reduction in total binding by 93% ± 1.7%, compared to wild-type animals (Figure 2C). Similarly, [^{125}I]α-bungarotoxin total binding (Figure 2B) was 96% ± 0.4% lower in α7 nAChR gene-deficient mice (Figure 2C). In wild-type mice, no difference in [^{125}I]Iodo-ASEM and [^{125}I]α-bungarotoxin binding was observed (Figure 2A,B). However, traces of nonspecific binding were again noted in white matter structures (arrowheads in Figure 2A).

[^{125}I]Iodo-ASEM binding in β2 nAChR gene-deficient mice was different compared to [^{125}I]α-bungarotoxin. An overall 58% ± 2.7% lower specific [^{125}I]Iodo-ASEM binding was observed, as compared to corresponding wild-type controls (Figure 2C). In contrast, [^{125}I]α-bungarotoxin binding was reduced by 23% ± 0.2%, being less affected by β2 nAChR gene-deficiency as compared to the reduction in [^{125}I]Iodo-ASEM binding.

Saturation binding in rat and pig brain sections indicated that [^{125}I]Iodo-ASEM binding was saturable. In the rat, non-linear regression analysis revealed an equilibrium dissociation constant (K_d) of 1.14 nM (cortex, Figure 3B) and 1.17 nM (hippocampus, Figure 3A) with corresponding receptor density (B_{max}) of 0.70 fmol/mg protein (cortex) and 1.44 fmol/mg protein (hippocampus), respectively (Figure 3A,B). In comparison, the pig cortex showed a K_d of 1.21 nM with a B_{max} of 5.47 fmol/mg protein (Figure 3C). The non-specific binding of [^{125}I]Iodo-ASEM at concentrations near the K_d was low (rat hippocampus, 20%; rat cortex, 30%; pig cortex, 10%).

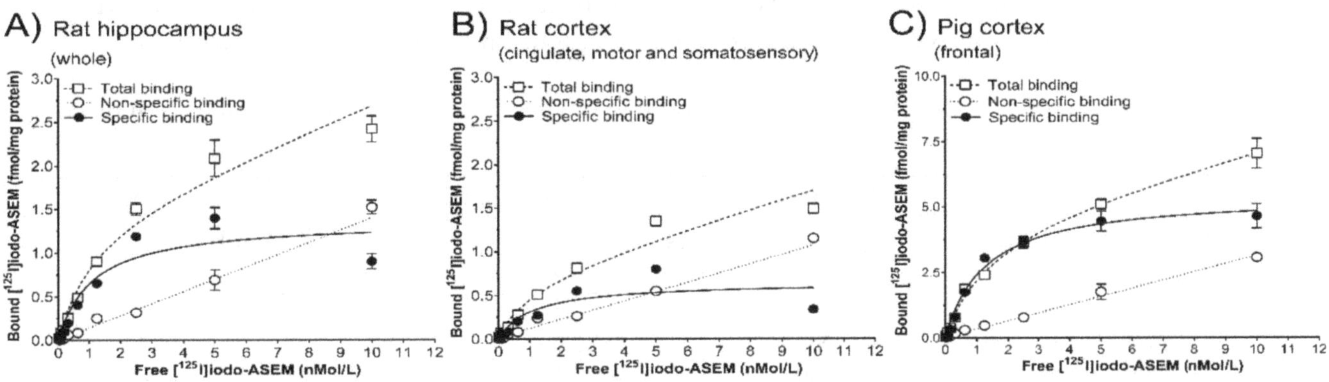

Figure 3. Saturation binding of [^{125}I]Iodo-ASEM (0.02-10 nMol/L) to 12 µm sections from the rat hippocampus and cortex (**A**, **B**, $n = 1$) and pig frontal cortex (**C**, $n = 1$) brain. Non-specific binding was determined in the presence of 10 µMol/L SSR-180,711. Optical density of the autoradiograms was converted into ligand binding (fmol/mg protein ± S.E.M.) from a representative experiment. Data from saturation binding experiments were analysed by non-linear regression. Individual K_d and B_{max} values are indicated in Section 2.1. All autoradiographic experiments and quantifications are carried out in 2–4 sections per animal using 10 radioligand concentrations.

A range of selective α7 nAChR ligands (10 µMol/L each), including the α7 nAChR preferring antagonist methyllycaconitine (MLA), were used to test whether in vitro [^{125}I]Iodo-ASEM binding (0.5 nMol/L) could be blocked in the pig cortex (Table 2). The partial agonists, NS14492, TC-5619, EVP-6124, A-582941, and SSR-180,711, showed almost complete (>90%) blocking of [^{125}I]Iodo-ASEM binding in receptor dense areas of the cortex, e.g. layers 1–3. In contrast, GTS-21 (weak α7 nAChR agonist, ~70% reduction) and MLA (α7 nAChR preferring antagonist, ~80% reduction) exhibited less efficacious blockade of [^{125}I]Iodo-ASEM binding in the pig cortex.

Table 2. Blocking of [^{125}I]Iodo-ASEM binding in the pig cortex by a series of $\alpha 7$ nAChR ligands.

Ligand (10 μMol/L)	[^{125}I]Iodo-ASEM Binding in the Pig Cortex, Layers 1–3 (%, mean ± S.E.M.)	[^{125}I]Iodo-ASEM Binding in the Pig Cortex, Layers 4–6 (%, mean ± S.E.M.)
NS14492	4.04 ± 0.55	9.25 ± 0.83
TC-5619	7.88 ± 1.65	7.60 ± 0.30
EVP-6124	2.50 ± 0.20	5.50 ± 0.07
A-582941	3.22 ± 0.28	4.44 ± 0.93
SSR-180,711	2.92 ± 0.35	3.53 ± 0.50
GTS-21	30.92 ± 2.55	31.39 ± 2.15
MLA	20.46 ± 2.18	18.16 ± 2.41

Results are given in % remaining binding of total binding (mean ± S.E.M.).

2.2. *In Vivo PET Imaging in the Pig Using [^{18}F]ASEM*

[^{18}F]ASEM readily entered the pig brain and highest tracer accumulation was found in the thalamus followed by cortex, striatum and cerebellum (Figure 4A,C). [^{18}F]ASEM uptake in the white matter was initially lower than in the grey matter regions, however the tracer kinetics were also slower, resulting in lower grey to white matter ratio at the end of the scans. The metabolism of [^{18}F]ASEM in pigs was relatively slow, with 60% of the radioactivity at 120 min still being parent radioligand (data not shown). Kinetic modelling was performed to quantify the tracer uptake. Baseline V_T values varied between animals but after correcting for free fraction in plasma(f_P), there was only a 5% difference in V_T/f_P values between the two baseline animals (Table 3). This also suggest that V_T/f_P values are unaffected by relatively large differences in injected mass (0.35 μg and 1.78 μg).

Table 3. Kinetic modelling of [^{18}F]ASEM with the Logan Graphical Analysis model in different pig brain regions.

Comparison of Baseline V_T Values.				
Kinetic Modelling	**Animal 1**		**Animal 2**	
0–90 min	V_T	V_T/f_P	V_T	V_T/f_P
Frontal cortex	7.87	43.70	3.75	41.66
Somatosensory cortex	8.33	46.27	4.15	46.14
Occipital cortex	8.03	44.63	3.77	41.86
Remaining cortex	7.63	42.37	3.78	41.94
Thalamus	8.83	49.06	4.12	45.73
Striatum	7.41	41.17	3.77	41.94
Hippocampus	7.53	41.83	3.59	39.93
Cerebellum	6.66	36.99	3.16	35.07
Comparison of V_T Values at Baseline and After Pre-treatment with SSR-180,711				
Kinetic Modelling	**Animal 1**		**Animal 3**	
0–150 min	V_T	V_T/f_P	V_T	V_T/f_P
Frontal cortex	6.73	37.38	3.61	22.57
Somatosensory cortex	7.26	40.35	3.94	24.60
Occipital cortex	6.96	38.65	3.90	24.40
Remaining cortex	6.68	37.08	3.60	22.50
Thalamus	7.42	41.24	4.34	27.15
Striatum	6.51	36.19	3.83	23.92
Hippocampus	6.55	36.41	3.37	21.09
Cerebellum	5.55	30.82	3.39	21.17

In a third animal, we evaluated the specificity of [^{18}F]ASEM binding in vivo, by administering SSR-180,711 (1 mg/kg) prior to injection of [^{18}F]ASEM. Compared to the baseline studies, we found an increase in [^{18}F]ASEM uptake in all brain areas investigated (Figure 4A). Quantification of uptake and subsequent correction for f_P revealed that SSR-180,711 administration decreased the V_T/f_P compared to baseline (Table 3). Occupancy was computed with the Lassen plot using V_T/f_P values comparing baseline data from animal 1 and blocking data from animal 3 (0-150 min scan data). We found that the 1 mg/kg SSR-180,711 dose resulted in a 49% occupancy (Figure 4B).

From the Lassen plot, the volume of non-displaceable binding (V_{ND}/f_P) was found to be 9.2 mL/cm^3. When comparing the V_{ND}/f_P to the V_T/f_P in the thalamus, we found that 78% of the signal observed in the thalamus is specific binding, leaving 22% as non-displaceable binding.

In one animal, [^{18}F]ASEM acquisition time was 240 min, which allowed subsequent analysis of the time-stability of the parameters estimated with kinetic modelling. Again, the LGA model was used to determine V_T with different scan length and V_T values were found to decrease with more time included in the kinetic modelling. Using all data (0–240 min), V_T values were 5.4 mL/cm^3 (thalamus), 5.0 mL/cm^3 (frontal cortex) and 4.0 mL/cm^3 (cerebellum).

The upper half of the table shows the baseline distribution volumes (V_T) values with and without correction for free fraction in plasma (f_P) in two different animals. Bottom part of the table describes V_T values with and without correction for (f_P) at baseline (animal 1) and after pre-treatment with SSR-180,711 (animal 3). See Table 4 (Material and Methods) for f_P values in the individual animals. Because animal 2 was only scanned for 90 min, the acquisition time of animal 1 was truncated to 90 min to allow for comparison.

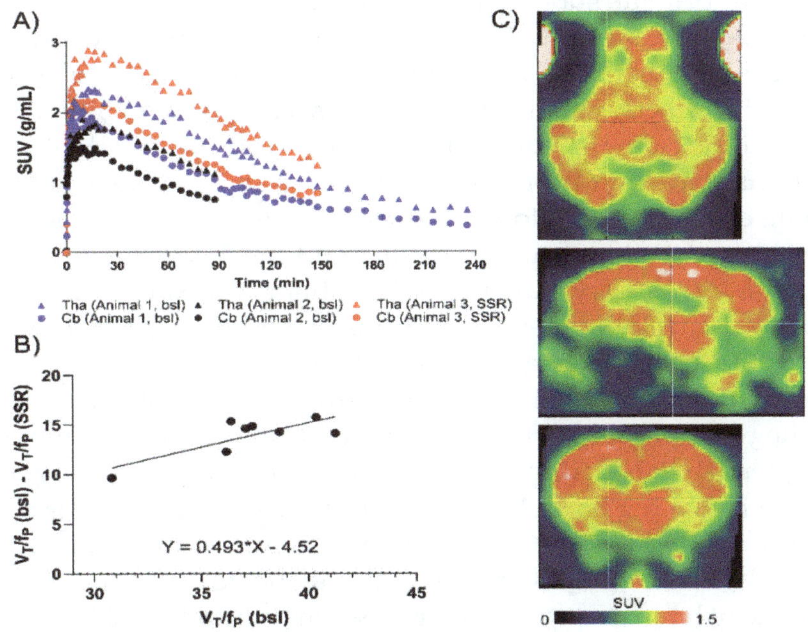

Figure 4. [^{18}F]ASEM binding in the pig brain. (**A**) Time-activity curves of [^{18}F]ASEM in three different animals: Animal 1, bsl, blue; Animal 2, bsl, black; Animal 3, SSR-180,711 pre-treated, red. The regions shown are: Thalamus (tha, triangles) and cerebellum (cb, circles). (**B**) Lassen plot with total distribution volumes (V_T) corrected for free fraction in plasma (f_P) using values from animal 1 and animal 3. Each point represents one region of interest (ROI), please refer to the method section for the complete list of ROIs. (**C**) Summed PET image (0–240 min) from animal 1 showing the distribution of [^{18}F]ASEM in the pig brain. SUV: standard uptake value. Bsl: baseline. SSR: SSR-180,711 (1 mg/kg).

3. Discussion

In this study, we investigated binding properties of radiolabelled ASEM in vitro ([^{125}I]Iodo-ASEM] and in vivo ([^{18}F]ASEM). Autoradiography was used to determine the applicability of [^{125}I]Iodo-ASEM for in vitro assessment of $\alpha7$ nAChR receptor distribution and occupancy in the mammalian brain. [^{125}I]Iodo-ASEM showed high-affinity and specific binding to $\alpha7$ nAChR in the rat, mouse and pig brain. Specific binding was absent in $\alpha7$ gene-deficient mice, indicating high specificity and selectivity. Saturation binding experiments in rat and pig brain sections revealed low nanomolar K_d values (approximately 1 nM) in both species. B_{max} in the pig cortex was considerably higher as compared to the binding found in the mouse and rat brain cortex. Such species differences are well documented in the literature, e.g., for metabotropic glutamate 5 receptors and the 18 kDa translocator protein between monkey and humans [55,56]. As affinity and selectivity are major criteria for radiotracers, our data further substantiates the suitability of ASEM derivatives as favourable $\alpha7$ nAChR tracers [57,58]

We found that the affinity of [^{125}I]Iodo-ASEM in the pig brain as determined with autoradiography was in a similar range as [^{3}H]NS14492 [59]. In contrast, higher affinities and receptor densities are reported for radioligand binding assay in brain homogenates for a number of different $\alpha7$ nAChR ligands, such as [^{3}H]NS14492 and [^{3}H]A-585539 [60], including other dibenzothiophenes [26,38].

Across the brain and specifically regions with high $\alpha7$ nAChR expression, such as hippocampus and superficial cortical layers, non-specific binding of [^{125}I]Iodo-ASEM at concentrations near the K_d was low (10%–30% of total binding) and produced a robust specific signal. However, a consistent nonspecific binding component in white matter was observed in all investigated species, in particular the corpus callosum and subcortical tracts. This is supported by previously reported in vivo findings in human and non-human primate subjects [39,43], where tracer uptake was lowest in white matter structures, such as the corpus callosum. Furthermore, we also observed slower in vivo kinetics in white matter structures in the pig brain. This could be caused by lower perfusion or kinetics may be different when the tracer interacts with lipid membranes, compared to interaction with the receptor. As in vitro binding conditions are distinctly different due to absent metabolism and blood flow, it is possible that these effects may limit pronounced non-specific white matter binding in vivo or that the nonspecific binding exhibits much slower kinetics. Under the employed incubation conditions, [^{125}I]α-bungarotoxin shows no white matter residual binding. However, under the same conditions, the overall non-specific binding in grey matter for [^{125}I]α-bungarotoxin is approximately 45% in human (data not shown) and 55% in pig brain tissue, where it is much lower for [^{125}I]Iodo-ASEM (~10%–30%).

[^{125}I]Iodo-ASEM binding enables an important distinction between grey and white matter structures, e.g., the distinct cortical laminar binding pattern observable in the pig. While [^{125}I]Iodo-ASEM binding was prominent in the deeper cortical layers in the mouse and rat, superficial cortical layers were intensely labelled in the pig. Using in vitro autoradiography, similar laminar cortical binding pattern in the pig brain has also recently been reported for a structurally different $\alpha7$ nAChR radioligand, [^{3}H]NS14492 [61]. Binding of both tracers was matching the pattern of [^{125}I]α-bungarotoxin, the in vitro gold-standard radioligand for $\alpha7$ nAChR. However, the spatial binding pattern in the rodent brain was only similar between [^{125}I]Iodo-ASEM and [^{125}I]α-bungarotoxin, but not for [^{3}H]NS14492, suggesting different binding profiles of antagonists and agonists, or species differences in affinity.

[^{125}I]Iodo-ASEM proved specific to the $\alpha7$ nAChR, as evidenced by the lack of specific binding in $\alpha7$ nAChR gene-deficient mice and a virtually complete block of cortical [^{125}I]Iodo-ASEM binding by a wide range of structurally different $\alpha7$ nAChR selective ligands and MLA, with the rank order being NS14492=TC-5619=EVP-6124=A-582941=SSR-180,711>MLA>GTS-21. While this corresponds well with the individual high affinities in the nanomolar range (NS14492, TC5619, EVP-6124, A-582941, SSR-180,711) [31,62–65], as compared to the lower affinity of a partial agonist (GTS-21) [66], it could also reflect the general differences between antagonists and agonist in terms of binding sites and kinetics.

When comparing to $[^{125}I]\alpha$-bungarotoxin, the specific binding of $[^{125}I]$Iodo-ASEM was lower in the rat and mouse brain, but higher in the pig cortex. While species differences in receptor structure may account for the discrepancies, it should also be considered that different incubation protocols were used for the determination of optimal $[^{125}I]$Iodo-ASEM and $[^{125}I]\alpha$-bungarotoxin binding. Hence, a relatively high detergent concentration was required in the experiments to obtain optimal total tissue binding of $[^{125}I]$Iodo-ASEM, which may potentially affect binding of the radioligand in the mammalian species tested, e.g., through differences in lipid content and myelination. For example, $[^{125}I]$Iodo-ASEM showed some degree of non-displaceable binding to white matter structures, which could be caused by the ligands' lipophilicity and/or different kinetics in white matter structures.

Interestingly, radioligand binding in β2 nAChR gene-deficient mice was more strongly reduced for $[^{125}I]$Iodo-ASEM than $[^{125}I]\alpha$-bungarotoxin. This observation suggests different binding properties and subtype selectivity to heteromeric α7β2 nAChR, compared to the homomeric receptors. In the CNS, heteromeric α7β2 nAChR are identified in the mouse forebrain and hippocampal neurons, rat basal forebrain cholinergic neurons, as well as in the human basal forebrain and cerebral cortex. Importantly, α7β2 nAChR display distinct functional properties as compared to homomeric α7 nAChR [51,67], owing to their slower whole cell decay kinetics and current amplitudes in both transfected cell systems and native rodent neurons [53,54,68–70]. Accordingly, co-expression of α7 and β2 nAChR subunits in *Xenopus* oocytes also results in lower maximal responses (evoked current amplitudes) of selective α7 nAChR agonists but does not shift pharmacology to a more β2-like profile [52–54,71]. These in vitro studies in transfected cell systems therefore suggest that α7 nAChR agonists bind to the α7-α7 subunit interface, and β2 subunits likely do not contribute to the ligand binding site on heteromeric α7β2 nAChR [67,71]. When using selective α7 nAChR antagonists, including MLA and α-bungarotoxin, to alter the response to some nicotinic agonists in either homomeric α7 and heteromeric α7β2 nAChR, results have been less consistent, as they show unaltered [54] or reduced potency [52] and efficacy [53] in comparison to homomeric α7 nAChR expressed in *Xenopus* oocytes. The functional significance of heteromeric α7 nAChR expression is not well understood, with recent work suggesting that this subtype combination might be more sensitive to inhibition by oligomeric amyloid β_{1-42} [68,69] and isoflurane [72], as compared to homomeric α7 nAChR. Our finding that binding of $[^{125}I]$Iodo-ASEM, an antagonist, was markedly reduced in the forebrain of β2 gene-deficient mice therefore may suggest that $[^{125}I]$Iodo-ASEM binds to heteromeric α7β2 nAChR in the brain, as opposed to $[^{125}I]\alpha$-bungarotoxin. Whether this is due to different affinity for homomeric α7 and heteromeric α7β2 nAChR requires further in vitro studies. Although speculative, this may offer a chance to probe the binding of amyloid β_{1-42} to heteromeric α7β2 nAChR in vivo using PET.

In vivo uptake of $[^{18}F]$ASEM into the pig brain occurred rapidly within the first 10–20 min and a reversible but slower washout was found, as observed in human and non-human primate subjects [39,43]. The in vivo distribution of $[^{18}F]$ASEM found here is very similar to that of $[^{11}C]$NS14492 and importantly, also in accordance with the distribution of α7 nAChR in the pig brain [31,73]. Furthermore, our data with $[^{18}F]$ASEM matches previous reports with the structurally similar analogue $[^{18}F]$DBT-10 in piglets [40].

We found variations in brain uptake and f_P in the two baseline animals, and this result is consistent with the interpretation that lower f_P will lead to lower brain uptake [74]. Due to the limited number of animals in this study, this observation merits further investigations. Our finding is however supported by PET studies in non-human primates with $[^{18}F]$ASEM and $[^{18}F]$DBT-10, where V_T/f_P was shown to be a more stable outcome measure than V_T [44,45]. This has also been shown for radiotracers binding to other neurotransmitter receptors [75].

V_T was found to increase slightly when the scan time was prolonged. This phenomenon was most pronounced in the thalamus and least pronounced in the white matter and is evident from the TACs (Figure 4A), where the ratio between e.g., thalamus and cerebellum was lower at 240 min than at 90 min. This finding is in contrast with the non-human primate and human data, where V_T was underestimated when reducing the PET data from 180 to 60 min [44]. Given that ASEM is an antagonist, it is unlikely that internalization of the receptor-ligand complex is an explanation for the decrease in V_T. We cannot exclude that other receptor adaptations, such as (de)sensitization, could be responsible for this observation. Desensitization could occur if experiments were not conducted at tracer dose, i.e., but we did not attempt to identify the mass dose limit of unlabelled ASEM. Although the injected doses of ASEM varied in the two baseline animals, we only found a 5% difference in the calculated V_T/f_P, which suggest that the studies were conducted at tracer doses. The injected doses in this study (0.007–0.085 ug/kg) are higher than the doses used in the non-human primate evaluation of [^{18}F]ASEM, where injected doses ranged from 0.009 to 0.056 μg/kg [44]. Further studies are needed to identify the mass dose limit of unlabelled ASEM.

While pre-treatment with 1 mg/kg SSR-180,711 resulted in an increased uptake of [^{18}F]ASEM, kinetic modelling for quantification of tracer uptake showed that SSR-180,711 at this dose resulted in 49% occupancy. A similar phenomenon has also been reported in piglets when [^{18}F]DBT-10 was blocked by the weak agonist NS6740, which was ascribed to a potential blood flow-driven effect of NS6740 leading to greater central uptake of [^{18}F]DBT-10 [40]. The increased tracer uptake could also be a result of peripheral α7 nAChR binding sites having been blocked by SSR-180,771. The occupancy found by us is in line with previous work of Horti et al., reporting 39% and 81% occupancy for doses of 0.5 and 5 mg/kg SSR-180,711, respectively [39]. The occupancy computed in this study should be interpreted with care, as the baseline and blocking study is conducted in two different pigs. Due to the half-life of [^{18}F]ASEM, it was not possible to conduct the study in the same animal on the same day. A further limitation to this in vivo study is the low number of PET scans and animals and thus we can only provide a descriptive presentation of the data, without statistical evaluations.

From our results, [^{125}I]Iodo-ASEM therefore offers several advantages over [^{125}I]α-bungarotoxin: 1) low nonspecific binding, 2) similar high affinity and selectivity and 3) in vivo applicability and direct comparison of PET data with autoradiographic data. The lower nonspecific binding of [^{125}I]Iodo-ASEM is advantageous primarily in vitro, as it allows for a better signal-to-noise ratio over [^{125}I]α-bungarotoxin at very similar affinities. While a low nonspecific binding would also be favourable under in vivo conditions (e.g., PET), having two nearly identical molecules as tracers offers interesting avenues, especially for preclinical studies. In vivo PET/SPECT imaging data can be acquired through [^{18}F]ASEM, [^{18}F]DBT10 or [^{123}I]Iodo-ASEM and results can be validated or extended by using the advantages of in vitro autoradiography (e.g. resolution) with [^{125}I]Iodo-ASEM.

In conclusion, [^{125}I]-Iodo-ASEM is applicable for visualizing α7 nAChR binding in vitro, its binding is different between species, and may potentially bind to heteromeric α7β2 nAChR. In addition, [^{18}F]ASEM is demonstrated to have suitable kinetic properties for in vivo quantification of α7 nAChR in the pig.

4. Materials and Methods

4.1. Compounds and Radioligands

[^{125}I]Iodo-ASEM [(3-(1,4-diazabycyclo[3.2.2]nonan-4-yl)-6-(^{125}I-iododibenzo[b,d]thiopentene 5,5-dioxide)] was labelled according to previously published procedures [42]. Mean molar activity was 59.94 ± 6.25 TBq/mmol. [^{125}I]Tyr-54-mono-Iodo-α-bungarotoxin (81.4 TBq/mmol) was purchased from Perkin-Elmer (Skovlunde, Denmark). (-)-nicotine tartrate was purchased from Sigma-Aldrich (St. Louis, MO). Unlabelled ASEM and precursor for radiosynthesis was provided by DanPET (Malmoe, Sweden). The α7-selective ligands were purchased from Sigma-Aldrich (MLA) or provided by DanPET (NS11492) or NeuroSearch A/S (Copenhagen, Denmark) (SSR-180,711, TC-5619, EVP-6124, A-58294, and GTS-21.

4.2. *Tissue Origin and Sectioning for In Vitro Autoradiography*

All animal procedures were approved by the Danish Animal Experimentation Inspectorate (J. No. 2012-15-2034-00156) and treated in concordance with the European Communities Council Directive of 24th November 1986 (86/609ECC).

One female Sprague-Dawley rat (250 g, obtained from Charles River, Sulzfeld, Germany) was euthanized with an intraperitoneal overdose of pentobarbital, the brain was quickly removed and snap-frozen in −50 °C 2-methylbutane, then stored at −80 °C until further processing.

Mice deficient for the α7 subunits (The Jackson Laboratory) and β2 (Institut Pasteur, Paris, France) and their corresponding wild-type littermates were bred (C57BL/6J background) in an animal care facility at Virginia Commonwealth University. Brains from α7 and β2 gene-deficient mice and corresponding wild-type littermates were kindly provided by Dr. M. Imad Damaj (Dept. of Pharmacology and Toxicology, Virginia Commonwealth University, Richmond, VA, USA).

One two-month old female Danish domestic pig (Landrace x Yorkshire x Duroc, 22 kg) was euthanized with an intravenous injection of pentobarbital, the brain was quickly excised, separated in two hemispheres and frozen on dry ice, before being stored at −80 °C.

All brain specimens were cut in 12 μm serial sections on a cryostat (Microm HM 500 OM, Walldorf, Germany), thaw-mounted onto Super Frost slides (Thermo Scientific, Hvidovre, Denmark), briefly air dried and stored at −80 °C until further processing. Protein concentration was determined from single or three sections with the Bio-Rad Protein Assay (Bio-Rad, Hercules, CA, USA) based on the method of Bradford [76].

4.3. *In Vitro Autoradiography with [^{125}I]Iodo-ASEM*

Initial optimization of assay conditions was performed to maximize total binding while keeping non-specific binding low. Adjustments included buffer composition and pH, detergent concentration, wash and incubation time and temperature. An assay buffer with 50 mMol/L Tris-HCl pH 7.4, 21 °C (termed Tris-HCl buffer) provided best preserved tissue integrity and lowest non-specific binding, as compared to physiologic Tris, Tris-EDTA-EGTA or HEPES-KRH buffer (data not shown). For all further experiments, tissue from 1–2 animals was used, with experiments and quantifications carried out using 3–4 sections for pig and rat tissue and 3–6 sections for mouse tissue. Adjacent sections were used for autoradiography for all similar experiments (e.g. saturation binding). Sections were brought to room temperature and pre-incubated for 20 min in Tris-HCl buffer (pH 7.4, 21 °C), then incubated for 60 min in the same buffer (21 °C) containing 1.5% Triton X-100 (v/v) and 0.5-1.0 nMol/L [^{125}I]Iodo-ASEM in a humidified chamber. Non-specific binding of [^{125}I]Iodo-ASEM was assessed in the presence of 10 μMol/L SSR-180,711, added to the buffer. Blocking of [^{125}I]Iodo-ASEM binding was investigated with a series of individual α7 nAChR selective compounds (10 μMol/L) added to the incubation buffer, i.e., methyllycaconitine (MLA) [77], SSR-180,711 [63], NS14492 [31], TC-5619 [64], EVP-6124 [65], A-582941 [62], and GTS-21 [66]. Following incubation, slides were rinsed in Tris-HCl buffer (pH 7.4, 21 °C), washed 2 × 5 min in Tris-HCl buffer (pH 7.4, 4 °C) and rinsed (5 sec) in ice-cold distilled water. Slides were gently dried under an air stream and exposed to 4% paraformaldehyde vapour overnight at 4 °C, followed by another drying step in a desiccator for 1 h. Adjacent sections were used for autoradiography.

4.4. *In Vitro Autoradiography with [^{125}I]α-bungarotoxin*

Slides were thawed at room temperature (21 °C) for 30 min, followed by 30 min of rehydration in 50 mMol/L Tris buffer with 0.1% BSA (w/v), pH 7.3 (binding buffer). For assessment of α-bungarotoxin binding, the binding buffer contained 0.5 mMol/L [^{125}I]α-bungarotoxin and 4.5 nMol/L unlabelled α-bungarotoxin (Tocris, Denmark) yielding a total of 5 nMol/L α-bungarotoxin (incubation buffer). Total binding was determined using one set of slides incubated with the radioligand for 2 h at room temperature in a humidified chamber. Non-specific binding was determined in the presence of 1 mMol/L (-)-nicotine added to the incubation buffer. Afterwards, slides were briefly rinsed in binding buffer, followed by 2 × 30 min of washing in ice-cold binding buffer (4 °C). Finally, slides were briefly rinsed (5 sec) in ice-cold distilled water, dried under a gentle air stream and exposed to 4% paraformaldehyde vapour overnight at 4 °C. On the next day, the slides were dried for 1 h in a desiccator.

4.5. Saturation Binding and Kinetic Analysis Using In Vitro Autoradiography

Saturation binding was carried out in rat and pig brain sections as described above (Section 4.3). Sections were incubated with ten serial dilutions of [^{125}I]Iodo-ASEM ranging from 0.02 to 10 nMol/L, with concentrations measured by gamma-counting. Non-specific binding was determined in adjacent sections in the presence of 10 μMol/L SSR-180,711 for each radioligand concentration. Binding was terminated by washing the sections in ice-cold binding buffer. The equilibrium dissociation constant (K_d) and maximum number of binding sites (B_{max}) were determined by non-linear regression analysis of a one-site saturation binding model using GraphPad Prism 6.0 (GraphPad Software, Inc., San Diego, CA, USA).

4.6. Autoradiographic Image Acquisition and Analysis

BAS SR2040 phosphor imaging plates (Fujifilm, Toyko, Japan) were exposed to the samples along with [^{125}I] standards (ARI 0133A; American Radiolabeled Chemicals, St. Louis, USA) for 24-72 hours. Imaging plates were scanned using a Phosphor Imager BAS-2500 (Fujifilm Europe GmbH, Düsseldorf, Germany). Images were converted to TIF-files using the manufacturer's software and analysed in QuantityOne (BioRad, Waltham, MA, USA). Regions of interest (ROIs) were drawn over grey and white matter structures, depending on the investigated species. High intensity circular spots were occasionally observed in [^{125}I]Iodo-ASEM autoradiographs and were excluded from the analysis. For α7 and β2 gene-deficient mice, only one ROI was drawn over the whole brain, again excluding spots and irregular white matter binding. In the rat brain, the ROIs were drawn over cortex and hippocampus. From the pig brain, only frontal cortex sections were cut, the ROIs therefore contained the frontal cortex and white matter tracts. The mean values of optical density per mm^2 (averaged from the replicates) were converted to radioactive concentration using a linear regression derived from the [^{125}I] radioactive standards. A global background of the imaging plate and individual non-specific binding were subtracted. Final values were expressed as fmol/mg protein, based on the protein measurements from individual sections.

4.7. Radiosynthesis of [^{18}F]ASEM

The radiosynthesis of [^{18}F]ASEM was performed as previously published [26]. No-carrier-added aqueous ^{18}F-fluoride from the target was collected at a non-conditioned activated (10 mL ethanol, 20 mL water and dried with air) anion-exchange cartridge (QMA). A solution of 20 mg of 1,10-diaza-4,7,13,16,21,24-hexaoxabicyclo[8.8.8]hexacosane (Kryptofix-222) and 3.3 mg of K_2CO_3 dissolved in a 0.65 mL methanol-water mixture (97/3 v/v) was used to elute the ^{18}F-fluoride off the cartridge. The elute was thereafter dried by evaporation at 90 °C under nitrogen and then further dried twice with 1 mL dry acetonitrile. To the dried Kryptofix®222/[^{18}F]fluoride complex, 2.4 mg (0.006 mmol)/L of 3-(1,4-Diazabicyclo[3.2.2]nonan-4-yl)-6-nitrodibenzo[b,d]- thiophene 5,5-Dioxide dissolved in 0.8 mL DMSO was added. The reaction was performed at 160 °C for 15 min and afterwards the crude was quenched with 3.5 mL H_2O. Reactants and by-products were separated from [^{18}F]ASEM by semi-preparative HPLC [Luna column, Phenomenex Ltd. Aschaffenburg, Germany; 10 μm C18(2) 10×250 mm column, flow rate 6 mL/min, eluent: Ethanol/0.1% H_3PO_4 in water (25:75) with 6 mM ascorbic acid to prevent radiolysis]. The retention time for [^{18}F]ASEM was 400-450 s and the product was collected into a vial containing 9 mL of PBS (phosphate-buffered saline). The product was visually inspected for clarity, absence of colour and visible particles. Chemical and radiochemical purities were assessed by analytical HPLC [Kinetex column, Phenomenex Ltd. Aschaffenburg, Germany; 2.6μ C18

4.60 × 50 mm, eluent: ACN/0.1% H_3PO_4 in water (25:75) RT: [^{18}F]ASEM = 1.3 min; nitro precursor = 1 min; flow rate 1.5 mL/min]. Molar activity (A_m) of the radiotracer was determined as follows: the area of the UV absorbance peak corresponding to the radiolabelled product was measured (integrated) on the HPLC chromatogram. This value was then converted into a molar mass by comparison with an average of integrated areas (triplet) of a known standard of the reference compound.

4.8. *In Vivo Imaging in the Pig*

Three female pigs (21, 22 and 23 kg) were used for in vivo PET imaging on a HRRT PET scanner (Siemens Healthcare, Erlangen, Germany). All animal procedures were approved by the Danish Council for Animal Ethics (journal no. 2012-15-2934-00156).

4.8.1. Animal Procedures

Before scanning, anaesthesia was induced with i.m. injection of 0.13 mL/kg Zoletil veterinary mixture (Virbac, Kolding, Denmark; 10.87 mg/kg xylazine + 10.87 mg/kg ketamine + 1.74 mg/kg methadone + 1.74 mg/kg butorphanol + 10.87 mg/kg tiletamine + 10.87 mg/kg zolezepam). Hereafter, anaesthesia was maintained with constant propofol infusion (1.5 mg/kg/h intravenous (i.v.); B. Braun, Melsungen, Germany). An arterial i.v. catheter was employed for blood sampling from the right femoral artery and two venous i.v. catheters for injections were placed in the left and right mammary veins. During anaesthesia, animals were endotracheally intubated and ventilated. Vital parameters (heart rate, body temperature, blood pressure, oxygen saturation and end tidal CO_2) were continuously monitored during the scan.

4.8.2. PET Scanning

[^{18}F]ASEM was given as intravenous i.v. bolus, with experimental details described in Table 4.

Table 4. Experimental details of [^{18}F]ASEM PET scans in pigs.

Details	Animal 1	Animal 2	Animal 3
Type of experiment	Baseline	Baseline	SSR-180,711; 1 mg/kg
Scan length	240 min	90 min	150 min
Molar activity	20 GBq/μmol	345 GBq/μmol	388 GBq/μmol
Injected activity	99 MBq	335 MBq	189 MBq
Injected mass	1.78 μg	0.35 μg	0.18 μg
Free plasma fraction	18%	16%	9%

4.8.3. Blood Sampling

During the first 30 min of the scans, radioactivity in the whole blood was continuously measured using an ABSS autosampler (Allogg Technology, Mariefred, Sweden) counting coincidences in a lead-shielded detector. Concurrently, arterial whole blood was sampled manually at times 2.5, 5, 10, 20, 30, 40, 50, 70, 89, 91, 120 and 150 min after injection of [^{18}F]ASEM. Total radioactivity in plasma (500 μL) and whole blood (500 μL) was measured in a well counter (Cobra 5003; Packard Instruments, Meriden, CT, USA), which was cross-calibrated to the HRRT scanner and autosampler. All measurements of radioactivity were decay corrected to the time of radioligand injection.

4.8.4. Metabolite Analysis

Radiolabelled parent compound and metabolites were determined by direct injection of plasma into a radio-HPLC system (Dionex Ultimate 3000; Thermo Fisher Scientific, Hvidovre, Denmark) configured for column switching. Manually drawn arterial whole blood samples were centrifuged (1500 g, 7 min, 4 °C), and plasma was filtered through a syringe filter (Whatman GD/X 13 mm or 25 mm, PVDF membrane, 0.45 μm pore size; Frisenette ApS, Knebel, Denmark) prior to the analysis by HPLC as previously described [78]. To increase sensitivity on gamma counts from samples with low levels of radioactivity, eluent from the HPLC was collected into fractions (10 mL) using a fraction collector (Foxy Jr FC144; Teledyne, Lincoln, NE, USA) and counted offline in a well counter (2480 Wizard^2 Automatic Gamma Counter, Wallac Oy, Turku, Finland).

4.8.5. Determination of Free Fraction

The free, non-protein bound fraction of [^{18}F]ASEM in pig plasma, f_P, was estimated using an equilibrium dialysis chamber method as previously described [79].

4.8.6. Reconstruction and Pre-Processing of PET Data

150 -minute list-mode PET data were reconstructed in 58 dynamic frames (6×10, 6×20, 6×30, 6×60, 4×120, 14×300, 8×150, 8×300 s). One animal was scanned for 240 min using the mentioned framing protocol but adding 9 frames of 600 s). Images consisted of 207 planes of 256×256 voxels of $1.22 \times 1.22 \times 1.22$ mm. A summed picture of all counts in the 150-min scan was reconstructed for each pig and used for co-registration to a standardized MRI-based atlas of the domestic pig brain, similar to that previously published [80]. The time activity curveds (TACs) were calculated for the following volumes of interest (VOIs): thalamus, striatum, hippocampus, cerebellum, white matter, frontal cortex, somatosensory cortex, occipital cortex, rest of the cortex. Radioactivity in all VOIs was calculated as the average of radioactive concentration (Bq/mL) in the left and right sides. Outcome measure in the TACs was calculated as radioactive concentration in VOI (in kBq/mL) normalized to the injected dose corrected for animal weight (in kBq/kg), yielding standardized uptake values (g/mL).

4.8.7. Kinetic Modelling of PET Data

The PET imaging data were analysed with the Logan graphical analysis (LGA) model, using the metabolite corrected arterial plasma concentration to calculate the primary outcome measure: total distribution volume (V_T). The secondary outcome measure was V_T values corrected for free fraction in plasma (V_T/f_P). The parent fraction curve for [^{18}F]ASEM was fitted with a Watabe fit. Both curves were constrained to 1.0 at time = 0. Kinetic modeling was performed in PMOD version 3.0 (PMOD Technologies).

Author Contributions: Conceptualization: C.K.D., J.D.M., A.G.H., M.G.P., D.P; Methodology: C.K.D., H.D.H., G.M.K., M.M.H.; Formal analysis: C.K.D.; H.D.H., H.H.H.; Investigation: C.K.D.; H.D.H., E.T.L.; Resources: D.P., R.C.M., M.M.H., A.G.H.; Writing—original draft preparation: C.K.D.; H.H.H., H.D.H.; Writing—review and editing: C.K.D., H.D.H., J.D.M., A.G.H., M.G.P., G.M.K., M.M.H.,; Visualization: C.K.D., H.D.H.; Supervision: J.D.M., G.M.K.; Funding acquisition: J.D.M., G.M.K., M.G.P.; All authors have read and agreed to the published version of the manuscript.

Acknowledgments: The authors would like to thank the animal facilities at the Department of Experimental Medicine, University of Copenhagen.

References

1. Marutle, A.; Zhang, X.; Court, J.; Piggott, M.; Johnson, M.; Perry, R.; Perry, E.; Nordberg, A. Laminar distribution of nicotinic receptor subtypes in cortical regions in schizophrenia. *J. Chem. Neuroanat.* **2001**, *22*, 115–126. [CrossRef]
2. Kulak, J.M.; Carroll, F.I.; Schneider, J.S. [125I]Iodomethyllycaconitine binds to alpha7 nicotinic acetylcholine receptors in monkey brain. *Eur. J. Neurosci.* **2006**, *23*, 2604–2610. [CrossRef] [PubMed]

3. Whiteaker, P.; Davies, A.R.; Marks, M.J.; Blagbrough, I.S.; Potter, B.V.; Wolstenholme, A.J.; Collins, A.C.; Wonnacott, S. An autoradiographic study of the distribution of binding sites for the novel alpha7-selective nicotinic radioligand [3H]-methyllycaconitine in the mouse brain. *Eur. J. Neurosci.* **1999**, *11*, 2689–2696. [CrossRef] [PubMed]
4. Quik, M.; Choremis, J.; Komourian, J.; Lukas, R.J.; Puchacz, E. Similarity between rat brain nicotinic alpha-bungarotoxin receptors and stably expressed alpha-bungarotoxin binding sites. *J. Neurochem.* **1996**, *67*, 145–154. [CrossRef] [PubMed]
5. Lendvai, B.; Kassai, F.; Szajli, A.; Nemethy, Z. alpha7 nicotinic acetylcholine receptors and their role in cognition. *Brain Res. Bull.* **2013**, *93*, 86–96. [CrossRef] [PubMed]
6. Picciotto, M.R.; Lewis, A.S.; van Schalkwyk, G.I.; Mineur, Y.S. Mood and anxiety regulation by nicotinic acetylcholine receptors: A potential pathway to modulate aggression and related behavioral states. *Neuropharmacology* **2015**, *96*, 235–243. [CrossRef] [PubMed]
7. Albuquerque, E.X.; Pereira, E.F.; Alkondon, M.; Rogers, S.W. Mammalian nicotinic acetylcholine receptors: From structure to function. *Physiol. Rev.* **2009**, *89*, 73–120. [CrossRef]
8. Dani, J.A.; Bertrand, D. Nicotinic acetylcholine receptors and nicotinic cholinergic mechanisms of the central nervous system. *Annu Rev Pharm. Toxicol* **2007**, *47*, 699–729. [CrossRef]
9. Maurer, S.V.; Williams, C.L. The Cholinergic System Modulates Memory and Hippocampal Plasticity via Its Interactions with Non-Neuronal Cells. *Front Immunol.* **2017**, *8*, 1489. [CrossRef]
10. Bosmans, G.; Shimizu Bassi, G.; Florens, M.; Gonzalez-Dominguez, E.; Matteoli, G.; Boeckxstaens, G.E. Cholinergic Modulation of Type 2 Immune Responses. *Front Immunol.* **2017**, *8*, 1873. [CrossRef]
11. Freedman, R.; Hall, M.; Adler, L.E.; Leonard, S. Evidence in postmortem brain tissue for decreased numbers of hippocampal nicotinic receptors in schizophrenia. *Biol. Psychiatry* **1995**, *38*, 22–33. [CrossRef]
12. Guillozet-Bongaarts, A.L.; Hyde, T.M.; Dalley, R.A.; Hawrylycz, M.J.; Henry, A.; Hof, P.R.; Hohmann, J.; Jones, A.R.; Kuan, C.L.; Royall, J.; et al. Altered gene expression in the dorsolateral prefrontal cortex of individuals with schizophrenia. *Mol. Psychiatry* **2014**, *19*, 478–485. [CrossRef]
13. Kunii, Y.; Zhang, W.; Xu, Q.; Hyde, T.M.; McFadden, W.; Shin, J.H.; Deep-Soboslay, A.; Ye, T.; Li, C.; Kleinman, J.E.; et al. CHRNA7 and CHRFAM7A mRNAs: Co-Localized and Their Expression Levels Altered in the Postmortem Dorsolateral Prefrontal Cortex in Major Psychiatric Disorders. *Am. J. Psychiatry* **2015**. [CrossRef] [PubMed]
14. Thomsen, M.S.; Weyn, A.; Mikkelsen, J.D. Hippocampal alpha7 nicotinic acetylcholine receptor levels in patients with schizophrenia, bipolar disorder, or major depressive disorder. *Bipolar Disord.* **2011**, *13*, 701–707. [CrossRef] [PubMed]
15. Sugaya, K.; Giacobini, E.; Chiappinelli, V.A. Nicotinic acetylcholine receptor subtypes in human frontal cortex: Changes in Alzheimer's disease. *J. Neurosci. Res.* **1990**, *27*, 349–359. [CrossRef]
16. Araud, T.; Graw, S.; Berger, R.; Lee, M.; Neveu, E.; Bertrand, D.; Leonard, S. The chimeric gene CHRFAM7A, a partial duplication of the CHRNA7 gene, is a dominant negative regulator of alpha7*nAChR function. *Biochem. Pharmacol.* **2011**, *82*, 904–914. [CrossRef]
17. Gillentine, M.A.; Lozoya, R.; Yin, J.; Grochowski, C.M.; White, J.J.; Schaaf, C.P.; Calarge, C.A. CHRNA7 copy number gains are enriched in adolescents with major depressive and anxiety disorders. *J. Affect. Disord.* **2018**, *239*, 247–252. [CrossRef]
18. Sinkus, M.L.; Graw, S.; Freedman, R.; Ross, R.G.; Lester, H.A.; Leonard, S. The human CHRNA7 and CHRFAM7A genes: A review of the genetics, regulation, and function. *Neuropharmacology* **2015**. [CrossRef]
19. Gillentine, M.A.; Berry, L.N.; Goin-Kochel, R.P.; Ali, M.A.; Ge, J.; Guffey, D.; Rosenfeld, J.A.; Hannig, V.; Bader, P.; Proud, M.; et al. The Cognitive and Behavioral Phenotypes of Individuals with CHRNA7 Duplications. *J. Autism Dev. Disord.* **2017**, *47*, 549–562. [CrossRef]
20. Hua, S.; Ek, C.J.; Mallard, C.; Johansson, M.E. Perinatal hypoxia-ischemia reduces alpha 7 nicotinic receptor expression and selective alpha 7 nicotinic receptor stimulation suppresses inflammation and promotes microglial Mox phenotype. *Biomed Res. Int.* **2014**, *2014*, 718769. [CrossRef]
21. Han, Z.; Li, L.; Wang, L.; Degos, V.; Maze, M.; Su, H. Alpha-7 nicotinic acetylcholine receptor agonist treatment reduces neuroinflammation, oxidative stress, and brain injury in mice with ischemic stroke and bone fracture. *J. Neurochem.* **2014**, *131*, 498–508. [CrossRef] [PubMed]

22. Dash, P.K.; Zhao, J.; Kobori, N.; Redell, J.B.; Hylin, M.J.; Hood, K.N.; Moore, A.N. Activation of Alpha 7 Cholinergic Nicotinic Receptors Reduce Blood-Brain Barrier Permeability following Experimental Traumatic Brain Injury. *J. Neurosci.* **2016**, *36*, 2809–2818. [CrossRef] [PubMed]
23. Mavropoulos, S.A.; Khan, N.S.; Levy, A.C.J.; Faliks, B.T.; Sison, C.P.; Pavlov, V.A.; Zhang, Y.; Ojamaa, K. Nicotinic acetylcholine receptor-mediated protection of the rat heart exposed to ischemia reperfusion. *Mol. Med.* **2017**, 23. [CrossRef] [PubMed]
24. Gatson, J.W.; Simpkins, J.W.; Uteshev, V.V. High therapeutic potential of positive allosteric modulation of alpha7 nAChRs in a rat model of traumatic brain injury: Proof-of-concept. *Brain Res. Bull.* **2015**, *112*, 35–41. [CrossRef] [PubMed]
25. Pike, V.W. Considerations in the Development of Reversibly Binding PET Radioligands for Brain Imaging. *Nicotin4* **2016**, *23*, 1818–1869.
26. Gao, Y.; Kellar, K.J.; Yasuda, R.P.; Tran, T.; Xiao, Y.; Dannals, R.F.; Horti, A.G. Derivatives of dibenzothiophene for positron emission tomography imaging of alpha7-nicotinic acetylcholine receptors. *J. Med. Chem.* **2013**, *56*, 7574–7589. [CrossRef]
27. Toyohara, J.; Hashimoto, K. α7 Nicotinic Receptor Agonists: Potential Therapeutic Drugs for Treatment of Cognitive Impairments in Schizophrenia and Alzheimer's Disease. *Open Med. Chem. J.* **2010**, *4*, 37–56. [CrossRef]
28. Hashimoto, K.; Nishiyama, S.; Ohba, H.; Matsuo, M.; Kobashi, T.; Takahagi, M.; Iyo, M.; Kitashoji, T.; Tsukada, H. [^{11}C]CHIBA-1001 as a novel PET ligand for α7 nicotinic receptors in the brain: A PET study in conscious monkeys. *PLoS ONE* **2008**, *3*, e3231. [CrossRef]
29. Rötering, S.; Scheunemann, M.; Fischer, S.; Hiller, A.; Peters, D.; Deuther-Conrad, W.; Brust, P. Radiosynthesis and first evaluation in mice of [(18)F]NS14490 for molecular imaging of alpha7 nicotinic acetylcholine receptors. *Bioorganic Med. Chem.* **2013**, *21*, 2635–2642.
30. Kim, S.W.; Ding, Y.S.; Alexoff, D.; Patel, V.; Logan, J.; Lin, K.S.; Shea, C.; Muench, L.; Xu, Y.; Carter, P.; et al. Synthesis and positron emission tomography studies of C-11-labeled isotopomers and metabolites of GTS-21, a partial alpha7 nicotinic cholinergic agonist drug. *Nucl. Med. Biol.* **2007**, *34*, 541–551. [CrossRef]
31. Ettrup, A.; Mikkelsen, J.D.; Lehel, S.; Madsen, J.; Nielsen, E.O.; Palner, M.; Timmermann, D.B.; Peters, D.; Knudsen, G.M. ^{11}C-NS14492 as a novel PET radioligand for imaging cerebral alpha7 nicotinic acetylcholine receptors: In vivo evaluation and drug occupancy measurements. *J. Nucl. Med.* **2011**, *52*, 1449–1456. [CrossRef] [PubMed]
32. Deuther-Conrad, W.; Fischer, S.; Hiller, A.; Becker, G.; Cumming, P.; Xiong, G.; Funke, U.; Sabri, O.; Peters, D.; Brust, P. Assessment of alpha7 nicotinic acetylcholine receptor availability in juvenile pig brain with [(18)F]NS10743. *Eur. J. Nucl. Med. Mol. Imaging* **2011**. [CrossRef] [PubMed]
33. Ouach, A.; Vercouillie, J.; Bertrand, E.; Rodrigues, N.; Pin, F.; Serriere, S.; Boiaryna, L.; Chartier, A.; Percina, N.; Tangpong, P.; et al. Bis(het)aryl-1,2,3-triazole quinuclidines as alpha7 nicotinic acetylcholine receptor ligands: Synthesis, structure affinity relationships, agonism activity, [(18)F]-radiolabeling and PET study in rats. *Eur. J. Med. Chem.* **2019**, *179*, 449–469. [CrossRef] [PubMed]
34. Huan, W.; Aiqin, W.; Jianping, L.; Qianqian, X.; Xia, L.; Lei, Y.; Yu, F.; Huabei, Z. Radiosynthesis and in-vivo evaluation of [125I]IBT: A single-photon emission computed tomography radiotracer for alpha7-nicotinic acetylcholine receptor imaging. *Nucl. Med. Commun.* **2017**, *38*, 683–693. [CrossRef] [PubMed]
35. Wang, S.; Fang, Y.; Wang, H.; Gao, H.; Jiang, G.; Liu, J.; Xue, Q.; Qi, Y.; Cao, M.; Qiang, B.; et al. Design, synthesis and biological evaluation of 1,4-Diazobicylco[3.2.2]nonane derivatives as alpha7-Nicotinic acetylcholine receptor PET/CT imaging agents and agonists for Alzheimer's disease. *Eur. J. Med. Chem.* **2018**, *159*, 255–266. [CrossRef] [PubMed]
36. Teodoro, R.; Scheunemann, M.; Wenzel, B.; Peters, D.; Deuther-Conrad, W.; Brust, P. Synthesis and radiofluorination of novel fluoren-9-one based derivatives for the imaging of alpha7 nicotinic acetylcholine receptor with PET. *Bioorg. Med. Chem. Lett.* **2018**, *28*, 1471–1475. [CrossRef]
37. Sarasamkan, J.; Scheunemann, M.; Apaijai, N.; Palee, S.; Parichatikanond, W.; Arunrungvichian, K.; Fischer, S.; Chattipakorn, S.; Deuther-Conrad, W.; Schuurmann, G.; et al. Varying Chirality Across Nicotinic Acetylcholine Receptor Subtypes: Selective Binding of Quinuclidine Triazole Compounds. *Acs Med. Chem. Lett.* **2016**, *7*, 890–895. [CrossRef]

38. Schrimpf, M.R.; Sippy, K.B.; Briggs, C.A.; Anderson, D.J.; Li, T.; Ji, J.; Frost, J.M.; Surowy, C.S.; Bunnelle, W.H.; Gopalakrishnan, M.; et al. SAR of alpha7 nicotinic receptor agonists derived from tilorone: Exploration of a novel nicotinic pharmacophore. *Bioorg. Med. Chem. Lett.* **2012**, *22*, 1633–1638. [CrossRef]
39. Horti, A.G.; Gao, Y.; Kuwabara, H.; Wang, Y.; Abazyan, S.; Yasuda, R.P.; Tran, T.; Xiao, Y.; Sahibzada, N.; Holt, D.P.; et al. 18F-ASEM, a radiolabeled antagonist for imaging the alpha7-nicotinic acetylcholine receptor with PET. *J. Nucl. Med.* **2014**, *55*, 672–677. [CrossRef]
40. Teodoro, R.; Scheunemann, M.; Deuther-Conrad, W.; Wenzel, B.; Fasoli, F.M.; Gotti, C.; Kranz, M.; Donat, C.K.; Patt, M.; Hillmer, A.; et al. A Promising PET Tracer for Imaging of alpha(7) Nicotinic Acetylcholine Receptors in the Brain: Design, Synthesis, and In Vivo Evaluation of a Dibenzothiophene-Based Radioligand. *Molecules* **2015**, *20*, 18387–18421. [CrossRef]
41. Horti, A.G. Development of [(18)F]ASEM, a specific radiotracer for quantification of the alpha7-nAChR with positron-emission tomography. *Biochem. Pharmacol.* **2015**, *97*, 566–575. [CrossRef] [PubMed]
42. Gao, Y.; Mease, R.C.; Olson, T.T.; Kellar, K.J.; Dannals, R.F.; Pomper, M.G.; Horti, A.G. [(^{125})I]Iodo-ASEM, a specific in vivo radioligand for alpha7-nAChR. *Nucl. Med. Biol.* **2015**, *42*, 488–493. [CrossRef] [PubMed]
43. Wong, D.F.; Kuwabara, H.; Pomper, M.; Holt, D.P.; Brasic, J.R.; George, N.; Frolov, B.; Willis, W.; Gao, Y.; Valentine, H.; et al. Human brain imaging of alpha7 nAChR with [(18)F]ASEM: A new PET radiotracer for neuropsychiatry and determination of drug occupancy. *WinnieBbb13* **2014**, *16*, 730–738.
44. Hillmer, A.T.; Li, S.; Zheng, M.Q.; Scheunemann, M.; Lin, S.F.; Nabulsi, N.; Holden, D.; Pracitto, R.; Labaree, D.; Ropchan, J.; et al. PET imaging of alpha7 nicotinic acetylcholine receptors: A comparative study of [18F]ASEM and [18F]DBT-10 in nonhuman primates, and further evaluation of [18F]ASEM in humans. *Eur. J. Nucl. Med. Mol. Imaging* **2017**, *44*, 1042–1050. [CrossRef]
45. Hillmer, A.T.; Zheng, M.Q.; Li, S.; Scheunemann, M.; Lin, S.F.; Holden, D.; Labaree, D.; Ropchan, J.; Teodoro, R.; Deuther-Conrad, W.; et al. PET imaging evaluation of [(18)F]DBT-10, a novel radioligand specific to alpha7 nicotinic acetylcholine receptors, in nonhuman primates. *Eur. J. Nucl. Med. Mol. Imaging* **2016**, *43*, 537–547. [CrossRef]
46. Wong, D.F.; Kuwabara, H.; Horti, A.G.; Roberts, J.M.; Nandi, A.; Cascella, N.; Brasic, J.; Weerts, E.M.; Kitzmiller, K.; Phan, J.A.; et al. Brain PET Imaging of alpha7-nAChR with [18F]ASEM: Reproducibility, Occupancy, Receptor Density, and Changes in Schizophrenia. *Int. J. Neuropsychopharmacol. /Off. Sci. J. Coll. Int. Neuropsychopharmacol.* **2018**, *21*, 656–667.
47. Coughlin, J.M.; Du, Y.; Rosenthal, H.B.; Slania, S.; Min Koo, S.; Park, A.; Solomon, G.; Vranesic, M.; Antonsdottir, I.; Speck, C.L.; et al. The distribution of the alpha7 nicotinic acetylcholine receptor in healthy aging: An in vivo positron emission tomography study with [(18)F]ASEM. *NeuroImage* **2017**, *165*, 118–124. [CrossRef]
48. Coughlin, J.; Du, Y.; Crawford, J.L.; Rubin, L.H.; Behnam Azad, B.; Lesniak, W.G.; Horti, A.G.; Schretlen, D.J.; Sawa, A.; Pomper, M.G. The availability of the alpha7 nicotinic acetylcholine receptor in recent-onset psychosis: A study using (18)F-ASEM PET. *J. Nucl. Med.* **2018**. [CrossRef]
49. Coughlin, J.M.; Rubin, L.H.; Du, Y.; Rowe, S.P.; Crawford, J.L.; Rosenthal, H.B.; Frey, S.M.; Marshall, E.S.; Shinehouse, L.K.; Chen, A.; et al. High availability of the alpha7 nicotinic acetylcholine receptor in brains of individuals with mild cognitive impairment: A pilot study using (18)F-ASEM PET. *J. Nucl. Med.* **2019**. [CrossRef]
50. Vetel, S.; Vercouillie, J.; Buron, F.; Vergote, J.; Tauber, C.; Busson, J.; Chicheri, G.; Routier, S.; Serriere, S.; Chalon, S. Longitudinal PET Imaging of alpha7 Nicotinic Acetylcholine Receptors with [(18)F]ASEM in a Rat Model of Parkinson's Disease. *WinnieBbb13* **2019**. [CrossRef]
51. Wu, J.; Liu, Q.; Tang, P.; Mikkelsen, J.D.; Shen, J.; Whiteaker, P.; Yakel, J.L. Heteromeric alpha7beta2 Nicotinic Acetylcholine Receptors in the Brain. *Trends Pharm. Sci.* **2016**, *37*, 562–574. [CrossRef] [PubMed]
52. Thomsen, M.S.; Zwart, R.; Ursu, D.; Jensen, M.M.; Pinborg, L.H.; Gilmour, G.; Wu, J.; Sher, E.; Mikkelsen, J.D. alpha7 and beta2 Nicotinic Acetylcholine Receptor Subunits Form Heteromeric Receptor Complexes that Are Expressed in the Human Cortex and Display Distinct Pharmacological Properties. *PLoS ONE* **2015**, *10*, e0130572. [CrossRef] [PubMed]
53. Moretti, M.; Zoli, M.; George, A.A.; Lukas, R.J.; Pistillo, F.; Maskos, U.; Whiteaker, P.; Gotti, C. The novel alpha7beta2-nicotinic acetylcholine receptor subtype is expressed in mouse and human basal forebrain: Biochemical and pharmacological characterization. *Mol. Pharmacol.* **2014**, *86*, 306–317. [CrossRef] [PubMed]

54. Zwart, R.; Strotton, M.; Ching, J.; Astles, P.C.; Sher, E. Unique pharmacology of heteromeric alpha7beta2 nicotinic acetylcholine receptors expressed in Xenopus laevis oocytes. *Eur. J. Pharmacol.* **2014**, *726C*, 77–86. [CrossRef]
55. Patel, S.; Hamill, T.G.; Connolly, B.; Jagoda, E.; Li, W.; Gibson, R.E. Species differences in mGluR5 binding sites in mammalian central nervous system determined using in vitro binding with [18F]F-PEB. *Pet§Cholin2* **2007**, *34*, 1009–1017. [CrossRef]
56. Fujita, M.; Imaizumi, M.; Zoghbi, S.S.; Fujimura, Y.; Farris, A.G.; Suhara, T.; Hong, J.; Pike, V.W.; Innis, R.B. Kinetic analysis in healthy humans of a novel positron emission tomography radioligand to image the peripheral benzodiazepine receptor, a potential biomarker for inflammation. *NeuroImage* **2008**, *40*, 43–52. [CrossRef]
57. Van de Bittner, G.C.; Ricq, E.L.; Hooker, J.M. A philosophy for CNS radiotracer design. *Acc Chem. Res.* **2014**, *47*, 3127–3134. [CrossRef]
58. Laruelle, M.; Slifstein, M.; Huang, Y. Relationships between radiotracer properties and image quality in molecular imaging of the brain with positron emission tomography. *Nicotin4* **2003**, *5*, 363–375. [CrossRef]
59. Magnussen, J.H.; Ettrup, A.; Donat, C.K.; Peters, D.; Pedersen, M.H.F.; Knudsen, G.M.; Mikkelsen, J.D. Radiosynthesis and in vitro validation of 3H-NS14492 as a novel high affinity $\alpha 7$ nicotinic acetylcholine receptor radioligand *Mol. Cell. Neurosci.* **2014**. [CrossRef]
60. Anderson, D.J.; Bunnelle, W.; Surber, B.; Du, J.; Surowy, C.; Tribollet, E.; Marguerat, A.; Bertrand, D.; Gopalakrishnan, M. [^{3}H]A-585539 [(1S,4S)-2,2-dimethyl-5-(6-phenylpyridazin-3-yl)-5-aza-2-azoniabicyclo[2.2.1]hept ane], a novel high-affinity alpha7 neuronal nicotinic receptor agonist: Radioligand binding characterization to rat and human brain. *J. Pharmacol. Exp. Ther.* **2008**, *324*, 179–187. [CrossRef]
61. Magnussen, J.H.; Ettrup, A.; Donat, C.K.; Peters, D.; Pedersen, M.H.; Knudsen, G.M.; Mikkelsen, J.D. Radiosynthesis and in vitro validation of (3)H-NS14492 as a novel high affinity alpha7 nicotinic receptor radioligand. *Eur. J. Pharmacol.* **2015**, *762*, 35–41. [CrossRef] [PubMed]
62. Bitner, R.S.; Bunnelle, W.H.; Anderson, D.J.; Briggs, C.A.; Buccafusco, J.; Curzon, P.; Decker, M.W.; Frost, J.M.; Gronlien, J.H.; Gubbins, E.; et al. Broad-spectrum efficacy across cognitive domains by alpha7 nicotinic acetylcholine receptor agonism correlates with activation of ERK1/2 and CREB phosphorylation pathways. *J. Neurosci.* **2007**, *27*, 10578–10587. [CrossRef] [PubMed]
63. Biton, B.; Bergis, O.E.; Galli, F.; Nedelec, A.; Lochead, A.W.; Jegham, S.; Godet, D.; Lanneau, C.; Santamaria, R.; Chesney, F.; et al. SSR180711, a novel selective alpha7 nicotinic receptor partial agonist: (1) binding and functional profile. *Neuropsychopharmacology* **2007**, *32*, 1–16. [CrossRef] [PubMed]
64. Hauser, T.A.; Kucinski, A.; Jordan, K.G.; Gatto, G.J.; Wersinger, S.R.; Hesse, R.A.; Stachowiak, E.K.; Stachowiak, M.K.; Papke, R.L.; Lippiello, P.M.; et al. TC-5619: An alpha7 neuronal nicotinic receptor-selective agonist that demonstrates efficacy in animal models of the positive and negative symptoms and cognitive dysfunction of schizophrenia. *Biochem. Pharmacol.* **2009**, *78*, 803–812. [CrossRef] [PubMed]
65. Prickaerts, J.; van Goethem, N.P.; Chesworth, R.; Shapiro, G.; Boess, F.G.; Methfessel, C.; Reneerkens, O.A.; Flood, D.G.; Hilt, D.; Gawryl, M.; et al. EVP-6124, a novel and selective alpha7 nicotinic acetylcholine receptor partial agonist, improves memory performance by potentiating the acetylcholine response of alpha7 nicotinic acetylcholine receptors. *Neuropharmacology* **2012**, *62*, 1099–1110. [CrossRef] [PubMed]
66. Meyer, E.M.; Tay, E.T.; Papke, R.L.; Meyers, C.; Huang, G.L.; de Fiebre, C.M. 3-[2,4-Dimethoxybenzylidene]anabaseine (DMXB) selectively activates rat alpha7 receptors and improves memory-related behaviors in a mecamylamine-sensitive manner. *Brain Res.* **1997**, *768*, 49–56. [CrossRef]
67. Nielsen, B.E.; Minguez, T.; Bermudez, I.; Bouzat, C. Molecular function of the novel $\alpha 7\beta 2$ nicotinic receptor. *Cell. Mol. Life Sci. Cmls* **2018**, *75*, 2457–2471. [CrossRef]
68. Liu, Q.; Huang, Y.; Shen, J.; Steffensen, S.; Wu, J. Functional alpha7beta2 nicotinic acetylcholine receptors expressed in hippocampal interneurons exhibit high sensitivity to pathological level of amyloid beta peptides. *Bmc Neurosci.* **2012**, *13*, 155. [CrossRef]
69. Liu, Q.; Huang, Y.; Xue, F.; Simard, A.; DeChon, J.; Li, G.; Zhang, J.; Lucero, L.; Wang, M.; Sierks, M.; et al. A novel nicotinic acetylcholine receptor subtype in basal forebrain cholinergic neurons with high sensitivity to amyloid peptides. *J. Neurosci.* **2009**, *29*, 918–929. [CrossRef]

70. Khiroug, S.S.; Harkness, P.C.; Lamb, P.W.; Sudweeks, S.N.; Khiroug, L.; Millar, N.S.; Yakel, J.L. Rat nicotinic ACh receptor alpha7 and beta2 subunits co-assemble to form functional heteromeric nicotinic receptor channels. *J Physiol* **2002**, *540*, 425–434. [CrossRef]
71. Murray, T.A.; Bertrand, D.; Papke, R.L.; George, A.A.; Pantoja, R.; Srinivasan, R.; Liu, Q.; Wu, J.; Whiteaker, P.; Lester, H.A.; et al. alpha7beta2 nicotinic acetylcholine receptors assemble, function, and are activated primarily via their alpha7-alpha7 interfaces. *Mol. Pharmacol.* **2012**, *81*, 175–188. [CrossRef] [PubMed]
72. Mowrey, D.D.; Liu, Q.; Bondarenko, V.; Chen, Q.; Seyoum, E.; Xu, Y.; Wu, J.; Tang, P. Insights into distinct modulation of α7 and α7β2 nicotinic acetylcholine receptors by the volatile anesthetic isoflurane. *J. Biol. Chem.* **2013**, *288*, 35793–35800. [CrossRef] [PubMed]
73. Teodoro, R.; Moldovan, R.P.; Lueg, C.; Gunther, R.; Donat, C.K.; Ludwig, F.A.; Fischer, S.; Deuther-Conrad, W.; Wunsch, B.; Brust, P. Radiofluorination and biological evaluation of N-aryl-oxadiazolyl-propionamides as potential radioligands for PET imaging of cannabinoid CB2 receptors. *Org. Med. Chem. Lett.* **2013**, *3*, 11. [CrossRef] [PubMed]
74. Innis, R.B.; Cunningham, V.J.; Delforge, J.; Fujita, M.; Gjedde, A.; Gunn, R.N.; Holden, J.; Houle, S.; Huang, S.-C.; Ichise, M.; et al. Consensus nomenclature for in vivo imaging of reversibly binding radioligands. *J. Cereb. Blood Flow Metab: Off. J. Int. Soc. Cereb. Blood Flow Metab.* **2007**, *27*, 1533–1539. [CrossRef] [PubMed]
75. Gallezot, J.-D.; Weinzimmer, D.; Nabulsi, N.; Lin, S.-F.; Fowles, K.; Sandiego, C.; McCarthy, T.J.; Maguire, R.P.; Carson, R.E.; Ding, Y.-S. Evaluation of [(11)C]MRB for assessment of occupancy of norepinephrine transporters: Studies with atomoxetine in non-human primates. *NeuroImage* **2011**, *56*, 268–279. [CrossRef]
76. Bradford, M.M. A rapid and sensitive method for the quantitation of microgram quantities of protein utilizing the principle of protein-dye binding. *Anal. Biochem.* **1976**, *72*, 248–254. [CrossRef]
77. Ward, J.M.; Cockcroft, V.B.; Lunt, G.G.; Smillie, F.S.; Wonnacott, S. Methyllycaconitine: A selective probe for neuronal alpha-bungarotoxin binding sites. *Febs Lett.* **1990**, *270*, 45–48. [CrossRef]
78. Gillings, N. A restricted access material for rapid analysis of [(11)C]-labeled radiopharmaceuticals and their metabolites in plasma. *Nucl. Med. Biol.* **2009**, *36*, 961–965. [CrossRef]
79. Kornum, B.R.; Lind, N.M.; Gillings, N.; Marner, L.; Andersen, F.; Knudsen, G.M. Evaluation of the novel 5-HT4 receptor PET ligand [11C]SB207145 in the Gottingen minipig. *J. Cereb. Blood Flow Metab.* **2009**, *29*, 186–196. [CrossRef]
80. Villadsen, J.; Hansen, H.D.; Jorgensen, L.M.; Keller, S.H.; Andersen, F.L.; Petersen, I.N.; Knudsen, G.M.; Svarer, C. Automatic delineation of brain regions on MRI and PET images from the pig. *J. Neurosci. Methods* **2018**, *294*, 51–58. [CrossRef]

Permissions

 Every chapter published in this book has been scrutinized by our experts. Their significance has been extensively debated. The topics covered herein carry significant findings which will fuel the growth of the discipline. They may even be implemented as practical applications or may be referred to as a beginning point for another development.

The contributors of this book come from diverse backgrounds, making this book a truly international effort. This book will bring forth new frontiers with its revolutionizing research information and detailed analysis of the nascent developments around the world.

We would like to thank all the contributing authors for lending their expertise to make the book truly unique. They have played a crucial role in the development of this book. Without their invaluable contributions this book wouldn't have been possible. They have made vital efforts to compile up to date information on the varied aspects of this subject to make this book a valuable addition to the collection of many professionals and students.

This book was conceptualized with the vision of imparting up-to-date information and advanced data in this field. To ensure the same, a matchless editorial board was set up. Every individual on the board went through rigorous rounds of assessment to prove their worth. After which they invested a large part of their time researching and compiling the most relevant data for our readers.

The editorial board has been involved in producing this book since its inception. They have spent rigorous hours researching and exploring the diverse topics which have resulted in the successful publishing of this book. They have passed on their knowledge of decades through this book. To expedite this challenging task, the publisher supported the team at every step. A small team of assistant editors was also appointed to further simplify the editing procedure and attain best results for the readers.

Apart from the editorial board, the designing team has also invested a significant amount of their time in understanding the subject and creating the most relevant covers. They scrutinized every image to scout for the most suitable representation of the subject and create an appropriate cover for the book.

The publishing team has been an ardent support to the editorial, designing and production team. Their endless efforts to recruit the best for this project, has resulted in the accomplishment of this book. They are a veteran in the field of academics and their pool of knowledge is as vast as their experience in printing. Their expertise and guidance has proved useful at every step. Their uncompromising quality standards have made this book an exceptional effort. Their encouragement from time to time has been an inspiration for everyone.

The publisher and the editorial board hope that this book will prove to be a valuable piece of knowledge for researchers, students, practitioners and scholars across the globe.

List of Contributors

Ananth Shankar
Children and Young People's Cancer Services, University College London hospitals NHS Foundation Trust, London NW1 2PG, UK

Jamshed Bomanji
Department of Nuclear Medicine, University College London hospitals NHS Foundation Trust, London NW1 2PG, UK

Harpreet Hyare
Department of Radiology, University College London Hospitals NHS Foundation Trust, London NW1 2PG, UK
Department of Brain Repair and Rehabilitation, Institute of Neurology, University College London, London WC1N 3BG, UK

Salvatore Annunziata
Nuclear Medicine Unit, IRCSS Regina Elena National Cancer Institute, 00144 Rome, Italy

Roberto C. Delgado Bolton
Department of Diagnostic Imaging (Radiology) and Nuclear Medicine, University Hospital San Pedro and Centre for Biomedical Research of La Rioja (CIBIR), 26006 Logroño, La Rioja, Spain

Christel-Hermann Kamani and John O. Prior
Department of Nuclear Medicine and Molecular Imaging, Lausanne University Hospital and University of Lausanne, CH-1011 Lausanne, Switzerland

Domenico Albano and Francesco Bertagna
Nuclear Medicine, University of Brescia and Spedali Civili Brescia, 25123 Brescia, Italy

Giorgio Treglia
Department of Nuclear Medicine and Molecular Imaging, Lausanne University Hospital and University of Lausanne, CH-1011 Lausanne, Switzerland
Clinic of Nuclear Medicine and PET/CT Center, Imaging Institute of Southern Switzerland, Ente Ospedaliero Cantonale, 6500 Bellinzona, Switzerland
Health Technology Assessment Unit, Academic Education, Research and Innovation Area, Ente Ospedaliero Cantonale, 6500 Bellinzona, Switzerland

Lars Jødal
Department of Nuclear Medicine, Aalborg University Hospital, DK-9000 Aalborg, Denmark

Anne Roivainen and Vesa Oikonen
Turku PET Centre, Turku University Hospital, FI-20520 Turku, Finland
Turku PET Centre, University of Turku, FI-20520 Turku, Finland

Sirpa Jalkanen
MediCity Research Laboratory and Institute of Biomedicine, University of Turku, FI-20520 Turku, Finland

Søren B. Hansen and Aage K. O. Alstrup
Department of Nuclear Medicine and PET, Aarhus University Hospital, DK-8200 Aarhus, Denmark

Pia Afzelius
North Zealand Hospital, Hillerød, Copenhagen University Hospital, DK-3400 Hillerød, Denmark

Ole L. Nielsen
Department of Veterinary and Animal Sciences, University of Copenhagen, DK-1870 Copenhagen, Denmark

Svend B. Jensen
Department of Nuclear Medicine, Aalborg University Hospital, DK-9000 Aalborg, Denmark
Department of Chemistry and Biosciences, Aalborg University, DK-9100 Aalborg, Denmark

Susann Schröder
ROTOP Pharmaka Ltd., Department of Research and Development, Dresden 01328, Germany

Thu Hang Lai, Magali Toussaint, Sladjana Dukić-Stefanović, Winnie Deuther-Conrad, Rodrigo Teodoro, BarbaraWenzel, Rareş-Petru Moldovan and Peter Brust
Helmholtz-Zentrum Dresden-Rossendorf (HZDR), Department of Neuroradiopharmaceuticals, Institute of Radiopharmaceutical Cancer Research, Research Site Leipzig, Leipzig 04318, Germany

Mathias Kranz
PET Imaging Center, University Hospital of North Norway (UNN), Tromsø 9009, Norway
Nuclear Medicine and Radiation Biology Research Group, The Arctic University of Norway, 9009 Tromsø, Norway
Helmholtz-Zentrum Dresden-Rossendorf, Institute of Radiopharmaceutical Cancer Research, Department of Neuroradiopharmaceuticals, 04318 Leipzig, Germany
Tromsø PET Center, University Hospital of North Norway, 9009 Tromsø, Norway

Alexandra Chovsepian
University Hospital Munich, Department of Psychiatry, Ludwig-Maximilians-Universität (LMU) Munich, Munich 80336, Germany

Francisco Pan-Montojo
University Hospital Munich, Department of Psychiatry, Ludwig-Maximilians-Universität (LMU) Munich, Munich 80336, Germany
University Hospital Munich, Department of Neurology, Ludwig-Maximilians-Universität (LMU) Munich, Munich 81377, Germany

Qi Shang
University Hospital Munich, Department of Neurology, Ludwig-Maximilians-Universität (LMU) Munich, Munich 81377, Germany
University Hospital Carl Gustav Carus, Clinic of Neurology, Technische Universität Dresden (TUD), Dresden 01307, Germany

Masoud Sadeghzadeh, Daniel Gündel, Steffen Fischer and Friedrich-Alexander Ludwig
Department of Neuroradiopharmaceuticals, Institute of Radiopharmaceutical Cancer Research, Helmholtz-Zentrum Dresden-Rossendorf, Permoserstraße 15, 04318 Leipzig, Germany

Shirisha Jonnalagadda, Sravan K. Jonnalagadda and Venkatram R. Mereddy
Department of Chemistry and Biochemistry, Department of Pharmacy Practice & Pharmaceutical Sciences, University of Minnesota, Duluth, MN 55812, USA

Gerrit Schüürmann
UFZ Department of Ecological Chemistry, Helmholtz Centre for Environmental Research, Permoserstraße 15, 04318 Leipzig, Germany
Institute of Organic Chemistry, Technical University Bergakademie Freiberg, Leipziger Straße 29, 09599 Freiberg, Germany

Lester R. Drewes
Department of Biomedical Sciences, University of Minnesota Medical School Duluth, 251 SMed, 1035 University Drive, Duluth, MN 55812, USA

Jan-Michael Werner
Department of Neurology, Faculty of Medicine and University Hospital Cologne, University of Cologne, Kerpener St. 62, 50937 Cologne, Germany

Philipp Lohmann
Institute of Neuroscience and Medicine (INM-3, -4), Research Center Juelich, Leo-Brandt-St., 52425 Juelich, Germany

Gereon R. Fink and Norbert Galldiks
Department of Neurology, Faculty of Medicine and University Hospital Cologne, University of Cologne, Kerpener St. 62, 50937 Cologne, Germany
Institute of Neuroscience and Medicine (INM-3, -4), Research Center Juelich, Leo-Brandt-St., 52425 Juelich, Germany

Karl-Josef Langen
Institute of Neuroscience and Medicine (INM-3, -4), Research Center Juelich, Leo-Brandt-St., 52425 Juelich, Germany
Department of Nuclear Medicine, University Hospital Aachen, 52074 Aachen, Germany

Christos Sachpekidis and Antonia Dimitrakopoulou-Strauss
Clinical Cooperation Unit Nuclear Medicine, German Cancer Research Center, 69120 Heidelberg, Germany

Hartmut Goldschmidt
Department of Internal Medicine V, University Hospital Heidelberg and National Center for Tumor Diseases (NCT), 69120 Heidelberg, Germany

Sladjana Dukic-Stefanovic and Matthias Scheunemann
Helmholtz-Zentrum Dresden-Rossendorf, Institute of Radiopharmaceutical Cancer Research, Research Site Leipzig, Department of Neuroradiopharmaceuticals, 04318 Leipzig, Germany

Rien Ritawidya
Helmholtz-Zentrum Dresden-Rossendorf, Institute of Radiopharmaceutical Cancer Research, Research Site Leipzig, Department of Neuroradiopharmaceuticals, 04318 Leipzig, Germany
Center for Radioisotope and Radiopharmaceutical Technology, National Nuclear Energy Agency (BATAN), Puspiptek Area, Serpong, South Tangerang 15314, Indonesia

Bernhard Sattler and Osama Sabri
Department of Nuclear Medicine, University Hospital Leipzig, 04103 Leipzig, Germany

Nalin T. Jain
Helmholtz-Zentrum Dresden-Rossendorf, Institute of Radiopharmaceutical Cancer Research, Department of Neuroradiopharmaceuticals, 04318 Leipzig, Germany

Tatjana Sattler
Department of Claw Animals, University of Leipzig, 04103 Leipzig, Germany

Liqun Kuang, Deyu Zhao, Fengguang Xiong and Xie Han
School of Data Science and Technology, North University of China, Taiyuan 030051, China

Jiacheng Xing
School of Software, Nanchang University, Nanchang 330047, China

Zhongyu Chen
School of Software, East China Jiaotong University, Nanchang 330013, China

Guillaume Becker, Sylvestre Dammicco, Mohamed Ali Bahri and Eric Salmon
GIGA-Cyclotron Research Center-in vivo imaging, University of Liège, Allée du 6 Août, B30, 4000 Liege, Belgium

Chiara Da Pieve and Graham Smith
PET Radiochemistry, Division of Radiotherapy and Imaging, the Institute of Cancer Research, 123 Old Brompton Road, London SW7 3RP, UK

Ata Makarem
Division of Radiopharmaceutical Chemistry, German Cancer Research Center (DKFZ), Im Neuenheimer Feld 280, 69120 Heidelberg, Germany

Stephen Turnock, Justyna Maczynska and Gabriela Kramer-Marek
Preclinical Molecular Imaging, Division of Radiotherapy and Imaging, the Institute of Cancer Research, 123 Old Brompton Road, London SW7 3RP, UK

Henrik H. Hansen, Hanne D. Hansen, Gitte M. Knudsen and Jens D. Mikkelsen
Neurobiology Research Unit, Copenhagen University Hospital, Rigshospitalet, DK-2100 Copenhagen, Denmark

Cornelius K. Donat
Neurobiology Research Unit, Copenhagen University Hospital, Rigshospitalet, DK-2100 Copenhagen, Denmark
Department of Brain Sciences, Imperial College London, London W12 0 LS, UK

Ronnie C. Mease, Andrew G. Horti and Martin G. Pomper
Russell H. Morgan Department of Radiology and Radiological Science, The Johns Hopkins University School of Medicine, Baltimore, MD 21287, USA

Elina T. L'Estrade
Neurobiology Research Unit, Copenhagen University Hospital, Rigshospitalet, DK-2100 Copenhagen, Denmark
Department of Drug Design and Pharmacology, University of Copenhagen, Jagtvej 162, 2100 Copenhagen, Denmark
Department of Clinical Physiology, Nuclear Medicine & PET, Rigshospitalet, Blegdamsvej 9, 2100 Copenhagen, Denmark

Matthias M. Herth
Department of Drug Design and Pharmacology, University of Copenhagen, Jagtvej 162, 2100 Copenhagen, Denmark
Department of Clinical Physiology, Nuclear Medicine & PET, Rigshospitalet, Blegdamsvej 9, 2100 Copenhagen, Denmark

Dan Peters
DanPET AB, 216 19 Malmö, Sweden

Index

www.ingramcontent.com/pod-product-compliance
Lightning Source LLC
LaVergne TN
LVHW060554210926
848485LV00005B/1310
* 9 7 8 1 6 3 9 2 7 7 5 1 3 *